THE FAMILY
AND HIV

OTHER TITLES AVAILABLE FROM CASSELL:

R. Bor, R. Miller and E. Goldman: *Theory and Practice of HIV Counselling*
E. King: *Gay Men Fighting AIDS*
R. Nelson-Jones: *Practical Counselling and Helping Skills, Third Edition*

THE FAMILY
AND HIV

Edited by Robert Bor and Jonathan Elford

CASSELL

Cassell

Villiers House	387 Park Avenue South
41/47 Strand	New York
London WC2N 5JE	NY 10016–8810

Compilation © Robert Bor and Jonathan Elford 1994

First published 1994.
See list of Acknowledgements for dates of original publication.

British Library Cataloguing-in-Publication Data
A catalogue record for this book is available from the British Library.

ISBN 0–304–33069–8 (hardback)
0–304–32985–1 (paperback)

Typeset by Litho Link Ltd, Welshpool, Powys, Wales

Printed and bound in Great Britain by
Redwood Books, Trowbridge, Wiltshire

CONTENTS

List of Contributors

Dimitris Anastasopoulos	Department of Psychological Paediatrics, Aghia Sophia Children's Hospital, Athens, Greece
E. Maxine Ankrah	Faculty of Social Sciences, Makerere University, Kampala, Uganda
Sophie Aroni	Department of Haemophilia, Aghia Sophia Children's Hospital, Athens, Greece
Line Asselin	Faculté des Sciences Infirmières, Université de Montréal, Canada
Cissy Bachengana	MRC Research Programme on AIDS in Uganda, Uganda Virus Research Institute, Entebbe, Uganda
Robert Bor	Psychology Department, City University, London, UK
Mary Boulton	Academic Department of Community Medicine, St Mary's Hospital Medical School, London, UK
Thomas J. Coates	Center for AIDS Prevention Studies, University of California, San Francisco, USA
Anthony P.M. Coxon	Department of Sociology, University of Essex, Colchester, UK

Peter M. Davies — Department of Sociology, University of Essex, Colchester, UK

Jill Dawson — Department of Community Medicine and General Practice, University of Oxford, Oxford, UK

Jonathan Elford — Department of Public Health and Primary Care, Royal Free Hospital School of Medicine, London, UK

Dwight L. Evans — Department of Psychiatry, University of Florida College of Medicine, Gainesville, Florida, USA

Ray Fitzpatrick — Department of Community Medicine and General Practice, University of Oxford, Oxford, UK

Heather George — Department of Clinical Psychology, South Downs Health NHS Trust, Hove, East Sussex, UK

Eleanor Goldman — Haemophilia Centre, Royal Free Hampstead NHS Trust, London, UK

Gill Green — MRC Medical Sociology Unit, Glasgow, UK

Graham Hart — Academic Department of Genito-urinary Medicine, University College London Medical School, London, UK

Robert B. Hays — Center for AIDS Prevention Studies, University of California, San Francisco, USA

Ford C.I. Hickson — Project Sigma, South Bank University, London, UK

Robert Hilliard — Center for AIDS Prevention Studies, University of California, San Francisco, USA

Colleen Hoff — Center for AIDS Prevention Studies, University of California, San Francisco, USA

Andrew J. Hunt — Project Sigma, South Bank University, London, UK

Ellen Kajura — MRC Research Programme on AIDS in Uganda, Uganda Virus Research Institute, Entebbe, Uganda

Christos Kattamis — Department of Paediatrics, Athens University Medical School, Athens, Greece

Margarita Koutsanellou-Meyer	Greek Council for Refugees, Athens, Greece
Vassilis Ladis	Thalassaemia Unit, Athens University Medical School, Athens, Greece
Sigrid Larson	National Centre in HIV Social Research, University of New South Wales, Sydney, Australia
Jane Leserman	Department of Psychiatry, University of North Carolina at Chapel Hill, North Carolina, USA
Carol Levine	The Orphan Project: The HIV Epidemic and New York City's Children, New York, USA
Monica Lubega	Makerere University, Kampala, Uganda
Kathy McCann	Institute for Social Studies in Medical Care, London, UK
John McClean	Academic Department of Community Medicine, St Mary's Hospital Medical School, London, UK
Janet W. McGrath	Department of Anthropology, Case Western Reserve University, Cleveland, USA
Leon McKusick	Center for AIDS Prevention Studies, University of California, San Francisco, USA
Thomas J. McManus	King's College Hospital, London, UK
Riva Miller	AIDS Counselling and Social Care Unit, Royal Free Hampstead NHS Trust, London, UK
Rebecca Mukasa	Department of Sociology, Makerere University, Kampala, Uganda
Daan Mulder	MRC Research Programme on AIDS in Uganda, Uganda Virus Research Institute, Entebbe, Uganda
Sylvia Nakayiwa	Department of Sociology, Makerere University, Kampala, Uganda
Lucy Nakyobe	Department of Sociology, Makerere University, Kampala, Uganda
Barbara Namande	Department of Sociology, Makerere University, Kampala, Uganda
S. Nkombi	Faculty of Social Sciences, Makerere University, Kampala, Uganda

Martin Okongo	MRC Research Programme on AIDS in Uganda, Uganda Virus Research Institute, Entebbe, Uganda
Dionysia Panitz	Department of Psychological Paediatrics, Aghia Sophia Children's Hospital, Athens, Greece
Jonnie Pearson-Marks	Department of Anthropology, Case Western Reserve University, Cleveland, USA
Diana O. Perkins	Department of Psychiatry, University of North Carolina at Chapel Hill, North Carolina, USA
Helen Platokouki	Department of Haemophilia, Aghia Sophia Children's Hospital, Athens, Greece
Lance Pollack	Center for AIDS Prevention Studies, University of California, San Francisco, USA
Elizabeth A. Preble	United Nations Children's Fund, New York, USA
Mary Reidy	Faculté des Sciences Infirmières, Université de Montréal, Canada
Michael Ross	National Centre in HIV Social Research, University of New South Wales, Sydney, Australia
Charles B. Rwabukwali	Department of Sociology, Makerere University, Kampala, Uganda
Debra A. Schumann	Department of Population Dynamics, The Johns Hopkins University, Baltimore, USA
Janet Seeley	MRC Research Programme on AIDS in Uganda, Uganda Virus Research Institute, Entebbe, Uganda
Aaron Stowe	National Centre in HIV Social Research, University of New South Wales, Sydney, Australia
Marie-Elizabeth Taggart	Faculté des Sciences Infirmières, Université de Montréal, Canada
Gillian Thomas	National Centre in HIV Social Research, University of New South Wales, Sydney, Australia

John Tsiantis   Department of Psychological Paediatrics, Aghia Sophia Children's Hospital, Athens, Greece

Emma Wadsworth   Department of Child Health, University of Bristol, Bristol, UK

Uli Wagner   MRC Research Programme on AIDS in Uganda, Uganda Virus Research Institute, Entebbe, Uganda

Peter Weatherburn   Project Sigma, South Bank University, London, UK

Alex Wodak   Alcohol and Drug Services, St Vincent's Hospital, Sydney, Australia

Acknowledgements

We would like to thank the following publishers for permission to reprint the papers indicated.

© 1990 Milbank Memorial Fund
Chapter 1

© Carfax Publishing Company
Chapters 2, 4, 5, 7, 8, 9, 10, 12, 14, 17, 18

© Current Science
Chapter 3

© 1992 American Psychiatric Association
Chapter 6

© 1990 Pergamon Press
Chapter 11

© 1993 Pergamon Press
Chapter 15

© The Guilford Press
Chapter 13

© Association for Family Therapy, UK
Chapter 16

LIST OF ALL ORIGINAL PUBLICATIONS, BY CHAPTER NUMBER

1 Levine, C. (1990) AIDS and changing concepts of family. *The Milbank Quarterly*, 68, Suppl. 1, pp. 33–58.

2 Ankrah, E. M. (1993) The impact of HIV/AIDS on the family and other significant relationships: the African clan revisited. *AIDS Care*, 5, pp. 5–22.

3 Hays, R. B., McKusick, L., Pollack, L., Hilliard, R., Hoff, C. and Coates, T. (1993) Disclosing HIV seropositivity to significant others. *AIDS*, 7, pp. 425–31.

4 McGrath, J., Ankrah, E. M., Schumann, D. A., Nkumbi, S. and Lubega, M. (1993) AIDS and the urban family: its impact in Kampala, Uganda. *AIDS Care*, 5, pp. 55–70.

5 Green, G. (1993) Editorial review: social support and HIV. *AIDS Care*, 5, pp. 87–104.

6 Leserman, J., Perkins, D. O. and Evans, D. L. (1992) Coping with the threat of AIDS: the role of social support. *American Journal of Psychiatry*, 149, pp. 1514–20.

7 Hart, G., Fitzpatrick, R., McLean, J., Dawson, J. and Boulton, M. (1990) Gay men, social support and HIV disease: a study of social integration in the gay community. *AIDS Care*, 2, pp. 163–70.

8 McCann, K. and Wadsworth, E. (1992) The role of informal carers in supporting gay men who have HIV related illness: what do they do and what are their needs? *AIDS Care*, 4, pp. 25–34.

9 Stowe, A., Ross, M., Wodak, A., Thomas, G. V. and Larson, S. A. (1993) Significant relationships and social supports of injecting drug users and their implications for HIV/AIDS services. *AIDS Care*, 5, pp. 23–33.

10 Seeley, J., Kajura, E., Bachengana, C., Okongo, M., Wagner, U. and Mulder, D. (1993) The extended family and support for people with AIDS in a rural population in south west Uganda: a safety net with holes? *AIDS Care*, 5, pp. 117–22.

11 Preble, E. (1990) Impact of HIV/AIDS on African children. *Social Science and Medicine*, 31, pp. 671–80.

12 Reidy, M., Taggart, M.-E. and Asselin, L. (1991) Psychosocial needs expressed by the natural caregivers of HIV infected children. *AIDS Care*, 3, pp. 331–43.

13 Hoff, C. C., McKusick, L., Hilliard, B. and Coates, T. J. (1992) The impact of HIV antibody status on gay men's partner preferences: a community perspective. *AIDS Education and Prevention*, 4, pp. 197–204.

14 Hickson, F., Davies, P. M., Hunt, A. J., Weatherburn, P., McManus, T. J. and Coxon, A. P. M. (1992) Maintenance of open gay relationships: some strategies for protection against HIV. *AIDS Care*, 4, pp. 409–19.

15 McGrath, J. W., Rwabukwali, C. B., Schumann, D. A., Pearson-Marks, J., Nakayiwa, S., Namande, B., Nakyobe, L. and Mukasa, R. (1993) Anthropology and AIDS: the cultural context of sexual risk behaviour among urban Baganda women in Kampala, Uganda. *Social Science and Medicine*, 36, pp. 429–39.

16 Miller, R., Goldman, E. and Bor, R. (1994) Application of a family systems approach to working with people affected by HIV disease. *Journal of Family Therapy* (in press).

17 Tsiantis, J., Anastasopoulos, D., Meyer, M., Panitz, D., Ladis, V., Platokouki, N., Aroni, S. and Kattamis, C. (1990) A multi-level intervention approach for care of HIV-positive haemophiliac and thalassaemic patients and their families. *AIDS Care*, 2, pp. 253–66.

18 George, H. (1990) Sexual and relationship problems among people affected by AIDS: three case studies. *Counselling Psychology Quarterly*, 3, pp. 389–99.

We gratefully acknowledge the help and support of the following people: Elaine Harris and Wendy Tompsett, who painstakingly helped prepare the manuscript; Henry Duckett, Carfax Publishing Company, for his encouragement in developing this text; our colleagues Graham Hart and Lorraine Sherr for their support; and Naomi Roth and Pat Gordon Smith at Cassell for their enthusiastic interest throughout the preparation of this book.

Introduction: The Impact of HIV on the Family

Robert Bor and Jonathan Elford

HIV disease is not solely a medical issue but also has profound implications for social and family relationships. Traditionally, when a person is ill the family is seen to provide emotional, practical and social support. Experience has shown, however, that HIV disease disrupts this pattern of support. On the one hand HIV disease, like any other serious illness, affects family members both from day to day and in the long term. What distinguishes HIV disease from so many other illnesses, however, is the associated social stigma and the fact that HIV may be transmissible, or may already have been transmitted, within a relationship.

Most psychological and social research has concentrated on the impact of HIV disease on individuals. Only recently has attention turned to the effect of HIV disease on the family. Researchers now recognize that while HIV *infects* individuals, it also *affects* their relationships. This is one of the first books to address HIV disease in the family and draws on the work of experienced researchers and practitioners from around the world. It is most fitting that the book should be published in 1994, which has been designated by the United Nations as International Year of the Family. Recognition of the family may mark a change in emphasis in future social research and policy in relation to HIV disease.

THE FAMILY

HIV disease challenges the conventional view that the family is solely determined by blood relationships. In the opening chapter, Levine suggests that the family is a social system comprising individuals 'who by birth, adoption, marriage or declared commitment share deep, personal connections and are mutually entitled to receive . . . and provide support . . . especially in times of need'. Thus, the family, both of origin and of affiliation, may embrace a matrix of relationships including same-sex couples and networks of close friends as well as parents, siblings, children and other relatives.

In Africa, according to Ankrah (Chapter 2), the disruption of traditional family relationships as a result of HIV disease may require new affiliations outside the traditional family structure. Indeed, in response to HIV disease in the United States, gay men have created supportive relationships with one another that are as strong and as meaningful as those found within the traditional biological family. Consequently, when disclosing their seropositivity to others, gay men found friends and lovers responded more helpfully than relatives (Hays *et al.*, Chapter 3). Similarly, a Ugandan study found that a third of people with HIV chose not to disclose their seropositivity to their biological family for fear of rejection and lack of understanding (McGrath *et al.*, Chapter 4). These studies highlight the importance of Levine's concept of the family as comprising people with a shared commitment to each other, regardless of whether they are blood relations.

SOCIAL SUPPORT

There is a growing evidence pointing towards the link between support provided by the family, in its broadest sense, and the psychological well-being of people with HIV disease. However, research to date has mainly focused on gay men and has lacked methodological rigour (Green, Chapter 5). None the less, some important insights have been made. In the United States, a study among gay men with asymptomatic HIV infection found that satisfaction with one's social support was related to healthy coping strategies. Interestingly, the same study found that black gay men were less likely to seek social support than their white counterparts (Leserman *et al.*, Chapter 6).

In the UK, a study revealed the extent to which gay men provide support to other gay men with AIDS; a quarter of men interviewed said they had provided practical help and support to at least one person with AIDS. The caring relationship may work both ways, with today's carers themselves requiring support in the future. It was encouraging that in the above study over 90% of the subjects interviewed reported having access to people they could turn to at times of illness, mostly friends or partners. This finding challenges the assumption that gay men do not have easy access to social support (Hart *et al.*, Chapter 7). According to research conducted in London, the informal carers of gay men with HIV infection at an inner city hospital were predominantly their male partners or friends (McCann and Wadsworth, Chapter 8). While carers provided both physical and emotional support to their friends with HIV, they themselves felt inadequately supported both practically and emotionally. Indeed, some of the carers expressed a desire for help from their own *biological* family in supporting the person with HIV. Injecting drug users in Australia also reported that they were more likely to turn to friends rather than the biological family for support should they have HIV infection (Stowe *et al.*, Chapter 9).

These three studies highlight the crucial role of one's family of affiliation at times of illness. In fact, the biological family may be limited in the extent to which it alone can provide support for a relation with HIV infection. In Uganda, Seeley *et al.* (Chapter 10) found that the impact of HIV disease in certain communities was so great that traditional extended family networks were unable to cope with the increased demands put upon them.

CHILDREN

There may be families where both parents, but not all the children, will have HIV infection. As a consequence, Preble (Chapter 11) estimates that one in ten children in Central and East Africa may be orphaned during the 1990s. Orphanhood on this scale will inevitably lead to deprivation, which in turn will require appropriate services to meet some of the children's needs. In a family, the presence of a child with HIV infection almost certainly implies an infected mother. Clearly, this has implications for the parent–child relationship. Another important consideration is that the parents themselves will also require support in their dual role of caring for someone with HIV disease while attending to their own needs (Reidy *et al.*, Chapter 12).

CHOICE OF PARTNERS

HIV appears to play a central role in the way people make choices about personal relationships. In the United States, gay men who either were HIV-negative or had not been tested expressed a strong preference for HIV-negative romantic partners, while men with HIV infection had no such serostatus preference (Hoff *et al.*, Chapter 13). In most casual sexual encounters, however, the HIV status of those involved may not be known. Rules for negotiating safer sexual behaviour by gay men in casual encounters have been studied by Hickson *et al.* in the UK (Chapter 14). Against a background of HIV infection, gay couples have developed sets of rules for maintaining intimacy with their regular partners while minimizing the risk of transmitting HIV in casual encounters. By way of comparison, according to McGrath *et al.* (Chapter 15) Ugandan women appear to have been less able to influence their husbands' sexual behaviour *vis-à-vis* relationships outside marriage. While the women interviewed in this study said they complied with HIV risk reduction messages, they believed they were still at risk since they thought their husbands had not responded in the same way.

COUNSELLING

Psychotherapeutic work with people affected by HIV has traditionally focused on the individual. However, many problems experienced by any one person with HIV may be successfully addressed by involving the family. An innovative approach to working with an infected individual in the context of his or her family – of origin and affiliation – is illustrated in two case examples described by Miller *et al.* in the UK (Chapter 16). Another study, in Greece, describes how HIV-infected haemophilic and thalassaemic patients were helped to improve relationships with their families, and to cope with the anxiety associated with terminal illness (Tsiantis *et al.*, Chapter 17). Clearly, formal evaluation of these approaches is required. Since HIV is transmitted sexually, people may experience problems in relation to their sexual functioning regardless of their own, or their partners', HIV status. In a UK study, the range of problems seen in a number of patients included loss of libido, increased sexual drive as well as problems relating to sexual performance. Counselling for sexual problems in relationships is illustrated in three case studies (George, Chapter 18).

This book draws upon research conducted in a variety of settings, using different groups and applying a range of methodologies. Despite their differences, the chapters in this book provide an important insight into the impact of HIV disease on families and social networks. Inevitably, in an area of research that is still in its infancy, there are significant gaps in our knowledge. In particular, attention could usefully be paid to examining the relationship between the families of origin and affiliation and how this is mediated by the ever-changing cultural and social context. Of equal importance is the need to consider the application of these research findings to both policy and practice, for the ultimate benefit of all those infected with, and affected by, HIV.

THE
FAMILY

ONE

AIDS and the Changing Concept of the Family

Carol Levine

A few years ago, after my daughter's marriage, a friend remarked that the wedding had been very unusual. 'It was a first marriage,' she explained, 'and the parents of both the bride and groom were still married to their original partners.' Pointing out that my husband and I, unlike most of our friends, had avoided the exquisitely delicate questions of etiquette that complicate the weddings of children of divorced or 'blended' families, she asked, 'How does it feel to be an anomaly?'

This anecdote may reveal only a glimpse of life among a certain segment of the middle class in New York City in the mid-1980s. There can be no doubt, however, that across the nation American families have changed, are changing and will continue to change. A statistical snapshot of American families today documents the shifts. Data from the 1980 United States census show a sharp rise from the 1970 figures in the number of single-parent families, nearly all of them headed by women. Almost 20% of minors live with one parent, an increase from 12% in 1970. The number of people living alone also increased by 64% over the previous census. The number of unmarried couples living together almost tripled from 523,000 in 1970 to 1.56 million in 1980, and increased another 63% from 1980 to 1988 (US Bureau of the Census, 1981, 1988). In 1988, the proportion of households accounted for by married-couple families with children under the age of 18 present in the home had declined by 13% since 1970 (US Bureau of the Census, 1988). According to the US Department of Labor, by 1987 64% of married mothers with children under the age of 18 were working or seeking work, compared with 30% twenty years earlier, and less than 10% in 1940 (Levitan, Belous and Gallo, 1988). As Toffler (1980, pp. 211–12) has pointed out, 'If we define the nuclear family as a working husband, housekeeping wife, and two children, and ask how many Americans still live in this type of family, the answer is astonishing: 7% of the total United States population.' That percentage is undoubtedly lower ten years later.

Behind these statistics lie sweeping historical, economic, scientific and cultural trends. Families are no longer primarily units of production and procreation; they have become instead centres of emotional and social support. Procreation is separated from sexual behaviour and is an act of choice rather than necessity. Women, freed from constant childbearing, may choose to enter the labour force. Since they are frequently divorced or never married and are often the sole support of their children, they may have no choice but to enter the labour force.

These statistics are only numerical representations of the extraordinary diversity of family life today. They are based on 'household' composition, only one factor used to describe 'family'. They do not convey the complex and varying arrangements whereby individuals create, dissolve and re-create supportive and intimate bonds. Tolstoy's (1981 [1877]) famous dichotomous description of families, expressed in the opening lines of *Anna Karenina* – 'Happy families are all alike; every unhappy family is unhappy in its own way' – is only half true today. While the second half of the dictum is certainly valid, it is now the case that happy families are not all alike.

In this diverse and shifting milieu a major medical and social crisis encompassing AIDS and HIV disease (hereafter referred to as 'AIDS' for simplicity) heightens processes of change already under way and sets in motion new, particularized responses. This article is intended to describe some of these changes and to explore their potential impact on current and future families. It is an observational, speculative, non-empirical attempt to call attention to a largely unrecognized aspect of the epidemic rather than to provide a systematic sociological, historical or anthropological analysis.

While the subject of 'family' is difficult to confine with rigid boundaries, this article focuses on key intersections where families and societal institutions meet. At these intersections – such as medical decision making, custody decisions and housing law – definitions of family and rights of family members are straining to accommodate the new situation of AIDS. As Donzelot (1979) pointed out in *The Policing of Families*, the family is not a 'point of departure . . . a manifest reality, but . . . a moving resultant, an uncertain form whose intelligibility can only come from studying the system of relations it maintains with the sociopolitical level'. In this view families are social as well as biological constructs. In today's world both dimensions of family are being challenged.

WHO COUNTS AS FAMILY?

The answer to this apparently simple question is by no means easy. It depends on why the question is being asked and who is giving the answer. 'Family' can be used in many ways, from the narrowest interpretation to the most metaphorical, from description to polemic. Consider the recent case of Nancy Klein, a comatose and pregnant Long Island woman. With her parents' agreement, Mrs Klein's husband,

Martin, sought court permission for an abortion, which doctors hoped would improve her chances of recovery. John Short, an anti-abortion advocate, sought legal guardianship of Mrs Klein and her fetus. He claimed, 'We are all members of the human family. If we see someone being manipulated into killing a child, we have to step in' (*New York Times*, 1989b). In this case, the metaphor of 'family' was used to further a political agenda and to override the legal and ethically justifiable decision of a real-life family. The judge rules in favour of Mr Klein's request, this rejecting the claim that strangers who do not approve of medical decisions have a legal right to take decision-making power from traditional family members.

In this article I use a definition of 'family' that is broad but not unlimited. If everyone counts as family, then family loses its special meaning. If only a few count as family, then our understanding of human relationships is impoverished. What separates family from friends and strangers is not just blood or legal ties but an emotional quality of relationality, continuity and stability. Individuals are born and marry into families; they also choose to enter relationships that are family-like, even if they are called by other names. The essential characteristics of these relationships are: permanence (at least in intention); commitment to mutuality of various forms of economic, social and emotional support; and a level of intimacy that distinguishes this bond from other, less central attachments. Thus, my working definition is: *Family members are individuals who by birth, adoption, marriage or declared commitment share deep, personal connections and are mutually entitled to receive and obligated to provide support of various kinds to the extent possible, especially in times of need.* It is perhaps no accident that in the traditional marriage vows, the pledge to remain constant places 'in sickness' before 'in health'; sickness tests family strength and resiliency as few other crises do. In this context AIDS is the supreme test of family devotion.

This definition both respects traditional notions of family and recognizes non-traditional forms of commitment. Who would be excluded? People in intentionally transitory relationships; individuals who claim status as a family member solely as a convenience to obtain benefits otherwise not available; persons who by abandonment or other actions give up their claims to the benefits of family status. (While a father remains a father, no matter how he treats his child, the recognition that society gives to his status will diminish if he fails to fulfil the minimum obligations of parenthood.) This working definition will undoubtedly be problematic at the boundaries; the central core of deep, long-term, emotional commitment, however, should hold firm.

This definition has some traditional elements. Biological definitions are the most familiar (a word that itself is derived from 'family', and connotes shared associations). Dictionary definitions of 'family' stress the parent–child relationship. Thus, Webster's dictionary defines family as 'the basic unit in society having as its nucleus two or more adults living together and cooperating in the care and rearing of their own or adopted children'. Even this definition is being challenged by surrogate parenting, in which a couple commissions a woman to bear the man's child and secures her agreement to give up her maternal rights to the adoptive mother. New reproductive technologies create situations in which a child may have two different 'mothers' – one who supplies the genetic material and another who gestates the fetus. It is possible to add a third mother to this complex, if still another woman raises the child.

This working definition further delineates the functional definition offered by the Task Force on AIDS and the Family convened by the Groves Conference on Marriage and the Family: 'Families should be broadly defined to include, besides the traditional biological relationships, those committed relationships between individuals which fulfill the functions of family' (Anderson, 1988).

Individuals may count as family members people who are unrelated to them in any traditional way; for some purposes self-definition is more important than legal ties. But public policy definitions of family, which determine eligibility for various benefits and privileges, vary considerably from self-definitions. Thus, biologically and statutorily unrelated individuals are usually not eligible for the benefits accorded to spouses and children, regardless of the depth or duration of their emotional or economic attachments.

Legislatures, courts and governmental agencies differ in defining 'family'. For example, according to the US Bureau of the Census (1988), 'A family or family household requires the presence of at least two persons: the householder and one or more additional family members related to the householder by birth, adoption or marriage.' A householder who lives alone or exclusively with persons who are not related is defined as living in a 'nonfamily household'. Thus, non-traditional functional and relational coupling of two consenting and committed adults – for example, gay or lesbian couples – are by this definition specifically excluded from the designation of family.

The census bureau's definitions do not directly affect individuals' access to benefits, as do the definitions of some other agencies. There is no single, national legal definition of family; family law is administered by the states, and each state has different definitions. Moreover, definitions adopted by governmental agencies vary, with some being more restrictive than others. For example, the California corrections law limits the people who are entitled to overnight prison visitation with eligible inmates to persons who are related by blood, marriage or adoption (City of Los Angeles Task Force on Family Diversity, 1988, p. 22). On the other hand, the more broadly construed New York State definition of family in the Domestic Violence Prevention Act includes 'persons related by consanguinity or affinity', 'persons formerly married to one another regardless of whether they still reside in the same household', 'persons who have a child in common regardless of whether such persons are married or have lived together at any time', 'unrelated persons who are continually or at regular intervals living in the same household or who have lived in the past continually or at regular intervals', as well as a catch-all category of 'other individuals deemed to be a victim of domestic violence as defined by the department in regulation' (New York State, Social Services Law, Section 49(2)).

Some people in non-traditional relationships, and some gay and feminist social critics, reject the term 'family' because of its historical association with particular arrangements of economic, political and sexual power that they view as oppressive. Yet the alternatives, such as 'bonding groups' and 'friendship networks', fail to convey the notion of deep personal connectedness that is suggested by 'family'. 'Community' in some cases – for example, religious communities – does convey this sense, at least for its members. The word is used more commonly, however, to mean a much less central association. While it is important to recognize that family ties can constrain as well as bolster, most people share an understanding of family that suggests a special and enduring, if not necessarily happy, relationship.

As more and more people live in non-traditional arrangements, the distance between their needs and interests and official designations widens. This discrepancy is apparent in many areas, but appears with particular force in AIDS, which, at the same time, heightens the summed impact and lays bare the multiple parts of dysfunctional designations and categories. Those most affected by AIDS and HIV infection – gay men, intravenous drug users and their sexual partners, largely from poor, minority communities – are also those most likely to have non-traditional living or family arrangements. Even if they lived in traditional families before they became ill, the stigma of AIDS and the stress of coping with terminal illness may have created deep intrafamilial rifts. The person with AIDS may thus have to acquire a new family for emotional and economic support. This family may be made up of some traditional family members and friends; increasingly, health care workers and volunteers for social service agencies fulfil the functions of family. In its most extreme and metaphorical version, the hospital becomes the surrogate family. 'For many [babies with AIDS], Harlem Hospital is their mother and father. We're all they have,' says Margaret Heagarty, MD, director of paediatrics at the hospital (Breo, 1988, p. 33). Dr Heagarty, as *mater familias*, views her wards as claimants to both her relational and functional commitment.

AIDS is a catalyst in efforts to expand the definitions of 'family' to reflect the reality of contemporary life. A movement to recognize 'family diversity' has emerged in response to the problems experienced by members of non-traditional families, particularly some politically active gay and lesbian couples and elderly unmarried couples, in obtaining benefits such as medical insurance and bereavement leave for their 'domestic partners'. Starting in Los Angeles, and now spreading to other cities, the organizers call for expanded definitions of the family. The City of Los Angeles Task Force on Family Diversity's (1988) final report concluded:

> No legitimate secular policy is furthered by rigid adherence to a definition of family which promotes a stereotypical, if not mythical, norm. Rather, the appropriate function of lawmakers and administrators is to adopt policies and operate programs that dispel myths and acknowledge reality.

In May 1989 the City of San Francisco passed the nation's first law allowing unmarried homosexual and heterosexual couples to register publicly as 'domestic partners', thus paving the way for them to obtain health benefits, hospital visitation rights and bereavement leave. For a fee of $35, domestic partners, defined as 'two people who have chosen to share one another's lives in an intimate and committed relationship' can file a 'Declaration of Domestic Partnership' (*New York Times*, 1989i).

The boundaries and utility for public policy of expanding definitions of family are being tested. AIDS is stretching the boundaries and, by so doing, may change more than definitions. The structures and services of institutions may change in response to the differing arrangements that will be officially counted as 'family'.

FAMILIES IN CRISIS

AIDS throws families into crisis. Crises in family relationships are often the occasion for bringing private intrafamilial matters to the notice of social institutions that are designed to respond with services and assistance. Because the two groups most seriously affected by AIDS – gay men and intravenous drug users – are generally (and often inaccurately) considered to be isolated from family life, the impact of AIDS on internal family functioning and mental health has not been fully appreciated. Public policy has barely begun to recognize the enormous future needs for mental health and social services of persons with AIDS and their families, however defined. Families are implementers of public policy, sometimes by design, more often by default. A public policy that reduces hospital length of stay for AIDS patients by establishing diagnosis-related groups as the basis for reimbursement assumes that discharged patients will go 'home' and that families will provide care. Yet there are few supports in place to make it possible for families to implement that policy. 'Paco', a person with HIV disease, describes this plight: 'To me the problem is that I'm not getting help from anybody else. My parents are everything and they can't do it all. And Social Security opens my case and they close it and they open it again' (Citizens Commission on AIDS, 1989). This circumstance is not unique to AIDS. For example, there are no explicit employment or tax policies to enable adult children to care for frail, dependent, elderly parents.

Traditional families that have already developed internal ways of coping with crises may be totally unprepared for the stress created by external pressures, such as stigma. Whether the response is rejection or acceptance, as Gary Lloyd (1988), a sociologist of the family, states: 'Families with a member discovered to have HIV infection or diagnosis with AIDS will experience high levels of stress, and disruption in all areas of family life.'

Some families, however, react by mobilizing to fight the stigma and are able to transcend their initial fears and prejudices. They may speak publicly about the disease, raise money for research and care, and become advocates for their ill family member and all those affected. One suburban family with seven children was transformed by the experience of caring for a dying gay son; the mother became less concerned with other people's opinions; a sister became politically active; a son who is a physician altered the way he cared for his patients (Tiblier, Walker and Rolland, 1989).

Cultural or religious differences may affect family views. For example, some families have deeply held views against homosexuality or drug use. Nevertheless, in black families a tradition that reveres the mother–child bond may transcend negative attitudes towards these behaviours. Mildred Pearson, a black woman whose son Bruce died of AIDS in 1987, says: 'He was a wonderful son. My son was gay. I didn't like that, but he was. He did not leave me any babies or a whole lot of money, but he left me his strength. My son died with dignity' (*New York Times*, 1988).

Some Hispanic families, imbued with the concept of *familismo*, accept responsibilities of care for their sick family member, but may be wary of accepting the help of outsiders such as social workers. A counsellor in Chicago says, 'Latino people are hiding their children and loved ones with AIDS.' Part of their reluctance is based on unsatisfactory experiences with non-Spanish-speaking health care workers and, in some cases, a fear of discovery of illegal entry into this country. In addition, many Hispanic families have a deep distrust of doctors and the medical system (*Chicago Tribune*, 1987; Nelson Fernandez, personal communication).

Abandonment by families of their sick or disgraced members is a familiar theme in life and literature. Silas, the hired man in Robert Frost's (1971 [1914]) poem 'The Death of the Hired Man', goes back to Warren and Mary, his employers, to die. Warren asks his wife: 'Silas has better claims on us you think/Than on his brother? . . ./Why didn't he go there? His brother's rich./A somebody – a director in the bank.'

While many families have not abandoned a relative with AIDS, irrational fear of transmission added to religious or cultural stigma have led to rejection. Even among Jewish families, often stereotyped as the most protective and supportive of their children, AIDS creates divisions. In 1989, eight years into the HIV epidemic, a New York City congregation held a special, separate Passover *seder* for its members with AIDS because some of their families were afraid to invite them to the family gathering and risk the wrath of those who wanted no association with AIDS (*Newsday*, 1989a).

Because non-traditional families are more commonly socially and psychologically similar to the patient, having been deliberately formed around shared interests, they may be better equipped to respond to external pressures such as stigma, but not to the dependency and level of care occasioned by illness. Most of these family members are young; caring for someone their own age who is dying may be particularly traumatic. Where a number of people are involved, competition for the ill person's reliance and trust may erupt. Susan Sontag's (1986) short story, 'The Way We Live Now', depicts such a web of complex interrelationships:

> According to Lewis, he talked more often about those who visited more often, which is natural, said Betsy, I think he's even keeping a tally. And among those who came or checked in by phone every day, the inner circle as it were, those who were getting more points, there was still a further competition, which was what was getting on Betsy's nerves, she confessed to Jan; there's always that vulgar jockeying for position around the bedside of the gravely ill.

In some cases only certain family members are involved in the care and support of the person with AIDS; in others, the roles and functions are shared and rearranged to meet the needs of the moment. In still others, families are in conflict, occasionally or permanently, over issues such as treatment decisions, disposition of property and funeral arrangements. Within all families, relationships may shift over time, as individuals move in and out of different roles and functions.

NON-TRADITIONAL FAMILIES AND SOCIAL INSTITUTIONS: SLOUCHING TOWARDS FLEXIBILITY

While some families have demonstrated remarkable capacities to adjust to the stress of AIDS, the institutions that serve as their formal social support – the law, welfare systems, health care, insurance, housing – are less flexible. AIDS is only one of many situations revealing the inadequacies of these institutions in responding to the needs of non-traditional families, but because of its high visibility and urgency, it could be a catalyst for change.

American social institutions were constructed with a particular vision of the family that was a dim reflection of the reality of many minority, immigrant, poor or other families out of the white middle-class mainstream. These institutions are ill-prepared to deal with the complex, novel and highly charged issues presented by AIDS. Their inadequacy is apparent at many points between diagnosis of AIDS and death, and even beyond. Courts and other agencies have, however, already had to confront the problem in three areas: (a) decisions about medical treatment; (b) housing; and (c) custody decisions.

Decisions about Medical Treatment

A central focus of the field of biomedical ethics, which began in the 1960s as a response to the biological revolution and the prevailing norm of medical paternalism, has been patient autonomy – the right of competent individuals to make health care decisions for themselves. When the person is unable to make those decisions, because of either illness or legal incompetence, the classic quotation has been: 'Who decides?'

Legal efforts to ensure the rights of individuals to make treatment decisions or to designate a particular person as a proxy have centred on some form of advance directive or 'living will'. These documents set out the patient's wishes concerning what kinds of treatment are acceptable and under what conditions, and they may designate a person to act as proxy. Thirty-eight states and the District of Columbia now recognize advance directives for treatment decisions (Society for the Right to Die, 1987). Eighteen states have legalized the patient's appointment of a durable power of attorney in health care to express the patient's wishes if the patient becomes incompetent (Cohen, 1987). While durable powers of attorney are well established in financial matters, their status in health care is less certain, and decisions made by a person designated in this capacity may be challenged.

Although not legally entitled to make treatment decisions, 'the family' has generally been considered the appropriate surrogate. In the hierarchy of decision makers, parents are normally considered surrogates for minor children, spouses take on the surrogate role after marriage and children act as surrogates for widowed, elderly parents. When the family structure does not conform to these patterns, or is not defined by traditional relationships, conflicts among family members, and between family members and physicians or hospitals, may arise. Controversies concerning termination of life support have been at the centre of biomedical ethics discourse.

Bringing a new set of actors – lovers and non-traditional family members – into the equation complicates the decision-making process and sets the stage for conflict. A Minnesota case involving two lesbians has become a symbol for advocates for the rights of women, gay people and the disabled. Sharon Kowalski, a former high-school physical-education teacher, became paralysed and suffered brain damage after an automobile accident in November 1983. After the accident the woman with whom she had lived, Karen Thompson, told Ms Kowalski's parents about their lesbian relationship. Mr Kowalski was named his daughter's guardian in an out-of-court settlement that allows Ms Thompson broad visiting rights to Ms Kowalski, who was in a nursing home. In July 1985 Mr Kowalski received unconditional guardianship and barred Ms Thompson and other friends from any contact with his daughter. In September 1988, Ms Kowalski was moved, by a court order, to a different nursing home for an evaluation of her competency, and there she was reunited with Ms Thompson. The final determination of her competency, placement and guardianship are still unsettled (*New York Times*, 1989a).

Similar cases arise when one partner has AIDS. When the disease involves neurological impairments and dementia as an end-stage complication, the issue of a patient's competence is further clouded. Molly Cooke, a physician at San Francisco General Hospital, describes a typical case. A 27-year-old man with AIDS designated his lover as proxy and stated clearly that he did not want 'heroics' when he reached the terminal stage of his illness. The physician understood him to mean that he refused intubation and mechanical ventilation. When the patient's parents arrived to visit him from out of town, they learned that he was gay at the same time that they learned he had AIDS. Angry and upset, they insisted that 'everything be done' and threatened to sue the hospital. The lover withdrew as proxy and the physicians felt obliged to continue aggressive treatment. The patient died after 22 days on a respirator in the intensive care unit (Cooke, 1986).

In another San Francisco case, a 32-year-old gay man with Kaposi's sarcoma had been abandoned as a child by his parents and was raised by his grandmother. She refused to care for him when she learned of his diagnosis. His siblings refused to visit him, and his parents wrote to tell him that God was punishing him for being gay. The patient designated his partner as his durable power of attorney for health care, and affirmed his refusal of intubation should he become incompetent. After his death, the patient's father insisted that the body be flown to the Midwest for burial, even though the patient had stated his desire for cremation and a local funeral. In this case the patient's wishes were honoured, because of the durable power of attorney (Steinbrook *et al.*, 1985).

In still another case which reached the courts, Thomas Wirth, an AIDS patient at Bellevue Hospital in New York City, signed a living will refusing extraordinary treatment and naming a friend, John Evans, as guardian. The physicians challenged the directive, however, because it did not clearly specify which treatments were being refused. Evans took the case to court, but the court upheld the physicians. They argued that the particular condition that they were proposing to treat – a brain infection – was not by itself fatal. Mr Wirth died soon after the decision. See *Evans* v. *Bellevue Hospital (re Wirth)*, 16536 NY Supp. (27 July 1987).

These cases illustrate common dilemmas but they are atypical in one respect: in each case the patient had clear preferences and had taken some steps to implement them. Unfortunately, as Cooke (1986, p. 345) points out, 'many patients will be admitted to the hospital unable to express their wishes, without a previous documented discussion and without having appointed a proxy with durable power of attorney'. If this is true among the predominantly gay patient population of San Francisco, it is even more the case among the drug users and their sexual partners who now make up the majority of cases in New York City.

Kevin Kelly (1987), a psychiatrist at New York Hospital, has raised another possibility:

> Until now, the prevailing practice has been that, when a decision cannot be made by the patient or responsible others, physicians feel obliged to proceed as if the patient had given consent for all possible measures, but this epidemic may force us to reconsider this practice, and to substitute an alternative model in which the patient is assumed to have withheld consent unless it is specifically given.

Acknowledging that this model would sharply conflict with legal precedent, Kelly suggests that it would be applicable only when the patient is known to have an irreversibly terminal illness, his or her wishes cannot be determined and there is no one else to make the decision. Such a model may hold considerable appeal for physicians, especially since some of the life-prolonging interventions, which are generally futile anyway, involve an additional, albeit small, level of risk of HIV exposure to health care workers through needle sticks and blood splashes. It would, however, result in withholding care from a particular class of patients on the basis of their social status. The category of patients most likely to be affected would be the poor, probably minority, drug user, isolated from both family and friends. These patients would also be more likely to enter the health care system at a later stage of disease, thereby being more likely to have diminished competence. To deny care to such patients when care would be provided to similar patients who were fortunate enough to have social supports would be discriminatory.

Thus, AIDS is having an impact on treatment decisions. Physicians who regularly care for gay AIDS patients, as well as many patients themselves, are moving towards early, specific and ongoing discussions about treatment, including its termination. The *AIDS Legal Guide* encourages persons with AIDS to 'sign a Living Will if it represents their sentiments on the matter, because it serves as a communication of one's intent at a later time when one is no longer able to communicate' (Rubenfeld, 1987, sec. 9, p. 4). The New York State law on 'orders not to resuscitate', passed in April 1988, specifically included 'a close friend' among those who may be designated to act as surrogate on behalf of the patient to acknowledge the rights of gay partners to participate in 'do not resuscitate' (DNR) decisions (New York State Public Health Law, Article 29–B (Orders not to resuscitate), L. 1987, ch. 818. Effective 1 April 1988; Nancy Dubler, personal communication, 1988). This trend clearly strengthens the force of advance directives in non-AIDS cases and sets an example for physician/patient communication for other life-threatening illnesses.

But autonomous decision making in matters of health care may be neither as important nor as easy to implement for patients from poor, minority backgrounds. A sense of fatalism, powerlessness, religious traditions, acquiescence to the wishes of others – whether they are family or physicians – all may work against patient self-determination. Intravenous drug users are not generally interested in talking about living wills and durable powers of attorney; they just want to be treated, hoping and praying for the best. Here too, AIDS will test boundaries, in this case those of personal autonomy and family control.

AIDS may change the boundaries to include serious considerations of euthanasia or 'assisted suicide', thus creating an enormous additional potential for conflict within families. AIDS may even test the validity of informed consent as the basis of medical decision making. At the very least it will require renewed attention to the importance of communication among and between patient, physician and family. Physicians and hospital ethics committees may need special help in understanding, accepting and dealing with non-traditional family members as participants in this process. When the appointed surrogate – for information or for decision making – does not bear the usual relationship to the patient, traditional norms of professional practice may be threatened.

Housing

All families need shelter, and non-traditional families have particular difficulties in obtaining and retaining housing, because of restrictive zoning ordinances and tenancy laws. Zoning laws established in the post-Second-World-War building boom reflected the expectation that the typical family would consist of parents and children. Furthermore, zoning ordinances were intended to protect property values; deviations from the norm of the traditional family constellation are seen as economic threats. Such ordinances typically prohibit non-related individuals from sharing a single-family home. Thus, in addition to gay couples or young unmarried heterosexual couples, elderly couples who cannot afford to marry because their Social Security payments will be reduced may have difficulty in finding a place to live.

In Denver in May 1989, after considerable discussion, the city council voted to amend its 36-year-old ordinance and allow two adults unrelated by blood, marriage or adoption to live in the same house. The new ordinance also eliminates a $20 room-and-board permit for an unrelated couple living together. The earlier prohibition affected mainly unmarried couples living together, as well as single parents who rent out rooms to tenants to help defray expenses (*New York Times*, 1989f, g). Councilwoman Mary de Groot applauded the ruling: 'Zoning should be used for regulating land use and density, not relationships.' An opponent of the change, Councilman Bill Roberts, who is black, saw the move, however, as threatening Afro-American family stability: 'The most stable environment in which to raise children is in a house with a mother and a father who have a commitment to each other.'

New York's highest court, the State Court of Appeals, upheld a lower court that ruled that the town of Brookhaven's zoning law violated the state constitution by restricting the number of unrelated people who could live together as a 'functionally equivalent family'. The decision will make it easier for unrelated individuals to live together in areas previously restricted to single-family use (*New York Times*, 1989e).

In 1974, the US Supreme Court had, however, upheld a law in the village of Belle Terre, also in Long Island, that defined a family as people related by blood, marriage or adoption, or not more than two unrelated people. Recent amendments to the Federal Fair Housing Act, extending governmental protections against housing discrimination to disabled people and families with children, may have a powerful impact on the rights of people with AIDS and their families to obtain housing (*New York Times*, 1989d).

In urban areas, a common problem arises when the person named on a lease dies and the surviving partner or family member claims the right to remain as a tenant in a rent-controlled or rent-stabilized apartment. The case of *Braschi* v. *Stahl Associates Company* (74 NY 2d 201 (1989)) in New York City is the most significant legal challenge to the practice of limiting survivors' rights to traditional family members. Although the case involves a gay couple, the precedent it sets will be important for many people affected by the disease in low-income, minority communities, as well as for unmarried heterosexual couples and other non-traditional families. The situation is particularly dire for survivors who themselves are HIV-infected or have AIDS or who have responsibility for caring for another family member with AIDS. Eviction from an apartment upon the death of the primary tenant can lead to homelessness for the survivors.

Miguel Braschi lived with his life-partner Leslie Blanchard in Blanchard's rent-controlled New York City apartment for ten years, until Blanchard died of AIDS. Braschi, who was Blanchard's primary caregiver throughout his illness, was informed by the landlord that he was being evicted. The Supreme Court of New York County granted a preliminary injunction, halting the eviction. The judge found that, on the basis of the ten-year relationship, Braschi was a 'family member' within the meaning of the rent control law, Section 56(d) of the New York City Rent, Rehabilitation and Eviction Regulations. This section provides that 'family members who reside continuously for at least six months with the tenant of record, continue as rent-controlled tenants even after the tenant of record dies or vacates the premises'.

The landlord appealed, and the appellate division unanimously reversed the decision. While it recognized that Braschi had proved that the relationship with the tenant had been 'marked by love and fidelity for each other', it interpreted the rent control law 'as only protecting surviving spouses and family members within traditional, legally recognized familial relationships'. Braschi received permission for a direct appeal to the Court of Appeals, which decided in his favour in July 1989. Writing for the majority, Judge Titone said: 'The term family . . . should not be rigidly restricted to those people who have formalized their relationship by obtaining, for instance, a marriage certificate or an adoption order. The intended protection against sudden eviction should not rest on fictitious legal distinctions or genetic history, but instead should find its foundation in the reality of family life.' Further cases will undoubtedly seek to extend the ruling to rent-stabilized apartments and other types of housing, and some difficulties can also be expected in defining whether a particular couple meet the criteria for 'family' set out in the decision – 'two adult lifetime partners whose relationship is long-term and characterized by an emotional and financial commitment and interdependence'.

Custody Decisions

Parents are normally responsible for the care and nurturing of their children. But when circumstances prevent one or both parents from fulfilling this obligation, courts determine who shall have custody of the child. The state's interest is in seeing that the child is protected, as much as possible, from the harmful effects of divorce, separation or death. Traditionally, judges have wide latitude in determining a child's 'best interests'. Until recently the traditional presumption has favoured, however, the biological mother. The *Baby M* case in New Jersey marked a deviation from this traditional course: the biological or 'surrogate' mother, Mary Beth Whitehead, was defeated in her bid for custody by the biological father William Stern and the adoptive mother Elizabeth Stern. In general, courts are becoming much more responsive to paternal claims for custody.

Against this background, conflicts about custody of children related to AIDS or

HIV infection arise in two broad contexts: visitation rights in separation and divorce cases, where one parent is lesbian or gay or is HIV-infected or has AIDS; and the placement of children following the death of a parent with AIDS.

As homosexuality has become more openly discussed and, arguably, more accepted in society, homosexual or bisexual parents have become more willing to seek custody of their children when a marriage or sexual relationship dissolves. And in general more courts have been willing to accept these non-traditional relationships. But to the already volatile atmosphere of a failed relationship, the question of HIV infection adds an explosive charge.

How will judges weigh HIV status in making custody decisions? A judge who might have been willing to grant custody to a gay parent may not be so amenable if he is misinformed about the possibilities of HIV transmission in a family setting. In the Indiana case of *Stewart* v. *Stewart* (521 N.E. 2d 956 (Ind. Ct. App. 1988)), Mr Stewart sought to regain visitation rights to his one-year-old daughter after his former wife refused to let him see her. Mrs Stewart was addicted to drugs and alcohol, and had lost custody of her first two children before she met and married Mr Stewart. A trial court held that Mr Stewart could be denied all visitation rights to his daughter because he was HIV positive, although asymptomatic. An appeals court ruled, however, that HIV infection *per se* was not a reason to deny custody or visitation.

A New York court ruled, in *Jane and John Doe* v. *Richard Roe* (526 N.Y. Sup. 718 (14 March 1988)), that a father who had custody of his two children did not have to undergo HIV antibody testing as a condition of retaining custody, as the children's maternal grandparents had requested. The court in *Ann D.* v. *Raymond D.* (528 N.Y. 2d 718 (1988)) made a similar finding, ruling that 'a positive test result may not automatically be a "determinant factor" with respect to plaintiff's ability to be a custodial parent'.

Courts in other jurisdictions, however, have restricted the visitation rights of a parent with AIDS. For example, a New Jersey court ordered that a father with AIDS could not visit his child without supervision (*Jordan* v. *Jordan*, FV 12–1357–84 (Middlesex County, N.J., Sup.)).

On the basis of a review of the scientific and legal literature, Nancy Mahon (1988) concludes:

> A court's use of a parent's HIV infection as per se evidence of parental unfitness contravenes the best interests standard . . . unless judges perform a factually specific examination of how a particular parent's HIV infection affects a child, the child's best interests cannot be served.

Will future courts follow this standard? It will depend on judges' level of understanding and education. Hard cases, however, will inevitably arise, in which a parent's desire for custody must be weighed against the ability of that parent to provide appropriate care if he or she is seriously ill and likely to die or engaging in behaviour like drug use that undermines the stability of the child's life.

A second category of custody case is arising as increasing numbers of mothers become ill with AIDS. These cases now occur where there are substantial numbers of infected and ill women, especially in New York, New Jersey and Florida; as the epidemic progresses, they may be expected to arise elsewhere. The New York City Task Force estimates that 'over the next few years a minimum of 60,000–70,000 children in New York City will lose at least one parent to AIDS. Of these, maybe 10,000 will lose both parents to the disease' (New York City AIDS Task Force, 1988).

The surviving children, some of whom may be HIV-infected but many of whom are not, must be placed in someone's care. Whose should it be? The options for these children, the majority of them from poor minority families, are few and frequently bleak: placement with a member of the extended family who may be beset by the same social and economic problems as the natural mother; foster care, with its inherent impermanence; adoption, which is unlikely to be available for older children.

Frequently, decisions about custody are made by a dying mother; her wishes may conflict with those of surviving family members, the child or the professional team caring for her. Sometimes a child may wish to live with a relative whom the professionals consider ill-equipped for the responsibility but who may be the only biological relative. The legal options available to confer guardianship, such as testamentary provisions or deeds, are fraught with uncertainties (C. Zuckerman, personal communication, 1988).

As family courts become overwhelmed with these cases (not just as a result of AIDS, but of drug, particularly crack, addiction as well), it is likely that the decisions will be based more on which party has the most effective legal representation and not on the ill-defined concept of 'best interests of the child'. In addition to effective representation for mothers, advocates for the children may be required to ensure that they do not become pawns in an intra- or interfamilial or agency–family dispute.

It is possible that courts' traditional preference for granting custody to biological parents, even those who have not demonstrated a high level of concern for their children, may collapse under the weight of the caseload of orphaned children and drug-addicted parents. The foster care systems in affected communities may also be unable to accommodate a huge number of children with multiple problems, because many of the potential foster parents may also be affected by the disease. If the foster care system collapses, it is possible that some children may be placed in states far from their communities of origin, rather like the Asian children brought to the United States by adoptive parents. It is also possible that the very foundation of child placement since the Progressive Era – that children are better off in families than in institutions – may be re-examined. In New York City, however, group homes set up to accommodate 'boarder babies' released from hospitals and awaiting foster care placements are understaffed, in disrepair, and violate health and safety regulations (New York Times, 1989h).

In the future, custody decisions may, from necessity as much as principle, accommodate a wide variety of non-traditional family placements. With increased flexibility in these arrangements, it seems likely that most children could be placed in families. But some children – those hardest to place or those living in areas where families able and willing to accept them are in short supply – may have to live in institutions. Lois Forer (1988), a retired family court judge in Philadelphia who has seen at first hand the failures of both families and foster care, has already called for a return of orphanages. She says:

> Public institutions are answerable to the public. They can be inspected regularly by public officials. Committees of private citizens can act as overseers and keep a careful eye on the operations of such orphanages. It is difficult and expensive for social workers to inspect at frequent intervals all foster homes.

The choice may come down to admittedly inadequate family placement and admittedly but differently inadequate institutional placement. A change in basic social work philosophy, which has favoured families over institutions, would be profound and disturbing, but is not unthinkable.

THE FORMATION OF NEW FAMILIES

The process of change and adaptation is incomplete. Just as existing families continue to adjust to the exigencies of AIDS, the formation of new families may also be affected by law and changing custom. Individuals do not ordinarily make the commitment that defines 'family' without considerable prior interaction with the potential partner. Families start out as relationships. If evidence for the impact of AIDS in the areas already described is scant, it is even more fragmentary the more one looks to the future for families. This final section is, therefore, largely speculative.

Some changes may reflect the epidemiology of AIDS. For example, in some minority communities, large numbers of men and women of childbearing age are HIV-infected. These communities place a high cultural value on reproduction; children are seen as proof of virility or femininity, sources of pleasure, links to the past and hope for the future. How will HIV infection, and the consequent threat of the birth of HIV-infected babies, affect the formation of new relationships in these communities? Will a partner's HIV status be an important determinant? Will the post-AIDS society envisioned in Margaret Atwood's (1986) *The Handmaid's Tale*, in which healthy women serve as breeders, come to pass? It is not implausible that the wives of haemophiliacs or other men with HIV infection will choose artificial insemination rather than risk unprotected sex, HIV transmission to themselves and infection of their fetuses. Nor is it far-fetched to think that some infected women would choose not to bear children themselves but would engage a surrogate for that purpose.

Even among groups where procreation is not a supreme value, HIV status may be influential in the formation of new relationships that might lead to procreation. Public policy and medical practice may play a significant role. The intent of mandatory premarital HIV screening (which was tried and abandoned in Louisiana and later in Illinois), as well as of less coercive efforts to encourage voluntary testing among couples about to be married or women considering pregnancy, is to discourage marriage and reproduction among HIV-infected partners. For example, two epidemiologists reviewing data about heterosexual transmission concluded that 'societies may soon have to wrestle with many difficult questions, including the suitability of infected individuals for marriage and natural parenthood' (Haverkos and Edelman, 1988). In challenging this 'incautiously worded' comment, Ronald Bayer (1989) declared: 'Both moral sensibilities and our constitutional tradition revolt at the notion that classes of adults – defined in terms of biologic factors – be barred from marriage.' The authors replied: 'We personally do not support criminalized marriage, criminalized childbirth, coerced abortion, or compulsory sterilization . . . Nevertheless . . . we can predict that as the pandemic widens and deepens in our society, increasingly powerful voices will be heard calling for such state-imposed restrictions' (Edelman and Haverkos, 1989).

So far only one state (Utah) has passed a law invalidating marriages involving an HIV-infected partner. This law has not been tested. While the intent of the Utah law may be to protect traditional family norms, another source of opposition to sex involving HIV-infected partners comes from the Rajneesh religious communities, which reject exclusive, monogamous relationships. In their view, AIDS confirms their belief that illness is the result of sexual repression. One Rajneeshee explained: 'What they [all those Christians and bourgeoisie] can't see is that the family is what drove all those people to rebel in the first place – to become homosexuals and junkies. So, returning to the family would only worsen the situation!' (Palmer, 1989).

While organized opposition to marriage or sex involving an infected person may be limited, personal choices of sexual and especially marriage partners, only recently (and incompletely) freed from considerations of religion, race and economic or social status, may be tempered by disease. Even though AIDS is becoming a chronic illness, the HIV-infected person has a shorter life span than a healthy person. Those involved in a sexual relationship, which includes the vast majority of married couples, must always be constrained by concerns about transmission. An attorney with haemophilia described a failed romance:

> Not long after I was diagnosed as carrying the virus, I began dating a bright, attractive woman. I wanted to kiss her – certainly no big thing under normal circumstances. But I felt I must first tell her about the virus. . . . On a rational basis, she grasped that kissing me would almost certainly not be dangerous. But AIDS has taken on an identity of its own. . . . It was a world of which she wanted no part. Recreational sex was not worth risking one's life for, she explained, and what was the point of developing strong emotions for someone who could not lead a normal sex and family life? (*New York Times Magazine*, 1989a)

Disagreeing that life with HIV infection was inevitably asexual, the wife of a haemophiliac who died of AIDS nevertheless responded in a way that seemed to bear out the attorney's fears:

> I married my husband . . . after he was diagnosed with AIDS. It is true that we had a pre-existing relationship. However, it is also true that we had a romantic and sexual life after he was diagnosed. . . . I admit that the latter made me and my husband anxious, and that the anxiety could not be overcome completely. (*New York Times Magazine*, 1989b)

Although the stigma and discrimination surrounding the disease may diminish, they will not disappear. While existing relationships may survive and even be strengthened by knowledge of a partner's HIV infection, the formation of new relationships may well be deterred by the realities of the situation. On the other hand, there may be greater interest in, and social acceptance of, the legalization of marriages between homosexual partners (*New York Times*, 1989c). The City of San Francisco's registry of 'domestic partners' is a step towards legalization. Even in the absence of a formal mechanism, gay couples may announce their commitment in other ways. In New York City, Michael Feierstein, who works on AIDS programmes in the Department of Health, and his lover, Luke Denobriga, a hairdresser, announced their plans to hold a 'commitment ceremony' and to change their name to Mr and Mr Stanton (Luke's actual first name). In a memo to his colleagues, Mr Feierstein said:

> There is no mechanism in our society for gay people to publicly announce their relationships or 'marriage'. We're not permitted, by law, to marry. A recent trend in the Gay and Lesbian Community has been toward commitment ceremonies, wedding-like events for family and friends similar to those heterosexual people have been enjoying for centuries. (*Newsday*, 1989b)

In this explication the differences between non-traditional and traditional families seem less important than their similarities. AIDS is both heightening the creation of non-traditional families and presenting special problems for them. AIDS threatens the intimacy and acceptance that ideally undergird family relationships, while at the same time making them all the more powerful and necessary.

REFERENCES

Anderson, E. A. (1988) AIDS public policy: implications for families, *New England Journal of Public Policy*, 4, pp. 411–427.

Atwood, M. (1986) *The Handmaid's Tale* (New York, Fawcett).

Bayer, R. (1989) The suitability of HIV-positive individuals for marriage and pregnancy, *Journal of the American Medical Association*, 261, p. 993.

Breo, D. L. (1988) Harlem pediatrician's concern: fighting for children with AIDS, *American Medical News*, 21 October, 3, p. 33.

Chicago Tribune (1987) Obstacles for AIDS victims: Hispanics hampered by poverty, language barrier, by J. L. Griffin. 1 December.

Citizens Commission on AIDS (1989) *The Crisis in AIDS Care: A Call to Action* (New York).

City of Los Angeles Task Force on Family Diversity (1988) *Strengthening Families: A Model for Community Action*. Final Report.

Cohen, E. N., (1987) *Appointing a Proxy for Health-Care Decisions: Analysis and the Chart of State Law* (New York, Society for the Right to Die).

Cooke, M. (1986) Ethical issues in the care of patients with AIDS, *Quality Review Bulletin*, 12, pp. 343–346.

Donzelot, J. (1979) *The Policing of Families* (New York: Pantheon).

Edelman, R. and Haverkos, H. W. (1989) The suitability of HIV-positive individuals for marriage and pregnancy, *Journal of the American Medical Association*, 261, p. 993.

Forer, L. G. (1988) Bring back the orphanage, *Washington Monthly*, 20 (3), pp. 17–24.

Frost, R. (1971 [1914]) *Poems* (New York, Washington Square Press).

Haverkos, H.W. and Edelman, R. (1988) The epidemiology of AIDS among heterosexuals, *Journal of the American Medical Association*, 260, pp. 1922–1929.

Kelly, K. (1987) AIDS and ethics: an overview, *General Hospital Psychiatry*, 9, pp. 331–340.

Levitan, S. A., Belous, R. S. and Gallo, F. (1988) *What's Happening to the American Family?: Tensions, Hopes, Realities*, rev. edn (Baltimore, Johns Hopkins University Press).

Lloyd, G. A. (1988) HIV-infection, AIDS, and family disruption, in: A R. Fleming *et al.* (eds) *The Global Impact of Aids* (New York, Alan R. Liss).

Mahon, N. B. (1988) Public hysteria, private conflict; child custody and visitation disputes involving an HIV-infected parent, *New York University Law Review*, 63, pp. 1092–1141.

Newsday (1987) AIDS: trouble in a permissive society, by A. Peracchio. 10 November.

Newsday (1989a) AIDS patients' seder held by synagogue. 18 April.

Newsday (1989b) And you think your life is complicated?, by J. Nachman. 30 April.

New York City AIDS Task Force (1988) *Models of Care Report* (New York).

New York Times (1988) Mother of AIDS victim shares her story to teach others, by T. Morgan. 25 November.

New York Times (1989a) Woman's hospital visit marks gay rights, by N. Broznan. 8 February.

New York Times (1989b) Two men who fought L.I. abortion, by E. Schmitt, 13 February.

New York Times (1989c) Gay marriages: make them legal, by T. B. Stoddard, 4 March.

New York Times (1989d) The new truth in the fair housing law: H.U.D. officials now will sue in cases of discrimination, by T. J. Lenck. 12 March.

New York Times (1989e) Court upsets Long Island zoning law on unrelated people in home, by P. S. Gutis. 24 March.

New York Times (1989f) Denver zoning fight turns on defining a family. 26 March.

New York Times (1989g) Denver kills law that barred homes with unwed couples. 3 May.

New York Times (1989h) Health violations cited at child group homes, by S. Daley. 20 May.

New York Times (1989i) San Francisco votes legislation recognizing unmarried partners. 24 May.

New York Times Magazine (1989a) A life in limbo, by P. Bayer. 2 April.

New York Times Magazine (1989b) A life in limbo, by M. B. Ockey. 23 April.

Palmer, S. J. (1989) AIDS as metaphor, *Society*, 26, pp. 44–50.

Rubenfeld, A. R. (1987) *AIDS Legal Guide*, 2nd edn (New York, Lambda Legal Defense and Education Fund).

Society for the Right to Die (1987). *Handbook of Living Will Laws* (New York).

Sontag, S. (1986) The way we live now, *New Yorker*.

Steinbrook, R., Lo, B., Tirpack, J., Dilley, J. W. and Volberding, P. A. (1985) The ethical dilemmas in caring for patients with the acquired immunodeficiency syndrome, *Annals of Internal Medicine*, 103, pp. 787–790.

Tiblier, K. B., Walker, G. and Rolland, J. (1989) Therapeutic issues when working with families of persons with AIDS, in: E. Macklin (ed.) *AIDS and Families*, pp. 81–128 (Binghamton, N.Y., Harrington Park).

Toffler, A. (1980) *The Third Wave* (New York: Bantam Books).

Tolstoy, L. (1981 [1877]) *Anna Karenina* (New York, Bantam Books).

US Bureau of the Census (1981) *Marital Status and Living Arrangements: March 1980* (Washington, DC).

US Bureau of the Census (1988) *Households, Families, Marital Status and Living: March 1988*. Advance report (Washington, DC).

TWO

The Impact of HIV/AIDS on the Family and Other Significant Relationships: The African Clan Revisited

E. Maxine Ankrah

INTRODUCTION

Mrs Noreen Kaleeba, founder of The AIDS Support Organization (TASO) of Uganda, has described AIDS as a 'family burden', signifying the central role the African family plays in the management of disease and sickness and in the provision of health care. However, AIDS poses an extraordinary challenge. The African family unit must cope with a disease that threatens to inflict unprecedented levels of morbidity and mortality across sub-Saharan Africa by the turn of this century, according to World Health Organization projections. On the other hand, the changes that will ensue in its structure because of AIDS may, concomitantly, disrupt its functioning and weaken its capacity to respond to the health care needs of its sick members. However, African families over millennia of coping have developed an extensive repertoire of treatment and patient management approaches.

This review article first highlights aspects of the many traditional patterns of treatment and care that predate AIDS, but that with the multiple opportunistic infections associated with the disease are likely to be indispensable to the effective handling of the sick. This rich inheritance, despite the infusion of modern medicines and practices, constitutes more than an 'alternative' approach. For most African families, particularly among the rural and the poor, it is often the sole and critical resource available for easing the suffering of a family member with AIDS. Knowing the African experience of healing should help interveners to better appropriate the traditions of African families in their own AIDS strategies of care.

The explanation for the resilience of a people in environmental contexts that are prone to ill-health and disease can be found in their social organization. The crucial factor to the sustenance of the African family in the midst of AIDS is the social structure, which includes the nuclear family, the extended family and the clan. Understanding its functioning in contemporary Africa should provide clues to the potential of the African society to successfully withstand the adversities of AIDS. This social structure has hitherto been a neglected area in AIDS literature and research as well as in the strategies designed for family coping. Yet it is the context in which families are sustained, reorganized or created in wholly new forms. Therefore, we revisit this ancient and ubiquitous African structure with the hope that sufficient interest will be generated to spur a more rigorous examination of the theses proffered in this review.

AIDS is expected to facilitate or to vitalize totally new associations. Within such, individuals and/or families are emotionally bonded to others unrelated by blood or kinship ties, but who come together because of a common experience of suffering and death. These act to create institutional ties that serve to support persons who are vulnerable owing to AIDS. In effect, we conclude that the traditional African support system's resilience will remain a constant, despite AIDS.

THE AFRICAN FAMILY: TRADITIONAL AND MODERN, DIVERGENCE AND CHANGE

Defining 'the Family'

The African family is of interest to many disciplines. Varied interpretations have been given to its history, structure and functioning. Its potential for persistence, transformation and change, especially in times of crises such as war, famine or disease, has been studied. Belonging to a family is propagated through numerous bonds, ranging from consanguinity, affinity, adoption and propinquity, to surname identification. The African family is thus an extensive social network with a diversity of assured contacts.

Although seemingly broad, the entity we define as the 'African family' is not without limits. Murdock's definition of the family as a social group characterized by common residence, economic cooperation and reproduction is a useful point of departure. Perhaps looking at the family as a kin-based group of people living in a dwelling(s), occupying a single compound and including members temporarily resident elsewhere, but who recognize a common household head, according to Jaensen *et al*. (1984), is to be more strict.

While challenging each other's meanings of 'family', sociologists nevertheless seem to agree on its essential characteristics, including permanence – at least in intention – and commitment to mutuality in various forms of economic and social support (Levine, 1990), although some of the members may be temporarily dispersed for occupational, social or political reasons (Okediji, 1974; Kayongo-Male and Onyango, 1984; McGrath *et al*., 1991).

There are various types of African families, depending on the structure of each. A family at its simplest level includes a man, woman and their offspring; these constitute the nuclear or elementary family. The extended family, on the other hand, consists of a number of joint families. This can take the form of parents, their children with their families, all living in one compound or several contiguous compounds. Cousins of anyone in the nuclear family and other kin maintaining ties with the nuclear family through visiting or socio-economic support may also be included (Okediji, 1974; Kayongo-Male and Onyango, 1984). An extended family can, therefore, cover several generations.

The traditional extended family was a unit wherein basic production and distribution of material goods and services took place. This was an important socio-economic mechanism owing to its relatively big size and composition (Sudarkasa, 1982). It acted as a socializing agent for the new members of society. The larger kinship group, through extended family and clan elders, provided the know-how based on experience; young members provided the labour to get various tasks accomplished (Nahenow, 1979; Sudarkasa, 1982; Marwick, 1988). These institutions acted as effective agents of social control and social security.

Changing Families

Africa today is witnessing a process of radical change in the family as an institution – in its extended and conjugal form. The nature and extent of this change have been widely documented (Kayongo-Male and Onyango, 1984; Ankrah, 1978; Kilbride and Kilbride, 1990; Richards, 1966; Colson, 1970). The cooperative and caring obligations widely cherished between and among kin which were essential for stable and secure traditional family life are being gradually circumvented by the exigencies of economic stress, urbanization, education, Christianity and neo-colonial culture influences. The function of families as joint economic units of production is being rapidly altered. A man may no longer easily afford to adopt his brother's children. Only when one family in a kinship is seriously hit by famine, disease or death (as in the case of AIDS) do the traditional social obligations of sharing and support become evident. With increasing mobility and migration to the growing urban settings, the conjugal family takes up the role of defining expected behaviour of individual members and their tasks. Therefore, structural isolation of the conjugal family affects both the role performance and social relationships.

The trend towards nuclearization of the family is noted especially among the educated and urban populations. With continued influence of Western culture, African societies will increasingly focus more on conjugal relationships, and, thus, change the role and structure of their families.

Reduction in size of families in Africa has already been reported (Kayongo-Male and Onyango, 1984; Mbithi, 1978). Many people employed in urban settings and those conducting business have sought smaller families owing to economic pressures and their separation from their rural settings. With increased market as opposed to subsistence production, it becomes comparatively difficult to cater for a large number of relatives; hence the quest for more isolated conjugal units. This, together with the influence of Christianity, has meant a steady change towards monogamous marriages in many African families.

On family composition, Mbithi (1978) and others indicated in the 1970s that the majority of families had absentee male adults with a reduction in the degree of influence the father has in the rearing of children. Changes in sex ratios in urban areas in East Africa over two decades ago showed about 153 men for every 100 women in Kenyan towns, 146 men for every 100 women in Uganda towns, and 131 for every 100 women in Tanzanian towns (Kayongo-Male and Onyango, 1984), with such imbalances leading to increases in temporary unions and high rates of illegitimacy. All these factors tend to have adverse effects on family stability.

Despite the waves of change, many studies have reported persistence and continuity of the African family to perform its significant roles, perhaps in slightly altered ways. For instance, Aldous (1962) reviewed a variety of studies of the cities of Brazzaville, Dakar, Lagos, Leopoldville and Stanleyville. He concluded that the extended family still functioned strongly in the urban environment in terms of the co-residence of two or more nuclear families and joint activities among individual relatives and friendship networks of kin. Though capable of considerable transformation and radical changes in function, the African family, therefore, retains strong internal and external kin ties, even when members are 'lifted' out of the context of more or less homogeneous, rural life. This continued connectedness is most clearly evident in the persistence of the African clanship system.

THE AFRICAN CLAN

Its Support Functions

Extensive ethnographic and anthropological data support the view that the clan is the major principle around which African kinship groupings are organized. It is a social unit with a common ancestor and a common totem. Clans have survived through the centuries, are found almost ubiquitously across sub-Saharan Africa, are still recognized, and thus help to explain the strong consciousness of kinship and lineage that still remain a dominant mindset among most African peoples (Bascom and Herskovits, 1959; Ayisi, 1980; Caldwell *et al.*, 1990a, b).

Fortes (1945) defined the clan as

> a set of locally united lineages, each of which is linked with all or most others by ties of clanship, which act together in the service of certain common interests indicated by the bond of exogamy, by reciprocal rights and duties in events such as the funeral of a member of any one of them, by the ban on internecine war or feuds, and which act as a corporate unit in respect of these common interests in relation to other such units. . . . This definition does not exhaust all the attributes of social relations based on clanship ties.

Other sociologists and anthropologists of that period (Sumner, 1906, 1959; Radcliff-Brown, 1950; Richards, 1950; Fortes, 1957; Bascom and Herskovits, 1959; Linton, 1959, Titiev, 1959; Mandelbaum, 1960) included some or all of these dimensions in their analysis of data, usually derived from field studies of primitive cultures. Most of these sources note that clan membership is sanctioned by religious observance, such as an ancestral cult (Caldwell *et al.*, 1990a, b; Linton, 1959).

Mandelbaum's (1960) discussion of the subject brings into sharp focus the support function of the clan. He observes that a specific clan includes persons related by blood, mostly, but there are others in the grouping for whom kinship appears not to exist except in the possession of the clan name. This is sufficient, though, to compel persons to 'treat each other as though they all actually were blood relatives'. Members share with clanmates something of the 'pattern of mutual helpfulness' (Titiev, 1950; Fortes, 1945), and thus, the individual is 'strengthened' by the relationship with a group much larger than the immediate family. He compares the short duration in time with a stable and long passage of time of clans – usually through many generations. It is 'a corporation that outlasts its individual members'. In its corporate role (Mandelbaum, 1960; Fortes, 1945) the clan frequently executes certain services for the larger public such as providing leadership by, for example, chiefs and priests. Mandelbaum (1960) asserts:

> This very collective responsibility of the clan for the deeds of its individual members makes it a strong force for social order. Since all the clan members know they will bear a share of the trouble if one of their clan-mates go astray, they try to see to it that a potentially erring member is kept within socially approved limits.

Change and Continuity

Mandelbaum's work presents perhaps a picture of the ideal functioning of the clan. On the other hand, Fortes's detailed study of the Tales, Caldwell *et al.* (1990 a, b) and Sumner (1906, 1959) highlight many of the features of clan structure and operations that are pertinent to this assessment. Fortes (1957) points out that spatial distance and genealogical distance are the main factors upon which the incidence and variance of the rights and duties of clanship depend. The farther apart are these distances, the less likely there will be cooperation in those situations and events that mobilize clan ties. He contends that the closer the genealogical links – actual, putative or fictional, between two lineages – the more effectively do members assert the rights and perform the duties of clanship.

Mandelbaum (1960) concludes that clan solidarity is strengthened by proximity and by limited mobility. Where there is common residence, common efforts are both feasible and advantageous. Whether in the 1990s the African clan will act as a 'corporate' body with a sense of obligation towards members may well be a function of geographical more than social factors. Given that from 60 to 90% of most African populations still reside in rural communities and with extended families living contiguously, the social network of the clanship system may well still be largely intact. Although rapid urban growth in parts of sub-Saharan Africa has caused many members to scatter – with reduction of clan consciousness – this is not wholly the case in West Africa, where clan leaders as elders continue to provide guidance and support to members in urban communities (Ayisi, 1980).

Historically, with dispersal of clan members or other life conditions, social groupings or associations progressively take over functions of the clan. In time, these usually become more important than kinship ties (Sumner, 1906, 1959; Mandelbaum, 1960; Fortes, 1945) as social bonds. Such 'institutional ties' (Sumner, 1906, 1959) are formed in such diverse associations as trade unions, non-governmental social welfare, professional and civic organizations, cooperatives and the like. Those concerned with AIDS are frequently designated 'NGOs'. In these, people are held together by common interests and mutual participation in activities. These social networks are extensions of local groupings that expect the units to perform a variety of functions for members. Programme initiatives to deal with AIDS reflect a dominant trend towards utilization of such institutional ties and their relevant organizations.

These institutional ties (Sumner, 1906, 1959), nevertheless, have not replaced kinship ties among Africans. Transition to institutional ties is not yet complete, as is the case in industrialized countries. The associated ties and structures are more prominently an urban phenomenon and are subject to constraints, if not to reversals, in their impact on the AIDS problems in the 1990s. This could be brought on by socio-economic structural adjustment policies applied to the social sectors (Ankrah, 1991c). Consequently, AIDS portends a more, rather than a less, central role for the family and the clan.

Behavioural Change and Clan Influence

Bascom and Herskovits in the 1950s, Fortes (1962) and Caldwell *et al.* (1990a) noted the diminished capacity of the kinship system to exert control or to regulate the behaviour of members in the institutions of marriage and the family. The latter suggest that both were undermined by the colonial administration and law, the teachings of Christian missionaries about spousal relationships and modern education – all of which helped to change the relationship between the sexes. They argue that socio-economic change has also had an important impact, contending that this factor has radically altered the value of many, or any, wives and children for the African man in modern society, who might consider them both as economic liabilities. However, one thing still holds: he or she does not marry a clansman/ woman. He or she remains a brother or a sister.

Bascom and Herskovits (1959) maintain that in aspects of economics, religion, education and politics, kin groups have been displaced by such associations as just discussed. At the same time Caldwell *et al.* (1990b) suggest implicitly, as do Bascom and Herskovits (1959) directly, that change is not absolute. Continuity is also evident, particularly in the dimension of sexual and marital relationships. For example, polygyny has been sustained, despite other changes. These include reduction in the need for many wives or many children because of the emergence of states or nations that regulate interethnic conflict that formerly required many sons to fight tribal wars. They hold that polygyny is maintained because of the continued respect for old men that is embedded in the ancestral cult, which persists as a factor in African religious consciousness. Thus, 'elders' have retained their place in African social organization, with varying roles, responsibilities and degrees of authority to function for the good of the clan. In particular, they have retained their importance in matters of birth and death through their involvement with funerals and burials, the inheritance of widows and issues of succession and other rituals within the family and the clan. A phenomenon which threatens the survival of the clan system is undoubtedly a major concern for elders. AIDS poses such a threat.

Yet clans have been virtually neglected in AIDS strategies in Africa, ignoring the fact that traditional patterns nevertheless strongly impinge on contemporary living in Africa. However, the potential of a focus on kin structures to widen sectarian rifts in fragile nations (Ayisi, 1980) causes some social scientists to argue that to 'revive' the clan is to revive differences at a time when national unity is being sought. On the contrary, although the value of the collective may have been denigrated as a mechanism for positive social action because of the possibility of abuse, the African clan requires no reviving. It has never died; it only remains an ignored, but vital, resource for AIDS intervention. A more potent reason than 'politics' may explain the neglect of the clan. This lies in the conceptualization of the problems of AIDS from the perspective of the industrialized countries. An example of this is the notion of an 'AIDS orphan'. This conceptualization is seen in the increase in Africa of alternative associations based on institutional ties (Sumner, 1906, 1959), through which interventions are being designed, as we have already noted. But, since such associations in Africa have little or no base in the traditional relationship structure, they potentially lack authority over individual or collective behaviour that is sufficient to compel compliance with prescribed actions. Where these are creations of, or branches of, international organizations, they may even appear to be 'alien' to the local African culture and ways of behaving. Seeking legitimacy by the involvement of local professionals in positions of leadership often fails to convince the rural population, especially to become engaged in finding solutions, or to adopt the recommended changes in behaviour.

Therefore, the fact that the African clanship system has not rationally responded to the menace that AIDS is to its members may be explained more by the neglect of interveners in their preference for recently introduced models than by a lack of potential of the system to respond.

In brief, a broader understanding of the African kinship structure should, therefore, be sought, based on a reappraisal of the structure and functioning of the family, the clanship system and the links both have to other institutional networks that individuals choose to enter because of mutuality of interests and experiences. What families have done or do as treatment and care of sick members is the concern to which we next direct our attention.

TRADITIONAL PATTERNS OF TREATMENT AND CARE

Treatment

Disease prevention and medical practice in Africa are undoubtedly as old as the people themselves. In traditional medicine, relevant clan and family members knew about history-taking and physical examinations. Although they were limited in their ways of investigations, they nevertheless proceeded to the logical next steps of treatment by herbal or drug administration, exorcizing, incantations, suggestions or sacrifices (Sigarist, 1943; Straus and Mead, 1961; Maclean, 1982; Ruhakana, 1986).

Within families, drug treatment was perhaps the most important form of therapy. This was done through the application of herbs, grasses and special soil (Benjamin, 1955). Also used were insects, eggs, honey, alcohol, banana beer and bones (Mburu, 1973; Rutiba, 1982). In one case study, Maclean (1971) reports a Nigerian, experiencing general discomfort and malaise, instructing one of his wives to obtain the leaves of a particular plant which grew in profusion on a nearby path of waste land. Once gathered, the leaves were plunged into a pot of boiling water and the sufferer would take a drink of the infusion, sometimes washing with the liquid as well, while muttering short verses in Yoruba.

In these and other such cases, wives were inevitably the main health care givers of the family. However, knowledge of drug treatment, especially the empirical knowledge of herbs, including poisonous ones, was more available to boys. Traditionally, boys in the family were trained by their parents in the art of herding and hunting, during which basic herbal medicaments were shown to them (Mburu, 1973). Their female counterparts had the responsibility for care giving.

In many African societies, such as the Akamba (Ndeti, 1969), the Taita (Bostock, 1950), the Nyamwezi (Abrahams, 1959) and others (Sommerfelt, 1959; Perlman, 1959; Makhuba, 1978; Sargent, 1987), illness was not an isolated phenomenon, to be defined in its own terms. It was supposedly brought on by evil spirits or angry ancestors, ill-wishers or witch doctors. Among the Zulus, for instance, any disease associated with laboured breathing, pains in the chest, loss of weight and coughing up blood-stained sputum was attributed to the machinations of an ill-wisher (Benjamin, 1955). In most cases such diagnosis was made by members of the family, who consulted a diviner in case there arose some unanswered questions about the illness. Quite frequently, relatives were considered a source of disorder (Devisch, 1977).

Two traditional groups of healers, therefore, exist in most African societies: herbalists and diviners, who are often identified according to their clan attachments. They are still very potent and important members of their societies. For practical day-to-day medical needs, the family turns to the herbalist (Davies, 1959; Rutiba, 1982). Many of the herbalists specialize in particular disorders, such as infertility. Patients whose persistent symptoms require an understanding of deeper causes than the herbalist can fathom can appeal to diviners, who operate as psychotherapists. These often explore the patients' subconscious in order to unveil underlying causes of illness (Bostock, 1950).

Among the more traditional African societies of the past and still now in modern times, when families are experiencing a crisis the art of divination is called into play. It remains a sacred function, performed upon request by a supernaturally ordained person. There are a few gifted persons having the diagnostic skills needed to apprehend, reveal and protect against the evils of men and the personal sins of omission or commission. This implies that families recognize two causes of illnesses: the immediate or natural cause, often easily understood, and the ultimate or supernatural cause, with the latter necessitating divination. When AIDS appeared in the 1980s and presented a plethora of unusual symptoms, the natural response of families was to label it as a supernatural event and to solicit the help of both the herbal and the divination specialists. Their services continue to be sought.

Preventive Treatment

Various methods of prevention and care in traditional societies have also been reported (Weatherby, 1954; Benjamin, 1955; Maclean, 1971; Johnson *et al.*, 1990). Among the Yoruba, Maclean (1971) reveals, a husband may obtain material to construct a protective charm and see to it that his wife regularly drinks an infusion of herbal soup, containing specific plants highly regarded by herbalists. Among the Yoruba, Johnson *et al.* (1990) report, the 'shopanna' cult lays down strict regulations for public behaviour during an epidemic. For example, large gatherings of people are forbidden, and sweeping the compound and floor has to be done with a special soft and leafy branch instead of the usual bunch of stiff twigs. These measures, when taken in conjunction with the isolation of cases, and the disposal of bodies and personal effects, could have been instrumental in reducing the spread of diseases or in the avoidance of diseased AIDS patients today. Among the Sebei of eastern Uganda no person was permitted to walk over another person's legs for fear of contagion or infection of disease. In western Uganda, prevention of cough was through the avoidance of sharing drinking utensils with those having running noses.

Strong purgatives were avoided by pregnant women with intestinal worms for fear of miscarriage (Perlman, 1959). Otoo (1973) and Goodman (1951) also mention beliefs among the Ga of Ghana in the need for protective medicines being taken by women before going to the hospital for deliveries. Currently, many modern medical practitioners do not object to their patients visiting the traditional healer, or gaining the benefits of incantations, exorcizing and suggestions for conditions such as schizophrenia, chronic headaches and other diseases of no demonstrable organic cause.

Preventive medicine has, therefore, been part and parcel of traditional medical practice, with different societies setting their own norms of prevention of death through disease. This suggests that many African societies have precedents that, in effect, prepare them for eventual preventive drugs and vaccines, were these to be properly introduced. Traditional vaccination has also been widely reported (Oyebola, 1980; Makhuba, 1978; Green and Makhuba, 1984; Barkhuus, 1947). Among the Galla and Amhara of Ethiopia, Barkhuus (1947) reports vaccination for syphilis by cutting and rubbing in a mixture of herbal medicine and syphilitic pus. Green and Makhuba (1984) note the risk of tetanus and other infections due to the use of unsterilized cutting instruments and unhygienic procedures.

Some African societies had knowledge of surgery. Felkin (Davies, 1959), a European traveller in the early 1880s, is reported to have witnessed a local surgical operation in western Uganda, involving the extraction of a baby from the uterus by the abdominal route, an art that cannot have been a copied version of a Caesarian section. Among the Sebei of eastern Uganda, people coughing and spitting blood were successfully operated upon by the removal of part of the affected lung (Weatherby, 1954). The Kikuyu of Kenya performed the equivalent of a bore hole exploration long before modern neurosurgery reached Africa (Ruhakana, 1986).

Traditional African societies were, therefore, endowed with various forms of treatment. Where self-treatment within the family units, including consultations with clan leaders, failed, medicine-men were consulted. Some of these were, in effect, physicians, psychotherapists and social workers who used not one but a combination of natural herbs, magical instruments, counselling, punishment and regulations to remove deep-seated fear and anxiety as well as illnesses due to wholly natural causes.

Thus, a discussion of traditional patterns of treatment in the context of the AIDS epidemic is important, especially where the hitherto unrivalled efficacy of biomedicine is being challenged. Where there is yet no AIDS cure or vaccines, traditional medicine and practitioners do share the responsibility with the modern health care system in giving care to the family with an AIDS member (Ankrah, 1991a, b). The questioning of the efficacy of biomedicine is not a new phenomenon in Africa. In traditional societies illness was deeply embedded in the socio-cultural matrix, with the family and the clan as central.

As Mburu (1973) observes, it seems that from the African cosmological viewpoint, there are 'African' and 'non-African' maladies which require respective medical responses. The exogenous influences and unintended consequences of education have gradually had a negative impact on the trust earlier put in traditional medicine – and thus its erosion by modern practices. Nevertheless, traditional forms of treatment remain a major approach against familiar diseases, if not AIDS at present (Akerele, 1987; Hand, 1989; Maikere-Faniyo et al., 1989; Staugard, 1989; Anokbonggo et al., 1990; Goodgame, 1990).

The Management of Care

African traditional health care approaches reflect the centrality of the family and clan even more decisively than does treatment. Family members with special gifts directly provide not only herbal treatment, but other physiological, psychological, spiritual and case management needs as well (Zeichner, 1988; Mail and Matheny,

1989). At the nuclear family level, women are the primary health care givers (Ankrah *et al.*, 1989), while the men, as earlier noted, have tended to be the major herb collectors. The roles of these two are undergirded by the male household heads where they are still living. In cases that require assistance beyond the skills of the family, the immediate clan elders, herbalists or diviners are consulted. Referrals are then made within these clan networks and as necessary on an interclan basis until a remedy is found. This network also makes the material contributions for care as may specifically be required and available.

With urbanization on the increase, and the availability of modern medical facilities, medical professionals rather than family members tend to be the resource of choice for care to the degree that their services are accessible and affordable. This is not the case in the rural areas. And as socio-cultural patterns change slowly, the arrangement whereby the burden of care rests with the family and clan, as just briefly described, is expected to remain the norm rather than the exception. This eventually would undergird the current trend in the region to situate AIDS care in the home and community rather than in institutional settings.

Disruptions to the Family's Capacity to Care

The African family has shown a high degree of self-reliance in the past in coping with disease and illness. The assumption is that this will continue. However, AIDS does create wholly new social situations for the family. Studies emanating largely from developed countries show a wide range of responses that ensue at the discovery of the diagnosis of AIDS in a member. There are almost invariably profound and disruptive effects on the family. Lloyd (1988) notes that disruption, while expressed differently, occurs in all cultures and family structures.

We yet lack the breadth of empirical data that would give a comprehensive picture of the reaction to AIDS in the African family and the clan in general. We are thus left to construct the situation from a combination of studies and experiential sources, pending the anticipated increased focus in AIDS research on this area. Such material as is available, however, does adequately indicate the need to consider the entire kinship system in our assessment of impact and interventions against AIDS.

One manifested psychological impact of HIV/AIDS on families is stress (Lloyd, 1988; Murphy and Perry, 1988; Lovejoy, 1989). This arises partly from the reaction of the person with AIDS as perceived by the family. When the patient experiences shock and denial, anger, guilt, anxiety and suicidal tendencies, paranoid beliefs, personality change and sometimes psychosis (Lovejoy, 1989), the entire family is stressed.

Reactions of depression, mood swings and hostility directed towards caretakers are rarely understood by the family. As Lloyd (1988) observes, self-punishing behaviour, including arguments, threats, refusals to take medications or to follow medical procedures, and self-destructive abuse of drugs or alcohol, will be viewed as ingratitude by care-givers, who may themselves withdraw. Stress may thus breed alienation when finally the person with AIDS and the caretakers retreat from one another, often into silence. Feelings of isolation have been widely cited (Conant, 1988; Geis *et al.*, 1986), although actual abandonment of patients with AIDS has not been common. Cases of close family and social support due to fear have been reported (Mail and Matheny, 1989; Shine, 1985).

In a study of 22 urban families in Kampala, Uganda, McGrath *et al.* (1991) noted that family members tended to emphasize the implications of AIDS, including the fear of loss of a loved one, the burden of care for the patient and perhaps the care of the children that are left behind after the patient's death, and failure to realize future plans. Shock, disbelief and confusion over the diagnosis of AIDS are some of the immediate common responses (McGrath *et al.*, 1991; Lloyd, 1988). Therefore, once a member of the family is diagnosed as having HIV/AIDS, family members must face the stress of deciding whether to accept or to reject caretaking responsibilities. Whichever decision is taken, family concerns tend to show realism and to be positive; they are centred on issues of loss rather than on their fears or on the burden of caretaking (McGrath *et al.*, 1991; Miller *et al.*, 1989; Geis *et al.*, 1986).

Stigma attached to HIV/AIDS and its modes of transmission (Greif and Porembski, 1989) and shame (Lloyd, 1988) are strong emotions experienced by all members of the family facing AIDS. Such reactions of guilt and shame may greatly disrupt relationships with neighbours and this may aggravate patterns of family care. The stigma of AIDS, resulting from its association with promiscuity, and linked to the gradual physical weakening and loss of body weight, common to persons with AIDS in Africa, may heighten isolation from the community. Physical symptoms and the progression of AIDS increase family disruption, especially when neighbours and other acquaintances begin to suspect that AIDS exists in the family.

The Financial Burden of Care

Loss of family income through disruption of wage earnings outside the home due to demands for care has been widely reported. In a study of 33 families with symptomatic children, hospitalized in Mama Yemo Hospital, Kinshasa, Davachi *et al.* (1988) discovered that a single hospital admission of an infected child cost the equivalent of three months of a father's salary, and that the child's death cost the equivalent of 11 months of work.

Hassig *et al.* (1989), using a sample of adults in the same hospital, found that infected persons had spent twice as much for treatment prior to hospital admission than had the non-infected patients. McGrath *et al.* (1991) also observed that 14 of the 24 infected persons in their study relied solely on other family members' income for subsistence and medical care. Infection with HIV/AIDS, therefore, puts a financial burden on the immediate and the extended family of the person infected, especially when the illness curtails mobility and employment – both sources of the person's livelihood.

The impact may be felt more in urban than in rural settings where the kinship support structure is less genealogically and geographically cohesive, as noted earlier. Where the death of a breadwinner can mean the total breakdown of the nuclear family, as happens in the case of families in urban areas, choices will have to be made about residence. The bereaved survivors without financial support frequently must return to the village. The structure and the functioning of the family are, in such instances, disorganized.

Furthermore, the disruptions in African family life by HIV/AIDS will be felt very strongly at the level of material need (Ankrah, 1991c; Ankrah *et al.*, 1991), as at the level of psychological well-being. This is for yet another reason. Given the slow and sometimes long period of care needed by persons with AIDS before death, family expenditures on medicines – both traditional and modern – as well as on special foods all affect the family budget (Ankrah *et al.*, 1989, 1991). The extended family as a social support system may not readily offer relief because other economic demands may have forestalled its capacity to execute this traditionally cherished role. Moreover, when relatives of the AIDS patient do not accept the hospital's diagnosis and its discharging the person with AIDS, families may spend large sums of money going from one traditional healer to another in search of a cure. In the process, household routines are severely interrupted while income for the needs of other family members dwindles.

In African families, women are the primary care-givers in the home and providers of basic needs to other members. Therefore, a woman with AIDS not only lives with her own psychological fears; she must endure the termination of her child-bearing and nurturing role. In addition, an alternative care-giver has to be found to care for and to replace her. Therefore, as she is a key provider for all her children, a mother's death has profound socio-economic consequences for her orphans and for her husband, if he survives. Alternative mother-like relationships must be established through the extended family or the clan. The latter may more readily shoulder that responsibility than the former, where the former is already weakened by the death of productive members.

Mourning the Bereaved

In heavily affected areas in Africa the traditional institution of mourning has changed. A bereaved family was traditionally assisted by the community to organize the funeral. Neighbours, kinsmen and significant other mourners were expected to contribute to funeral costs, including food, as well as comforting and sharing in the bereavement, while agricultural and other work was suspended for a considerable period of time – depending on the rituals.

Changes are now taking place in funeral practices. Between June 1989 and March 1990 there were a reported 73 funerals in the research area of the Rakai Project (Makerere University/Columbia University) in Rakai District, Uganda. During the busy planting and harvesting months of July–September and February–March, people were overwhelmed by the demands of agricultural work and by the neighbourly demands to spend three non-working bereavement days to mourn the death of the persons who had died in the village. The practice now is to keep the bereaved company on the night of death or the arrival of the body, assist with preparing the grave, feed the mourners and attend the funeral.

Food Production and Supply

AIDS will also have a profound impact on family welfare and food supply, particularly as the illness progresses in the person infected. Pressure will be applied for the woman as the prime care-giver in the family to withdraw from paid employment, if the job conflicts with that role (Ankrah *et al.*, 1991). Older children are taken out of school, not only to reduce pressure on the family budget, but also to help with the care of the sick member of the household.

With respect to the food supply available to the affected African families, the FAO (Kingman, 1991) estimates that up to one in four farming families in those parts of Africa most severely affected by AIDS will suffer extreme labour shortages during the next decade. Norse observes that as a coping mechanism families will have to switch to crops that need less work to grow and harvest; thus affected families will have to stop growing labour-intensive crops such as tobacco. They will need to change to those needing progressively less and less attention, such as groundnuts, maize and cassava. The effect the shortage of food and crop failure has on standards of living has also been estimated by Kingman (1991). Malnutrition, especially affecting children, anaemia in pregnant women and other harmful effects have been noted (Kingman, 1991), which result from the increasingly reduced quantity, as well as the quality, of food available to the family.

AIDS and Children

Africa's high and increasing number of children left without the care of one or both parents, called by some 'AIDS orphans', is one of the most striking outcomes of the AIDS epidemic. It is estimated that between 3.1 and 5.5 million children will be orphaned in ten Eastern and Central African countries alone (UNICEF, 1990). Neglected in terms of the disruption of a relationship with the most significant others, or as a result of death, the children in affected families undergo severe psychological trauma before the deaths of their parents, as well as the continued suffering from maternal deprivation of infants who survive their mothers.

When young adolescents have had to care for a parent during terminal illness, school performance suffers severely. This is because of irregular attendance and an increasing inability to cope at school and with home care-giving, simultaneously. When the parent finally dies, many young people find themselves with insufficient schooling and, thus, with poor employment prospects. Sometimes they have no immediate guardians, owing to the weakened family support network.

In effect, AIDS-related morbidity and mortality of one or both parents has a devastating impact on family structure, income, household food security and the quality of care given to survivors long before the death of a productive family member or parent. Children, in particular, will need to be placed in someone's care after a parent dies. Where grandparents or other biological relatives are too old, poor or overwhelmed, a new 'family' may need to be created for them. Neither the African state nor non-governmental or donor organizations will be able to fulfil this role on the scale required at the present time or in the foreseeable future. Hence, there is a need in this decade for a renewed interest in the African kinship structure, and for a perspective that clearly mobilizes it and links it to strategies designed to support those in dire situations, as just described.

RESILIENCE AND RESPONSE

Sickness and death test the strength and ability of the African family to develop coping mechanisms. However, two major social networks potentially facilitate the processes of resilience and recovery amidst the continued onslaught of AIDS. The first is the emerging, but highly publicized, non-governmental organizations (NGOs) being established to address the needs of persons with AIDS and their families for psychological and material support.

These organizations, though not the subject of this paper, nevertheless have a valid place in health care. Given the scale of the AIDS problem that exists in the African region and the family implications of its impact, such NGOs are needed, especially in the cities and towns of Africa. They will encompass a variety of interpersonal commitments based on affiliation, altruism, empathy and mutual sharing of resources. However, with the level of development most African countries have reached in their social service systems, with the current socio-economic stagnation in Africa and recession abroad, those social networks, derived from institutional ties of mutual interest, can only supplement or complement the contributions of family units. They cannot supersede the African kinship networks.

The second social network, the clan, possesses the capability to organize against a potential threat to its survival. The clan will need to assist the nuclear family unit in a reorganizational process. This, in many instances, will mean helping the nuclear family to alter its structure. New families will have to be created where both parents have died. This could take a variety of forms, but still be specific to a particular cultural context. Fortunately, there are traditional precedences by which clans may fashion the 'new' creations.

By an age-old arrangement, when one adult in the immediate African family dies and the surviving member is economically able to maintain an independent household, then a single-parent family could continue (Eberstein *et al.*, 1988). The family will only maintain this structure if the bereaved spouse survives. If the single-parent family is mother-headed, survivors will be entitled to all possible forms of psychological support from members of the clan.

The single parent, on the other hand, is absorbed into existent units. This was seen most clearly prior to the AIDS epidemic through widow-inheritance, the practice wherein the widow would be remarried to a clan member, often to avoid placing the burden of care and maintenance of all members in the bereaved family on another household, especially in the case where the deceased was the breadwinner. A young widow with few children would and still does opt to return to her natal home, thus permanently altering the structure of the family. Then, members of the clan could maintain a few of the children, who by lineage belong to the clan. A new member then assumes the role of the household head, hence forming a new unit for the purpose of continuity of the family. To ensure such continuity is an obligation of the clan. The young widow may, through migration, remarry and/or join another clan, perhaps along with the youngest children of the deceased, who, nevertheless, maintain their former membership within the clan of the dead parent.

Barnett and Blaikie (1990) have noted that widows who are young and attractive are sometimes assumed to be AIDS-free, giving rise to anxiety when marriage is being considered. Under this circumstance the original homestead will be maintained by appointed members of the clan or the property is sold. This responsibility is solely that of the clan leadership. Other widows may, however, opt to migrate to other areas where their kin or other clan members are established. In this way, social and economic support for the migrants is assured, at least at a minimal level and for a period of time. Some men and women who are known to have been bereaved by AIDS may have to live as celibates. All of these responses, however, have important implications for the further spread of AIDS, as well as the protection of bereaved widows, widowers and children. What new form of family structure the wider clan endorses is, therefore, a matter of considerable importance.

Traditionally, orphans were absorbed into the extended family network. Even when AIDS strikes, few African children are without the extended family as a 'resource' system (Onyango and Waiji, 1988; Conant, 1988). In fact, most children orphaned by AIDS have been fostered by grandparents and other relatives; over time, however, financial resources are severely strained. In addition, urbanization and Western education have affected the way in which extended families now organize the lives of surviving members. A unique form of family reorganization is emerging due to AIDS. This is variously termed, but is here called 'children-alone' families, a designation accorded by a Ugandan (Obbo, 1991). An increasing number of orphaned siblings are left on a plot of land and in their deceased parents' house. Depending upon their early rearing, these children – sometimes with other young people in the family – manage to cook, grow food and struggle to acquire income for basic subsistence needs, including school fees. However, to succeed, such 'children-alone' families must be near close relatives and other members of the clan who may, at least in the absence of adult labour and economic assistance, offer social and psychological support by recognizing them, and involving them in all social matters, gatherings and/or celebrations. This is also done through regular visits between households. This new form of family structure does survive and later the eldest member may assume the symbolic role of family head. Whether an 'heir' is appointed depends upon the collective decision of the clan elders.

Lastly, a now common form of family restructuring owing to terminal illness and consequent AIDS-related mortality is the grandparent-headed families (Beers *et al.*, 1988). Grandparents who would normally count upon adult sons to provide for their old age are, instead, losing their adult offspring. They now must care for large numbers of parentless children with no financial support or little strength to do so. Before the death of the adult, the grandparents would have been required over a long terminal period to nurse their sons and daughters, while often they themselves suffer from some illness.

AIDS-related mortality among youthful parents implies, therefore, that elderly parents will find themselves contributing the major share to costs of economic survival needs. Beers *et al.* (1988) suggest that they will also have to undertake the hierarchical and organizational burdens of the entire community and family structures as well. Support and encouragement from the wider social groups will be indispensable to their task.

AIDS has thus not only altered the health status profile of the productive younger adults of the African family. It has also affected the family roles and functioning (McGrath *et al.*, 1991), which require in many families a basic reorganization process. This process could succeed. The critical factor will be the quality of support that family members receive from the clan leadership and the clan's ability to survive as a context of social adaptation.

CONCLUSIONS

The African tradition of treatment and care in times of disease and illness shows remarkable richness. I have argued that such lore is not totally lost. This is evident by the ubiquitous, contemporary, traditional healing practitioners that complement the efforts of the modern health system and the African family in attending to the sick. In fact, it is a truism to say that they are inseparable since, unlike modern medical professionals, traditional practitioners are usually identified by the family, and receive much of their knowledge and skill from that source.

Thus, with the pressure of the AIDS epidemic, the African family is not and should not be thought to be without resources to combat the ravages of the disease. What is indicated is a closer linkage between the modern medical professionals and representatives of the existent family structure. This includes serious dialogues and sharing between health care givers, and those traditional healers and members of families who treat the persons directly infected by HIV and AIDS. It also necessitates a thorough reappraisal of the total African kinship system *vis-à-vis* the institutional social networks, such as government, non-governmental and donor organizations, as has been suggested earlier.

Multidisciplinary research into the prevailing clanship system is of utmost importance. What is currently known about the clan as a social support system is dated, as our references show. There is thus a need to update our theoretical underpinnings, as well as to come abreast of the contemporary functioning of this social structure. Research is called for that explores the capability of the clan to organize the fight against a modern medical and social crisis as it did in the past with such events as plagues, epidemics and warfare.

Studies are needed that will provide answers to other important questions. What are the contemporary obligations and responsibilities recognized as integral to clan membership? What is the degree of replacement of clan responsibilities by institutionally based social groupings? What is the pattern of distribution and use of social provisions by families directly affected by AIDS? What would be the circumstances that would underpin an enhanced, substantive, material and psychological response to the needs of families? Cross-cultural studies in differing African countries are required to enable the social and medical interveners to identify the most suitable way to utilize the clan, i.e. to incorporate this social network into AIDS strategies without the assumed negative political repercussions alluded to earlier.

Doing all the above implies two additional efforts. The appropriate entry points into the clan's social structure would need to be ascertained. Clan leadership as a function is intact, but with varying degrees of authority and prominence (Ayisi, 1980; Caldwell et al., 1990a, b), especially in the rural areas where populations are essentially genealogically as well as geographically close. Clan elders as spokesmen of those populations – and the ancestors – are sufficiently credible respresentatives to compel attention to their counsel, if such counsel were sought. Clan elder councils in high HIV prevalence communities can provide possible links to a network of families with responsibilities and obligations towards one another. Data are needed, therefore, to reveal the precise capacity of these entities – the leaders and councils and interlocked families – to be channels of resources on behalf of clan members as well as mobilizers on behalf of the external programming systems concerned with AIDS prevention and spread. Identifying the elders with the skills to engage and negotiate with formal associations and resource systems beyond the traditional structure is thus a required complementary action.

As Africa seeks to maximize the inherent and supreme values it has traditionally conferred on the family, it can ill afford to ignore the still viable kinship structure, the clan, in its search for channels through which to confront HIV and AIDS.

REFERENCES

Abrahams, R. G. (1959) *African Concepts of Health and Disease* (Kampala, East African Institute of Social Research).

Akerele, O. (1987) The best of two worlds; bringing traditional medicine up to date, *Social Science and Medicine*, 24, pp. 177–181.

Aldous, J. (1962) Urbanization, the extended family and kinship ties in West Africa, *Social Forces*, 41, pp. 6–12.

Ankrah, E. M. (ed.) (1978) *Family Welfare in Africa: Educational Strategies* (New York, International Association of Schools of Social Work).

Ankrah, E. M. (1991a) AIDS and the social side of health, *Social Science and Medicine*, 32, pp. 967–980.

Ankrah, E. M. (1991b) The impact of AIDS on the social, economic, health and welfare systems. AIDS: Preserving the Family of Mankind, in: G. Gaetano (ed.) *Science Challenging AIDS* (Basel, Karger).

Ankrah, E. M. (1991c) AIDS: Socio-economic decline and health – a double crisis for the African woman, in: W. Agyei (ed.) *Population, Health and Development in Sub-Saharan Africa* (New York, UNFPA).

Ankrah, E. M., (1992) *Uganda: Report of the National Survey*. AIDS control Programme/WHO/ Makerere University, Intercountry Social and Behavioural Research, Global Programme on AIDS.

Ankrah, E. M., *et al.* (1989) *The Family and Care Giving in Uganda. V International Conference on AIDS*, Abstract WGP 32 (Montreal, Canada).

Ankrah, E. M., *et al.* (1991) The impact of AIDS on urban families: an assessment of needs. *VIth International Conference on AIDS in Africa*. Abstract WA251 (Dakar, Senegal).

Anokbonggo, W. W., *et al.* (1990) Traditional methods in management of diarrheal diseases in Uganda, *Bulletin of the World Health Organization*, 69, pp. 359–363.

Ayisi, E. O. (1980) *An Introduction to the Study of African Culture*, 2nd edn (London, Heinemann).

Barkhuus, A. (1947) Public health in Ethiopia, *CIBA Symposia*, 9, pp. 698–728.

Barnett, T. and Blaikie, P. (1990) *Community Coping Mechanisms in the Face of Exceptional Demographic Change*, Report to ODA, London.

Bascom, W. R. and Herskovits, M. J. (eds) (1959) *Continuity and Change in African Cultures* (Chicago, University of Chicago Press.)

Beers, C., *et al.* (1988) AIDS: the grandmother burden, in: A. F. Fleming *et al.* (eds) *The Global Impact of AIDS*, pp. 171–174 (New York, Liss).

Benjamin, D. (1955) *Health, Culture and Community* (New York, Russell Sage Foundation).

Bostock, P. G. (1950) *The Peoples of Kenya: The Taita* (Nairobi, East African Publishing House).

Caldwell, J. C., Orubuloye, I. O. and Caldwell, P. (1990a) *Changes in the Nature and Levels of Sexual Networking in an African Society: The Destabilization of the Traditional Yoruba System*, Health Transition Working Paper No. 4 1990 (Canberra, Australian National University).

Caldwell, J. C., Caldwell, P. and Orubuloye, I. O. (1990b) *The Family and Sexual Networking in Sub-Saharan Africa: Historical Regional Differences and Present Day Implications*, Health Transition Working Paper No. 5 1990, Health Transition Centre (Canberra, Australian National University).

Colson, E. (1970) Family change in contemporary Africa, in: J. Middleton (ed.) *Black Africa: Its Peoples and Their Cultures Today*, pp. 152–158 (Toronto, Macmillan).

Conant, E. P. (1988) Soccial consequences of AIDS: implications for East Africa and the eastern United States, in: R. Kulstad (ed.) *An American Association for the Advancement of Science*, Symposia Papers (Washington, DC, AAAS).

Davachi, F., *et al.* (1988) The economic impact on families of children with AIDS in Kinshasha, Zaire, in: A. F. Fleming *et al.* (eds) *The Global Impact of AIDS*, pp. 167–169 (New York, Alan R. Liss).

Davies, J. N. P. (1959) The development of 'scientific' medicine in the African kingdom of Bunyoro Kitara, *Medical History*, 3, pp. 47–57.

De Gonzalez, N. and Sohen, L. (1965) The consanguinal household and matrilocality, *American Anthropologist*, pp. 1541–1549.

Destounis, N. P. (1987) AIDS: a medical disaster, *European Journal of Psychiatry*, 1 (4), pp. 44–49.

Devisch, R. (1977) Process for the articulation of meaning and ritual healing among the Northern Yaka (Zaire), *Anthorpos*, 72, pp. 683–708.

Eberstein, I.W., Serow, W. J. and Ahmad, O. B. (1988) AIDS: consequences for families and fertility, in: A. F. Fleming *et al.* (eds) *The Global Impact of AIDS*, pp. 175–182 (New York, Alan R. Liss).

Fortes, M. (1945) *The Dynamics of Clanship among the Tallensi* (London, Oxford University Press).

Fortes, M. (1957) Malinowski and the study of kinship, in: R. Firth (ed.) *Man and Culture: An Evaluation of the Work of Malinowski* (London, Routledge & Kegan Paul).

Fortes, M. (1962) *Marriage in Tribal Societies* (London, Cambridge University Press).

Geis, S. B., Fuller, R. L. and Rush, J. (1986) Lovers of AIDS victims: psychological stress and counselling needs, *Death Studies*, 10, pp. 43–53.

Goodgame, R. W. (1990) AIDS in Uganda – clinical and social features, *New England Journal of Medicine*, 323, pp. 383–389.

Goodman, I. (1951) Obstetrics in a primitive African community (the Gold Coast), *American Journal of Public Health*, Part II 41(11), pp. 56–64.

Green, E. C. and Makhuba, L. (1984) Traditional healers in Swaziland: toward improved cooperation between the traditional and modern health sectors, *Social Science and Medicine*, 18, pp. 1071–1079.

Greif, G. and Porembski, E. (1989) Implications for therapy with significant others of persons with AIDS, *Journal of Gay and Lesbian Psychotherapy*, 1, pp. 79–86.

Hand, R. (1989) Alternative therapies used by patients with AIDS. *The Lancet*, i, pp. 672–673.

Hassig, S. E. *et al.* (1989) The economic impact of HIV infection in adult admissions to internal medicine at Mama Yamo Hospital, *V International Conference on AIDS, Montreal, Canada*, Abstract THO 9.

Jaenson, C., *et al.* (1984) *Uganda Social and Institutional Profile* (Jinja, Uganda, USAID/EIL).

Johnson, J. M., *et al.* (1990) Juju soup: the witch herbalist's solution of infertility, *African Studies Review*, 33, pp. 39–64.

Kayongo-Male, D. and Onyango, P. (1984) *The Sociology of the African Family* (London, Longman).

Kilbride, P. L. and Kilbride, J. C. (1990) *Changing Family Life in East Africa: Women and Children at Risk* (Philadelphia, Pennsylvania State University).

Kingman, S. (1991) Epidemic threatens food supply in Africa. Interview with David Norse of FAO, Science Challenging AIDS, *International Conference on AIDS*, Newspaper (Florence, Italy), 16–21 June.

Levine, C. (1990) AIDS and the changing concept of the family, *Milbank Quarterly*, 68 (Suppl. 1), pp. 33–58.

Lévi-Strauss, C. and Mead, M. (1961) Cultural determinants, *American Journal of Public Health*, 51(10), pp. 150–153.

Linton, R. (1959) *The Tree of Culture* (New York, Vintage).

Lloyd, G. A. (1988) HIV-infection, AIDS, and family disruption, in: A. F. Fleming *et al.* (eds) *The Global Impact of AIDS* (New York, Alan R. Liss), pp. 183–190.

Lovejoy, N. C. (1989) AIDS: impact on the gay man's homosexual and heterosexual families, *Marriage and Family Review*, 14, pp. 285–316.

Maclean, C. M. V. (1971) *Magical Medicine: A Nigerian Case Study* (London, Penguin).

Maclean, C. M. V. (1982) Folk medicine and fertility: aspects of Yoruba medical practice affecting women, in: C. P. MacCormack (ed.) *Ethnography of Fertility and Birth* (New York, Academic Press), pp. 161–180.

Maikere-Faniyo, R., *et al.* (1989) Study of Rwandese medical plants used in the treatment of diarrhea, *International Journal of Ethnopharmacology*, 26, pp. 101–109.

Mail, P. D. and Matheny, S. C. (1989) Social services for people with AIDS: needs and approaches, *AIDS*, 3 (Suppl, 2), S273–277.

Makhuba, L. P. (1978) *The Traditional Healer* (The University of Botswana and Swaziland).

Mandelbaum, D. G. (1960) Social groupings, in: H. L. Shapiro (ed.) *Man, Culture, and Society* (New York, Oxford University).

Marwick, M. G. (1988) The modern family in a social anthropological perspective, *African Studies*, 17, pp. 137–158.

Mbithi, P. M. (1978) Responding to African family service needs, in: E. M. Ankrah (ed.) *Family Welfare in Africa: Educational Strategies*, pp. 35–39 (New York, International Association of Schools of Social Work).

Mburu, F. M. (1973) Traditional and modern medicine among the Akamba ethnic group, MA thesis (Kampala, Makerere University).

McGrath, J. W. *et al.* (1991) *AIDS and the Urban Family: Its Impact in Kampala, Uganda.*

Miller, R., *et al.* (1989) AIDS and children: some of the issues in haemophilia care and how to address them, *AIDS Care*, 1, pp. 59–65.

Murdock, G. P. (1949) *Social Structure* (New York, Macmillan).

Murphy, P. and Perry, K. (1988) Hidden grievers. Special issue. AIDS: principles, practices and politics, *Death Studies*, 12, pp. 451–462.

Nahemow, N. (1979) Residence, kinship and social isolation among the aged Baganda, *Journal of Marriage and the Family*, 41, pp. 171–183.

Ndeti, K. (1969) Elements of Akamba life, PhD thesis (Syracuse, Syracuse University).

Obbo, C. (1991) Reflections on the AIDS orphan in Uganda, Dossier, *The Courier*, 126, pp. 55–56.

Okediji, A. P. (1974) A psychosocial analysis of the extended family: the African case. Eighth annual convention of the National Association of Black Psychologists in Boston, Massachusetts (Boston).

Onyango, P. and Waiji, P. (1988) The family as a resource, in: A. F. Fleming *et al.* (eds) *The Global Impact of AIDS*, pp. 301–306 (New York, Alan R. Liss).

Otoo, S. N. (1973) The traditional management of puberty and childbirth among the Ga people, Ghana, *Tropical and Geographical Medicine*, 25, pp. 88–94.

Oyebola, D. D. O. (1980) Antenatal care as practiced by Yoruba traditional healers/midwives of Nigeria, *East African Medical Journal*, 57 (9), pp. 23–29.

Perlman, E. H. (1959) Preliminary inquiry into conceptions of health and disease in Toro, East Africa Institute of Social Research (eds) *Attitudes on Health and Disease*, pp. 47–59 (Kampala, Makerere College).

Radcliff-Brown, A. R. (1950) Introduction, in: A. R. Radcliff-Brown and D. Forde (eds) *African Systems of Kinship and Marriage* (London, Oxford University Press), pp. 1–85.

Richards, A. I. (1950) 'Some types of family structure amongst the central Bantu', in: A. R. Radcliff-Brown and D. Forde (eds) *African Systems of Kinship and Marriage* (Oxford, Oxford University Press).

Richards, A. I. (1966) *The Changing Structure of a Ganda Village* (East African Publishing House, Nairobi).

Ruhakana, R. (1986) Traditional medicine underdeveloped, in: *The New Vision*, pp. 8–9 Kampala, Uganda, Tuesday, December.

Rutiba, G. E. (1982) Traditional/modern therapy and Christian ministry of healing, with special reference to the Bafumbira of Kigezi, Ph.D. thesis (Kampala, Makerere University).

Sargent, C. (1982) *The Cultural Context of Therapeutic Choice: Obstetrical Care Divisions among the Bariba of Benin* (Reidel Publishing, Boston).

Shine, D. (1985) Diagnosis and management of AIDS in intravenous drug users, *Advances in Alcohol and Substance Abuse*, 5, pp. 25–34.

Sigarist, H. E. (1943) *Civilization and Disease* (Chicago, The University of Chicago).

Sommerfelt, K. (1959) The Bakonjo ideas of health and disease, in East African Institute of Social Research (eds) *Attitudes on Health and Disease*, pp. 35–37 (Kampala, Makerere College).

Staugard, F. (1989) *Traditional Medicine in a Transitional Society* (Gaberone, Ipelegeng Publishers).

Sudarkasa, N. (1982) African and Afro-American family structure, in: J. Cole (ed.) *Anthropology for the Eighties*, pp. 132–161 (New York, Free Press).

Sumner, W. G. (1906, 1959) *Folkways* (New York, Dover).

Titiev, M. (1959) *Introduction to Cultural Anthropology* (New York, Henry Holt).

UNICEF (1990) *Children and AIDS: An Impending Calamity. The Growing Impact of HIV Infection on Women and Family life in the Developing World* (New York, UNICEF).

Weatherby (1954) Sebei ideas of health and disease, in: East African Institute of Social Research (eds) *Attitudes on Health and Disease* (Kampala, Makerere College).

Zeichner, C. (1988) *Modern and Traditional Health Care in Developing Societies* (Lanham University Press).

THREE

Disclosing HIV Seropositivity to Significant Others

Robert B. Hays, Leon McKusick, Lance Pollack, Robert Hilliard,
Colleen Hoff and Thomas J. Coates

INTRODUCTION

Discovering that one is HIV seropositive brings with it a multitude of stressors, including confronting the possibility of a painful, debilitating illness, early death, stigmatization, discrimination and disruption of relationships with friends and family (Forstein, 1984; Christ and Weiner, 1985; Stulberg and Smith, 1988). Considerable research has demonstrated that support from significant others can buffer the impact of a wide variety of stressful life experiences (Cohen and Wills, 1985). An individual's social network can play a critical role in influencing coping, adaptation and recovery from serious illness (Wortman and Conway, 1985; Taylor *et al.*, 1986). Significant others may also play a crucial role in promoting an HIV-positive individual's adoption of vitally important medical practices, which can influence HIV disease progression (for example, monitoring T-cells, taking anti-viral medications).

However, disclosure of one's HIV seropositivity to significant others is a double-edged sword. It may open up the opportunity to receive social support. However, it may also lead to added stress, due to stigmatization, discrimination and disruption of personal relationships. Conversely, concealing one's HIV status from significant others may be stressful in itself and can interfere with obtaining and adhering to potentially critical medical treatments. Concealment can also have negative effects on significant others' well-being, since they may experience guilt, confusion or anger when they find out about the individual's illness (especially if this occurs after the individual is very sick or has died).

AIDS activists have urged HIV-seropositive individuals to 'come out' publicly about their serostatus as a means of personalizing HIV illness and decreasing stigma and stereotypes. For example, Magic Johnson's announcement that he was HIV positive has been heralded as a major breakthrough in destigmatizing the general public's view of HIV illness. However, little is known about the psychological consequences of disclosing one's seropositivity. Although self-disclosure literature generally indicates the positive, therapeutic effects of disclosure (Jouard, 1964; Derlega and Berg, 1987), it is clear that the tremendous amount of hysteria and irrationality surrounding AIDS issues can bring about highly unfortunate reactions. A disconcerting number of such incidents have been reported, including loss of job opportunities, ostracism in educational settings or by health-care workers, and even having one's house burned down by angry neighbours (Herek and Glunt, 1988). Clearly, HIV-positive individuals must be judicious in deciding whom to tell that they are HIV seropositive. Unfortunately, the existing research literature offers little to guide their decision-making process.

In this paper, we examine four questions. To whom are HIV-positive gay men likely to disclose their HIV status? At what point in the development of HIV illness is disclosure likely? What are the effects of disclosure to various individuals (gay friends, lovers, heterosexual friends, relatives, colleagues)? And what are the reasons for not disclosing to particular individuals?

Research on help-seeking and social support among gay men (Kurdek, 1988; Hays *et al.*, 1990a, b) has shown that gay men generally rely more on their gay peers than their relatives for support. We therefore hypothesized that HIV-positive gay men would be more likely to disclose their HIV status to gay friends than to relatives or co-workers. In addition, we expected that HIV-positive gay men would perceive the response of their gay friends to be more helpful than the responses of relatives or co-workers, because of their greater likelihood of empathy and knowledge about HIV issues.

METHODS
Participants and Procedures

ORIGINAL SAMPLE
The data for this study come from the AIDS Behavioral Research Project (ABRP), an ongoing longitudinal survey of San Francisco gay men who have been followed since 1984. The ABRP was designed initially to determine the impact of the AIDS epidemic on two groups of gay men: those at extreme risk of HIV and those whose behaviour potentially protected them from HIV infection. The details of the recruitment process and research design have been described in previous reports (McKusick, *et al.*, 1985a, b, 1990). Men were recruited initially in 1983 and 1984 at gay bars and bath-houses and by advertising for individuals in committed relationships and single, celibate men. A total of 754 men (51% of those approached to participate) were enrolled in the sample in 1984. Their ages ranged from 19 to 72 years (mean 35.71 years; s.d. 8.28). The majority of the sample were Caucasian (91%), had professional or white-collar occupations (77%) and had some college education (68%). Respondents have been mailed self-administered questionnaires at one-year intervals, which they are asked to complete and return by mail.

STUDY SAMPLE

At the sixth annual follow-up (November 1989), data were collected from 499 individuals (66% of those originally enrolled in the study). An additional 13% ($n = 101$) were known to have died (either through reports by their friends or through matching in the California Death Registry). Attrition analyses comparing respondents who remained in the sample between 1984 and 1989 with those who did not showed that men who were lost to follow-up reported experiencing more HIV-related physical symptoms ($\chi^2 = 7.28$; $P<0.01$) and greater depression ($t = 2.35$; $P<0.02$) than men who remained in the sample. Drop-outs were also less likely to be involved in a primary relationship than men who remained in the sample ($\chi^2 = 8.08$; $P<0.01$).

At the 1989 data collection, 81% ($n = 406$) of the men reported that they had been tested for HIV antibodies, of whom 40% ($n = 165$) reported that they were HIV positive. This analysis focuses only on HIV-antibody-positive men. The sample included 34 men who were diagnosed with AIDS, 54 who were HIV symptomatic (defined as experiencing two or more HIV-related symptoms, such as hairy leukoplakia, candidiasis or diarrhoea) and 77 who were asymptomatic. Ninety-six per cent of the men were white, 64% were college graduates, and the median annual income was US$35,000. Their ages ranged from 24 to 68 years (mean 39.6 years; s.d. 7.46).

ONE-YEAR FOLLOW-UP

The seventh annual data collection wave took place in November 1990. Of the 165 HIV-positive men who are the focus of the analyses presented here, 79% ($n = 130$) returned the follow-up. Fifty-one per cent ($n = 18$) of the men who did not return the follow-up (11% of the sample) were known to have died between the 1989 and 1990 assessments. We compared men who remained in the study for both 1989 and 1990 with men who were lost to follow-up after 1980 on demographic variables (age, education and income), depression, anxiety, HIV symptoms and disclosure patterns. Men who were lost to follow-up differed significantly from men who remained in the study on several variables. Drop-outs were more likely to have experienced HIV-related symptoms ($\chi^2 (1) = 17.91$; $P<0.001$) and to have been diagnosed with AIDS ($\chi^2 (1) = 25.80$; $P<0.0001$). They also reported more depression ($t(\text{d.f.} = 161) = 2.51$; $P<0.02$) and anxiety ($t(\text{d.f.} = 161) = 2.18$; $P<0.04$), had lower incomes ($t(\text{d.f.} = 163) = 3.23$; $P<0.01$) and were less educated ($t(\text{d.f.} = 163) = 2.43$; $P<0.02$). In addition, they reported having disclosed their HIV status to more people ($t(\text{d.f.} = 159) = 2.82$; $P<0.005$). Except for education, all these variables were associated with more advanced stages of HIV illness, so these differences mainly reflect the fact that individuals who were more sick in 1989 were less likely to continue with the study in 1990. This pattern is expected and unavoidable in studies with HIV-related individuals. Respondents who were lost to follow-up were included in all analyses except the longitudinal analyses.

Measures

The following measures from the 1989 data collection were included in the analyses reported here.

HIV STATUS

Respondents were asked whether they had obtained HIV-antibody testing and, if so, to indicate the test results. They were also asked to indicate on a checklist whether they had experienced a variety of physical symptoms commonly associated with HIV infection (for example, hairy leukoplakia, candidiasis, diarrhoea, fatigue) during the preceding 12 months (for at least two weeks) and whether they had been diagnosed as having AIDS. The sample was thus divided into three mutually exclusive groups: AIDS-diagnosed, symptomatic HIV positive (experiencing two or more HIV-related symptoms) and asymptomatic HIV positive (experiencing none or one HIV-related symptom).

RELATIONSHIP STATUS

Respondents indicated whether they were currently involved in a primary gay relationship, defined as 'a relationship with a man where you feel committed to him above anyone else and where you have had sex together'. They were also asked to indicate the HIV status of their partner, if known.

DISCLOSURE

Respondents were asked to indicate from the list of nine relationship categories (closest gay friend, closest heterosexual friend, lover/partner, mother, father, brother, sister, co-workers, boss/employer) those individuals to whom they had disclosed their HIV seropositivity. If the respondent did not have anyone within a particular relationship category, he was asked to circle 'not applicable' for that relationship.

HELPFULNESS RATINGS

For each individual to whom they had disclosed, respondents were asked to rate how helpful that individual's response had been on a five-point Likert scale, which ranged from very unhelpful (1) to very helpful (5). An overall mean helpfulness score of the respondent's significant others was computed by summing the helpfulness ratings of all individuals to whom the respondent had disclosed and dividing by the number of individuals told.

REASONS FOR NOT DISCLOSING

A free-response item asked respondents to provide reasons for not telling any of the people listed about their HIV status.

ANXIETY AND DEPRESSION

This measure was assessed in both 1989 and 1990. Respondents completed the Brief Symptom Inventory (BSI) (Derogatis and Melisaratos, 1983), which included six-item scales of anxiety and depression. For each scale, participants were asked to describe how much discomfort each of six symptoms caused during the previous month on a five-point Likert scale (0 = none, 4 = extreme). The scale score is the mean discomfort across the six items.

RESULTS

Group Comparisons

DEMOGRAPHICS

Analyses of variance (ANOVA) were performed to examine whether men at different stages of HIV infection differed from each other on demographic variables (age, education or income). The only significant difference found was for income ($F(2, 162) = 5.42$; $P<0.006$). Scheffe *post hoc* comparisons indicated that AIDS-diagnosed men reported lower incomes than the asymptomatic HIV-positive men ($P<0.05$). To control for differences in income between the groups, income was included as a covariate in all subsequent analyses that involved comparisons by HIV stage.

PSYCHOLOGICAL DISTRESS

Men at each stage of HIV infection reported relatively high levels of anxiety and depression in 1989. Published norms for the BSI depression and anxiety scales for adult male non-patient populations are 0.06 and 0.18, respectively (Derogatis and Melisaratos, 1983). For our sample, the mean depression score was 0.92 (T score = 67) for asymptomatic men, 1.24 (T score = 71) for symptomatic men, and 1.43 (T score = 71) for AIDS-diagnosed men. On the anxiety scale, the mean score for asymptomatics was 0.79 (T score = 64), 1.02 (T score = 69) for symptomatics and 1.30 (T score = 74) for AIDS-diagnosed men. To determine whether men at various stages of infection differed in levels of anxiety and depression, we performed analyses of covariance (ANCOVA) with income as a covariate. Significant group differences emerged for both depression ($F(2, 159) = 3.08$; $P<0.05$) and anxiety ($F(2, 159) = 4.14$; $P<0.02$). Planned comparisons indicated that asymptomatic HIV-positive men reported less depression ($t(160) = 2.48$; $P<0.02$) and less anxiety ($t(160) = 2.76$; $P<0.01$) than symptomatic HIV-positive or AIDS-diagnosed men.

Patterns of Disclosure

Table 3.1 shows the percentages of men who had disclosed their seropositivity to each category of individuals (respondents who did not have an existing individual within a particular relationship category were not included in calculating the percentage for that category). Virtually all the men disclosed their seropositivity to their lover/partner (98%) and to their closest gay friend (95%). Compared with gay friends, closest heterosexual friends were told less often (77%), but were still relatively likely to be told. χ^2 analyses showed that these patterns of disclosure did not differ for men at different stages of HIV infection (asymptomatic, symptomatic, AIDS-diagnosed). Disclosure to colleagues and relatives was less common: 60% had told co-workers, 47% had told their employer and 60% had told a family member – most often a sister (53%). Fathers were the least likely to be told (40%). Interestingly, as the significant χ^2 indicate, disclosure to relatives and colleagues was influenced by stage of HIV illness. Asymptomatic men were significantly less likely to disclose their status to relatives and colleagues than men experiencing HIV symptoms or those diagnosed with AIDS. On average, asymptomatics had told 54% (s.d. 27) of the people listed; symptomatics had told 66% (s.d. 29) and AIDS-diagnosed men had told 85% (s.d. 28). χ^2 and one-way ANOVA showed that there were no significant differences in demographic variables between men who did and did not disclose to various network members.

Table 3.1 Percentages of HIV-positive men at each stage of HIV illness who disclosed their HIV status to various others

	All men (n = 163)	Asympt. HIV + (n = 75)	Sympt. HIV+ (n = 54)	AIDS (n = 34)	χ^2 value
Lover/partner	98	98	97	100	n.s.
Friend					
Gay	95	95	96	94	n.s.
Hetero.	77	73	72	93	n.s.
Co-worker	60	52	60	77	5.81*
Sister	53	38	58	77	10.55†
Mother	48	30	58	79	19.71†
Boss	47	35	49	74	16.45†
Brother	43	30	54	71	10.58†
Father	40	26	45	71	11.58†

*$P<0.055$; †$P<0.01$. Asympt., asymptomatic; sympt., symptomatic; hetero., heterosexual; n.s., not significant.

Perceived Helpfulness of Network Members

The mean helpfulness ratings of the various individuals told are shown in Table 3.2. Multivariate ANCOVA (MANCOVA) with repeated measures was used to compare the perceived helpfulness of the various people to whom the respondents had disclosed. Since pairwise comparison *t* tests showed that ratings for lovers and gay friends did not differ significantly, their ratings were averaged into a single 'gay friend/lover' category. Similarly, the various relatives were averaged to form 'relatives', and employer and co-worker to form 'colleagues'. Thus, four general relationship categories were used: gay friend/lover, heterosexual friend, relative and colleague. The independent variables were (1) relationship category and (2) HIV stage (asymptomatic, symptomatic, AIDS-diagnosed). Income was included as a covariate. The dependent variable was the respondent's rating of the helpfulness of the person listed. The various relationship categories were not perceived to be equally helpful ($F(3, 59) = 4.58$; $P<0.01$). Planned comparisons, performed to identify the location of the difference, indicated that closest gay friends/lovers and closest heterosexual friends were perceived to be more helpful than relatives and colleagues ($F(1, 61) = 12.59$; $P<0.001$). There were no significant differences in helpfulness ratings between men at different stages of HIV infection (see Appendix).

Table 3.2 Helpfulness ratings* of people disclosed to by gay men at each stage of HIV illness

	Mean (s.d.)		
	Asymptomatic HIV+	Symptomatic HIV+	AIDS-diagnosed
Lover/partner	4.48 (0.99)	4.64 (0.70)	4.65 (0.79)
Gay friend	4.14 (1.19)	4.27 (0.99)	4.53 (0.94)
Heterosexual friend	3.98 (1.15)	4.18 (0.88)	4.12 (1.09)
Co-worker	3.97 (0.94)	3.68 (1.05)	3.83 (0.98)
Father	3.60 (1.18)	3.94 (0.87)	3.91 (1.45)
Mother	3.42 (1.26)	4.04 (0.91)	3.83 (1.15)
Boss	3.88 (1.12)	3.68 (1.32)	3.75 (1.25)
Sister	3.45 (1.40)	4.04 (0.96)	4.06 (1.20)
Brother	3.56 (0.92)	3.45 (1.19)	3.89 (1.05)

*1 = very unhelpful; 5 = very helpful.

Since respondents reported the HIV status of their primary partners, we were able to examine whether the partners' HIV status was related to their helpfulness ratings. We performed ANCOVA with the helpfulness ratings of the partners as the dependent variable. The independent variables were (1) partner's HIV status (positive, negative) and (2) respondent's HIV stage. Income was included as a covariate. The lack of significant effects indicated that HIV-negative and HIV-positive partners were rated equally helpful by HIV-positive men.

Correlations with Distress

Table 3.3 presents the Pearson correlations between helpfulness ratings of the men's significant others and their depression and anxiety scores, both cross-sectionally and longitudinally. As can be seen, the mean helpfulness of significant others was inversely associated with psychological distress (both depression and anxiety) cross-sectionally and one year later. The helpfulness ratings of friends (both gay and heterosexual) and colleagues all showed significant negative correlations with current depression (all r between -0.18 and -0.32; $P<0.03$), although only the helpfulness ratings of gay friends, lovers and bosses were significantly associated with depression levels one year later. Interestingly, the perceived helpfulness of mothers was positively associated with current depression ($r = 0.26$; $P<0.05$) and anxiety one year later ($r = 0.29$; $P<0.05$). Only the helpfulness of bosses showed a significant correlation with level of current anxiety ($r = -0.30; P<0.01$).

Table 3.3 Pearson correlations between helpfulness ratings and HIV-positive gay men's psychological distress cross-sectionally and one year later*

	Cross-sectional (1989)		Longitudinal (1990)	
	Depression	Anxiety	Depression	Anxiety
Mean helpfulness of significant others	−0.24†	−0.18‡	−0.21‡	−0.18‡
Lover/partner	−0.10	−0.11	−0.32†	−0.23
Gay friend	−0.18‡	−0.11	−0.18‡	−0.13
Heterosexual friend	−0.23‡	−0.12	−0.09	−0.02
Co-worker	−0.27†	−0.20	−0.05	−0.04
Sister	−0.14	−0.17	−0.22	−0.10
Mother	0.26‡	0.19	0.28	0.29‡
Boss	−0.32†	−0.30†	−0.31‡	−0.16
Brother	−0.21	−0.16	−0.02	0.03
Father	0.11	0.04	0.08	0.05

*The size of the coefficient necessary to reach 0.05 significance level varies because of the varying numbers of men who disclosed to each category of individuals.
†$P<0.01$; ‡$P<0.05$.

Reasons for Not Disclosing

In response to an open-ended question, respondents provided reasons why they had not disclosed their HIV status to the individuals listed. The most frequently mentioned reasons for not disclosing are listed below.

NOT WANTING TO WORRY OR UPSET OTHERS
Many men felt that disclosure would cause unnecessary or unhelpful emotional distress to those told, especially to family. By not disclosing, men felt that they were protecting significant others from pain or anxiety. As one man said,

> My parents are retired, live in their country club retirement village in Florida, and at this point in time, I do not want to make their lives complicated by having them shocked with something I know will freak them out, and make me uncomfortable as well. If the time comes that I need their assistance, I am certain that they will be compassionate and helpful; however at this time, I don't feel it is necessary.

Another man wrote, 'I'm not sick currently, and my family would constantly worry about me. We have an agreement. I've promised to tell them if I get sick.'

FEAR OF DISCRIMINATION
Many men feared that they would be treated in a discriminatory manner if others knew of their HIV status. This concern was most often expressed about co-workers and employers, concerning issues such as losing health insurance or opportunities

for advancement. As one man wrote, 'I feel vulnerable to discrimination based on their assumption that I wouldn't live long and therefore wouldn't be worth training (they haven't expressed this assumption but I fear it).' Others feared 'discrimination at work regarding long-term scheduling and staffing' or that 'health insurance costs could become a factor in their decisions about retaining or promoting me'.

FEAR OF DISRUPTING RELATIONSHIPS

Many men expressed the concern that knowledge of their HIV status would place a strain on their relationship with others or negatively affect how others interacted with them. As one man wrote, '[Disclosure] alters the status of the relationship. Creates worry, stress, sadness.' Others described the 'fear of being misunderstood and having family draw back', a desire to 'avoid tension in relationships', 'fear of rejection, fear of distancing', 'not wanting to focus too strongly on sad aspects'. As one man expressed it, 'I'm afraid of losing them.'

EMOTIONAL SELF-PROTECTION

The anticipated reactions and needs of others when told deterred many men from disclosing their HIV status. Many respondents were apprehensive that it would be draining to have to provide support to the person told or deal with their emotional reaction. As one man wrote, 'I don't need the heavy emotions, and I'm in no mood to have to support them and have to explain my health each time something new in the way of my condition comes up.' For many, concealing their HIV status protected them from the potentially draining reactions of others:

> I have not completely adjusted to the news myself, and I don't want the extra burden of handling their shock. Also, for as long as I appear healthy, I don't want to be treated any differently. To be given too much sympathy at this point would be depressing.

FEELING THAT THE PERSON WOULD HAVE LITTLE BENEFICIAL TO OFFER

Many men chose not to tell certain people because they felt that there was no benefit in doing so ('It would not, or may not, be helpful to me'). They frequently felt that others were not familiar enough with HIV issues to be able to provide helpful support: 'Most people who aren't dealing with HIV issues regularly don't have enough accurate information. There is still tremendous fear and discrimination.' 'My boss has made comments about AIDS that indicate he is poorly informed. Besides, it's none of his business.'

LACK OF INTIMACY WITH AN INDIVIDUAL

Unless they were sufficiently emotionally close to the person, many men did not feel it was worth while telling them ('Not close enough to matter. Not worth the hassle potential'). Many described a lack of intimate communication in their relationships with certain people that made discussing HIV status unlikely ('My brothers are Midwestern non-communicators. We don't generally discuss personal things'), although not necessarily unhelpful ('My father and I have never discussed personal things. We are distant in that way, although I'm sure he would support me if I did').

DESIRE TO CONCEAL ONE'S HOMOSEXUALITY

If men were not 'out of the closet' about being gay with certain people, they were often reluctant to tell them about their HIV status, since HIV and homosexuality are closely interconnected in many people's minds ('My parents don't know that I'm gay'; 'They need to conceal my homosexuality').

Many respondents reported that they planned to tell most of the people listed but that the timing was not yet right. Many asymptomatic men said that 'it wasn't relevant or necessary to tell people, it would only needlessly worry them', but that they would tell people if they started to become sick, or if it interfered with their work performance. Many men expressed ambivalent and conflicting emotions in wanting to be open with people, especially relatives, but not wanting to cause unnecessary stress to themselves or others; thus, many adopted a 'wait and see' approach to disclosing.

DISCUSSION

Gay men who are HIV positive are most likely to disclose their HIV status to their gay friends and lovers, and tend not to disclose to their relatives and colleagues until they become symptomatic. Friends and lovers are perceived to respond in a more helpful manner than relatives and colleagues. The helpfulness of significant others in response to disclosure was associated with less depression and anxiety (currently and one year later), demonstrating the potentially beneficial effects of disclosure. However, a wide range of compelling reasons for not disclosing HIV status to significant others were identified.

This pattern of findings is in agreement with other research that shows gay friends and lovers to be the first choice as a source of support for gay men dealing with HIV issues (Hays *et al.*, 1990a, b). This is probably owing to the considerable amount of trust, familiarity and empathy among gay peers. Although somewhat less likely to be disclosed to, the high helpfulness ratings given to close heterosexual friends suggest that disclosure to intimates who may be less familiar or directly involved with AIDS issues can also be valuable. Similarly, the finding that HIV-negative lovers were rated as helpful as HIV-positive lovers shows that characteristics of the relationship between an HIV-positive gay man and his significant others (for example, degree of understanding, quality of communication) may be more critical in determining the other's helpfulness than individual factors, such as whether the people disclosed to are themselves gay or HIV positive.

The finding that HIV-positive men tend to conceal their status from relatives and colleagues until they become symptomatic is important, but there may be several explanations for it. Disclosure may have been motivated by the men's increased support needs as they become symptomatic, reflected in the higher depression and anxiety scores of symptomatic compared with asymptomatic men. Alternatively, once symptoms emerge, the men may feel pressure that they cannot 'put off' telling others for much longer or that relatives and colleagues now 'have a right to know'. Or it may simply be more difficult to conceal one's status once symptoms emerge. It is likely that each of these factors operates to some degree. Would disclosing to family and colleagues earlier serve a useful purpose? One might argue that early disclosure is preferable, since it provides more opportunity for everyone involved to adapt to the individual's illness, reduces the stress HIV-positive individuals might experience from hiding their status, and increases the potential for receiving social support. Yet, as the participants expressed, early disclosure may also create needless worry among those told, may disrupt 'normal' functioning of relationships and may open up greater possibility for discrimination. An examination of the preferences and actual experiences of relatives and colleagues would be helpful. Do they necessarily want to be told? When? How does the knowledge influence their behaviour and psychological well-being? Insight into these questions would provide useful information for HIV-positive men wrestling with the decision of whether and when to tell certain individuals.

As these findings indicate, disclosing one's HIV seropositivity may contribute to improved psychological well-being if those disclosed to respond in a helpful manner. The beneficial effects of social support for gay men confronting HIV have been documented (Hays *et al.*, 1992). Significant others can provide HIV-positive individuals with a wide range of valuable resources – both tangible and emotional (for example, information about treatment options, financial assistance, sick care, sharing feelings, reassurance that one is loved and valued). However, before it is in the best interests of HIV-positive individuals to disclose their status to others, they must feel assured that the benefits of doing so will outweigh the potential costs. Safeguards against discrimination and stigmatization of HIV-infected individuals are an important first step. For example, the relation between boss helpfulness and lower anxiety may reflect the psychological benefits of employers assuring their HIV-infected employees that their job standing will not be jeopardized by their HIV status. Information about specific ways in which significant others can he helpful to HIV-infected individuals would also be useful in guiding the actions of those who interact with HIV-positive individuals. In this respect, the positive association between mother helpfulness and psychological distress is puzzling. Perhaps HIV-positive men who rely heavily on their parents for support may lack strong peer support networks and so feel more alienated in coping with their illness. However, receiving a considerable amount of help from parents may also have 'hidden costs' for adult men, by damaging egos and reducing self-esteem. Information about ways in which individuals can provide HIV-positive individuals with help that is not unintentionally 'victimizing' or counterproductive would be valuable. Whether the behaviours that are perceived as helpful vary depending on the relationship with the HIV-positive individual (relative versus friend versus co-worker) and the stage of illness are important questions for future research. The association between helpfulness and lower distress may also reflect the fact that it may be easier to help HIV-positive individuals who are less depressed and anxious. Thus information about ways for HIV positives to elicit effective support from others would be valuable.

Several factors may limit the generalizability of these findings. First, disclosure patterns and reasons for not disclosing may be different for non-gay populations and HIV-positive individuals who were infected through non-sexual means, such as injection drug use or blood tranfusion. Second, this sample was predominantly white, well-educated and middle-class. Disclosure patterns may differ for gay men from different ethnic or socio-economic groups. In addition, the disclosure patterns found here may reflect characteristics specific to San Francisco's gay community. Gay men who have moved here from other states may be less inclined to disclose to family members who are geographically distant and with whom they may have little opportunity to interact. There may also be more community services available to HIV-positive individuals in San Francisco than to individuals in other communities, who may turn more readily to relatives for support. Finally, an examination of the disclosure patterns and helpfulness ratings of individuals not assessed in this study, such as extended family members, casual friends, non-primary sex partners and health-care providers, would provide valuable supplementary information to help guide HIV-positive individuals through this difficult disclosure process.

APPENDIX

The discrepancy between the degrees of freedom of this analysis and those reported earlier is because of the repeated-measures design. Thus, only respondents who had disclosed to someone within each relationship category were included in this analysis. The mean ratings of these respondents were not significantly different to those of the men excluded from this analysis, so the respondents included in this analysis were judged not to be a biased representation of the total sample.

REFERENCES

Christ, G. H. and Weiner, L. S. (1985) Psychosocial issues in AIDS, in: V. T. De-Vita, S. Hellman and S. Rosenberg (eds) *AIDS: Etiology, Diagnosis, Treatment and Prevention*, pp. 173–179 (Philadelphia, J. B. Lippincott).

Cohen, S. and Wills, T. A. (1985) Social support, stress and the buffering hypothesis, *Psychological Bulletin*, 98, pp. 310–357.

Derlega, V. J. and Berg, J. H. (1987) *Self-disclosure: Theory, Research and Therapy* (New York, Plenum).

Derogatis, L. and Melisaratos, N. (1993) Brief symptom inventory: an introductory report, *Psychological Medicine*, 13, pp. 595–605.

Forstein, M. (1984) The psychosocial impact of the acquired immune deficiency syndrome, *Seminars in Oncology*, 11, pp. 77–82.

Hays, R. B., Catania, J. A., McKusick, L. and Coates, T. J. (1990a) Help-seeking for AIDS-related concerns: a comparison of gay men of various HIV diagnoses, *American Journal of Community Psychology*, 18, pp. 743–755.

Hays, R. B., Chauncey, S. and Tobey, L. (1990b) The social support networks of gay men with AIDS, *Journal of Community Psychology*, 18, pp. 374–385.

Hays, R. B., Turner, H. A. and Coates, T. J. (1992) Social support, HIV symptoms and depression among gay men, *Journal of Consulting and Clinical Psychology*, 60, pp. 463–469

Herek, G. M. and Glunt, E. K. (1988) An epidemic of stigma: public reactions to AIDS, *American Psychologist*, 43, pp. 886–891.

Jourard, S. M. (1964) *The Transparent Self* (New York, Van Nostrand).

Kurdeck, L. A. (1988) Perceived social support in gays and lesbians in cohabitating relationships, *Journal of Personality and Social Psychology*, 54, pp. 504–509.

McKusick, L., Coates, T. J., Morin, S. F., Pollack, L. and Hoff, C. (1990) Longitudinal predicators of reductions in unprotected anal intercourse among gay men in San Francisco: the AIDS Behavioral Research Project, *American Journal of Public Health*, 80, pp. 978–983.

McKusick, L., Horstman, W. and Coates, T. J. (1985a) AIDS and sexual behaviour reported by gay men in San Francisco, *American Journal of Public Health*, 75, pp. 493–496.

McKusick, L., Wiley, J. A., Coates, T. J. *et al.* (1985b) Reported changes in the sexual behaviour of men at risk for AIDS, San Francisco 1982–84: the AIDS Behavioral Research Project, *Public Health Reports*, 100, pp. 622–628.

Stulberg, I. and Smith, M. (1988) Psychosocial impact of the AIDS epidemic on the lives of gay men, *Social Work*, 33, pp. 277–281.

Taylor, S. E., Falke, R. L., Shoptaw, S. J. and Lightman, R. R. (1986) Social support, support groups and the cancer patient, *Journal of Consulting and Clinical Psychology*, 54, pp. 608–615.

Wortman, C. B. and Conway, T. L. (1985) The role of social support in the adaptation and recovery from physical illness, in: S. Cohen and S. L. Syme (eds) *Social Support and Health*, pp. 253–267 (New York, Academic Press).

FOUR

AIDS and the Urban Family: Its Impact in Kampala, Uganda

Janet W. McGrath, E. Maxine Ankrah, Debra A. Schumann, S. Nkumbi and Monica Lubega

INTRODUCTION

Uganda has become a locus of AIDS in East Africa and the world in the years since the discovery of the first case of AIDs ('slim disease') in Uganda (Serwadda *et al.*, 1985). Currently, Uganda is second only to the United States in number of AIDS cases reported to the World Health Organization (WHO, 1991). The areas of highest reported prevalence in Uganda are the city of Kampala and the rural Masaka and Rakai districts. Uganda will continue to bear a great burden resulting from AIDS morbidity and mortality in the foreseeable future. Maintenance of social group functions, including subsistence and economic activities, care for the sick and other vital activities, is important in mitigating the impact of epidemic disease (e.g. Neel *et al.*, 1970; McGrath, 1991), so it is critical to examine how social institutions in Uganda are responding to HIV and AIDS.

Because HIV infection is transmitted primarily through heterosexual intercourse in Uganda (Pattern II; Piot *et al.*, 1988) both male and female sexual partners in a union may be infected. When only one sexual partner is infected the other partner is also at risk. If a woman is infected and becomes pregnant her child is also at risk of becoming infected. In this way, HIV infection represents a risk to entire family units, not just individuals. Therefore, the epidemiological data strongly point to the need to examine the impact of this disease on the primary social institution affected by the HIV/AIDS epidemic: the family.

The tragedy of AIDS strikes not just the individual with the deadly infection, but his or her family and community as well. To date there has been little investigation of the impact of AIDS on household and family units, despite the fact that the diagnosis of AIDS has such far-reaching consequences (Eberstein *et al.*, 1988; Lloyd, 1988; Ankrah *et al.*, 1989, 1991; Macklin, 1989; Levine, 1990; UNICEF, 1990; Ankrah, 1991; McGrath *et al.*, 1991). Recently, attention has been paid to families after the death of their loved one, with special concern expressed for the fate of orphaned children (e.g. Hunter, 1990; Preble, 1990). However, the impact of AIDS on family units does not begin with the death of a parent: it begins with the infection and subsequent illness of the family member. Therefore, issues regarding AIDS must examine this impact within the family. This paper reports on a study undertaken in Kampala, Uganda, to investigate the impact of AIDS on families in which one or more adult members have AIDS (Ankrah, *et al.*, 1989, 1991; McGrath *et al.*, 1991). The study focuses on the Baganda, the most prominent ethnic group in the Kampala area.

The Dispersed Family as a Source of Assistance

Anthropologists and sociologists have extensively studied kinship, marriage and family in Africa concluding that:

> An institution at the core of African cultural patterns is the extended family, which subsumes the totality of how an African man relates to himself, his immediate family, his relatives, and other social beings and things in his environment. (Okediji, 1975, p. 93)

In urban Kampala, families are multiple households. It is necessary to consider the ability of a dispersed family to assist with and to accommodate to illness. In this respect LeVine (1970) notes that:

> African families do not have to be residentially intact in order to remain socially and psychologically real for their members, nor do the obligations of marriage and kinship diminish with prolonged absence. (p. 299)

With reference to AIDS, it is critical to examine the extent to which a dispersed network of kin can or does assist with care of AIDS patients and their families. (Terms such as 'AIDS patient' or 'AIDS victim' are terms that are used by the subjects in the study and have been retained for this purpose. Such terms, although objectionable to some advocates for persons with AIDS, are widely used in Uganda.)

The provision of health care is an important domain of family functioning (Janzen, 1978). In Uganda, as in much of Africa, the family is responsible for much of the nursing and health care, both in and out of the hospital (Muller and Abbas, 1990; Kalibala and Kaleeba, 1989). Illness and disease place burdens on the family in proportion to its ability to absorb an additional family member who may come to stay or who may be prevented from following normal patterns of mobility owing to illness. The extent to which persons with AIDS and their families perceive, and actually receive, support from the community impacts on the ability of the family to adapt to having a person with AIDS (PWA) in the household.

Several features of Baganda family structure have implications for the ability of the family as an institution to respond to AIDS. These features include household composition and post-marital residence patterns, cultural norms favouring independent living and high degrees of individual mobility.

Marriage residence patterns are a critical factor determining household composition. The traditional marriage residence pattern among the Baganda is neolocality, in which a married couple establish their own home instead of moving into the home of the bride's or groom's parents (Fallers, 1960; Southwold, 1965). In addition to establishing a separate household, married couples often moved to a village separate from their parents, but usually one in which the male had kin to help them get settled (Southwold, 1965). Extended family households *per se* were rare, even in rural areas where they might be expected to have been more common (Fallers, 1960). Residence patterns, therefore, contribute to a situation wherein families are dispersed across villages.

The cultural importance of independent living is demonstrated in a study of residential locations of urban elderly Baganda by Nahemow (1979), who reports that 63% of the respondents lived in households apart from adult children, while 30% lived with children still in school or 'otherwise dependent'. She notes, however, that older people, despite living alone, report that they receive considerable assistance from kin with regards to such needs as attending the market. Importantly, respondents report that this pattern of residential separation is the traditional pattern among the Baganda, with 99% of the respondents reporting that it is 'wrong and/or untraditional to live with one's adult married children'. Only 63% of the respondents say that it is, in fact, usual to live alone, because extenuating circumstances usually require joint living. Nevertheless, it seems that the separation of extended families into multiple households is not a recent development in Baganda social organization.

An important feature of Baganda social organization is mobility, both physical and social (e.g. Fallers, 1964; Southwold, 1965; Richards, 1966; Perlman, 1970; Kilbride and Kilbride, 1990). Physical mobility includes movements resulting from political affiliation as well as movement of family members according to the ability of the family to care for its members. Social mobility includes the ability to move up in social rank. In addition, many authors discuss the relationship of mobility to sexuality in general and marriage in particular, which is characterized by frequent partner change for both males and females (Southall and Gutkind, 1957; Obbo, 1980; Parkin, 1966; Mandeville, 1975, 1979).

AIDS among the Baganda, therefore, occurs within a social structure featuring mobility and dispersed kin networks. How the family as an institution responds to AIDS will depend to a large degree upon the extent to which the disease permits the maintenance of social function. We turn next to a consideration of this issue.

MATERIALS AND METHODS

Twenty-two families from urban and peri-urban Kampala were enrolled over a period of five months from March through July 1989. At that stage of the AIDS epidemic in Uganda, outpatient clinical and social services were newly established and patients were just beginning to use these facilities on a regular basis. For this reason there was no established study frame for the random selection of study participants, so that opportunistic sampling methods were used.

A family was eligible for recruitment if it had one or more adult members with a positive serologic test for HIV-1 infection, who was attending outpatient AIDS clinics at Mulago Hospital or St Francis Hospital at Nsambya, Kampala. Medical staff identified eligible persons with AIDS and introduced them to the interview team (ML, SN). Each person was invited to participate after being given a detailed description of the study. In obtaining informed consent, each person was told of the nature of the interviews and the methods of home visiting. Each was assured that their responses would remain confidential and that no other family or household member would be interviewed without the expressed consent of the person with AIDS.

An initial criterion for eligibility included the insistence that another adult member of the family be aware of the diagnosis of AIDS. This criterion was dropped when it was discovered that some patients chose to deny to themselves or their families that they were HIV infected or had AIDS. Seven persons would not allow contact with other family members, although they were willing to participate themselves. No differentiation was made between subjects based on the stage of the disease or how long they had been sick. Although it is recognized that this may influence both whom a patient informs of the diagnosis and how the family responds to the diagnosis, this initial study did not attempt to account for these variations.

All subjects were visited in their homes for four days within one week for periods of about six hours each day. The time of the visit was varied to permit interviewers to be present for different family functions, and to observe the interactions between the person with AIDS and other family members. If an individual was too ill to sustain a full day of visiting, periods were broken down to shorter lengths, but extended over more days, until an equivalent period of time was achieved. The discussions took place in varying contexts such as taking tea, sitting in the open compound, meeting in a scheduled location and conversations within the home. The choice of the context for discussion was left to the subject in order to maximize his or her control over the interview situation. In cases of extreme need, the interviewer provided small items, such as sugar for tea, as a gesture of concern.

Interviews were conducted in Luganda when this was the principal language shared by the researcher and the subject. English was used when this was not the case or when the educational level of the family permitted. All interviews were conducted by graduates in social work from Makerere University (SN, ML). Interviews were taped by consent and transcribed into English within 24–48 hours after the end of the day's visit. Each interview was reviewed with a senior investigator (EMA) and clarified where required.

Three interview schedules were employed. The first consisted of 26 open-ended questions concerned with the demographic information about the infected person, including marital status, household and family composition, and the identification of other 'significant others' to be involved in the study discussions. The second schedule consisted of 46 items focused on knowledge of AIDS, HIV infection and sexual relationships. Religious beliefs, practical issues of planning for survivors, health seeking behaviours, community reactions and support, and identification of specific needs were also expected.

The third schedule included 42 questions directed towards the family group for the purpose of ascertaining the family's concepts of the disease and treatment; perception of AIDS' impact with respect to the social interaction within and between members of the household; beliefs about the aetiology of AIDS in general; beliefs about how the person with AIDS became infected; material needs; and the family and community responses to the diagnosis of AIDS, with particular reference to stigma.

Individual family members' responses are the unit of analysis (as opposed to the entire family group). The major themes contained in the interview guides were analysed by coding each response to correspond to a theme and sorting text into constituent themes. These themes were tabulated and the trends observed are presented here.

RESULTS AND DISCUSSION

Seven families were recruited from Mulago Hospital and 15 families from St Francis Hospital at Nsambya. In two of the 22 families included in the study both the husband and wife were infected, resulting in a total of 24 infected individuals in the sample. The description of the subject population is presented in Table 4.1. The sample included 14 females and 10 males, ranging in age from 18 to 55 years (mean 31 years, standard deviation 9.8). Eighteen of the subjects are Baganda, two are Ankole, and there is one each of Luo, Teso, Kiga, Munyoro and unknown. Twelve subjects are Catholic, nine Protestant, two Muslim and one Jehovah's Witness. This distribution is approximately equivalent to the distribution of the general population with respect to these religions (Kaijuka *et al.*, 1989).

Table 4.1 Description of study subjects (*n* = 24)

Males	42% (10)
Females	58% (14)
Age	
Range	18–55 years
Mean	31 years
Ethnic group	
Ganda	75% (18)
Ankole	8% (2)
Luo, Teso, Kiga, Munyoro	4% (1) each
Religion	
Catholic	50% (12)
Protestant	38% (9)
Muslim	8% (2)
Jehovah's Witness	4% (1)

Five families in this sample are nuclear families; eight families contain the person with AIDS and a parent or parents, in combination with other relatives, including siblings, step-relations and in-laws; and nine families contain the person with AIDS and relatives, including siblings, step-relations and in-laws, but not a parent.

The impact of HIV/AIDS on families can be discussed from two perspectives: the psychosocial impact on the individuals within the family and the direct impact of the disease on family functioning. The psychosocial impact of AIDS is examined by asking persons with AIDS and family members about social relationships within the household and within the neighbourhood. That is, they were asked about their *own* reactions to the presence of AIDS and their *perceptions* of the reactions of others around them, including other members of the household and neighbours and friends. The direct impact of AIDS on the family was explored through examination of the impact of the disease on the economic well-being of the family.

Psychosocial Impacts

WITHIN THE HOUSEHOLD

Persons with AIDS and their family members do not always share the same perception as to the impact of AIDS on their family. Therefore, we must consider the perceptions of the patient separately from the perceptions of other family members.

Historically, ostracism and rejection of the diseased, or those thought to be at risk of becoming diseased, has been a common response to epidemic disease (e.g. McGrath, 1991; Nelkin and Gilman, 1988). None of the subjects in this study report having been thrown out of their homes or ostracized by their families. Three important things should be noted, however. First, four of the patients do not state that they have AIDS. Despite being told of the diagnosis by the clinic physician these individuals either do not understand their diagnosis or do not acknowledge it. Second, of the remaining 20 persons, only four had informed everyone in the household of the diagnosis of AIDS, seven have told no one about the diagnosis and eight have told some of their family and household (Table 4.2). Finally, we don't know to what extent criteria for inclusion in this study may have prevented contact with families in which rejection or ostracism had occurred, so that our sample may be biased towards families that have accepted the patient.

Among those who withheld the information about their diagnosis from all some of their families (*n* = 16), a prominent reason provided for not telling family members (seven responses) is that they would worry.

> The only people I could have told would have been my parents but I know that if I tell them now they will panic, they will be sick with worry. I have thought it wise to leave them out of it. (Ankole male, aged 26)

Table 4.2 Household and family members who have been informed of the diagnosis of AIDS

Who has been told	Number of households
Everyone in household	4
No one	8*
Aunts only	2
Mother only	2
Wife only	2
Brother only	1
Sister was told but did not understand	1

Four subjects with TB don't believe/understand that they have AIDS. *In one household the other family members have guessed that the subject has AIDS, but they did not think that she was aware of it herself.

One determinant of whom patients inform of their diagnosis is their perception of the likelihood that the family would reject them because of their disease. Three persons specifically feared that they would be asked to leave the household if it became known that they have AIDS.

> Nobody knows but I do not know what will happen if they come to know. Please do not let my sister know of it. Because she will let everybody around here know. She is a person who cannot keep a secret. And it may affect my staying here. (Ganda female, aged 28)

> I am afraid that if they learn that I have AIDS they may decide to send me home to die. They may fear to keep me in their house any longer let alone paying out money for a patient without any hope of permanent recovery. (Ankole male, aged 35)

Therefore, the anticipation of stigma may result in a desire not to tell family members or others.

Other reasons for not telling family members include the feeling that it is none of their business ($n = 2$) and that they wouldn't be understanding ($n = 1$). An individual may have different reasons for not telling different people. For example, one woman did not tell her father because she felt he would not understand, but she did not tell her mother because she did not want to worry her. These reasons may reflect fear of becoming dependent and/or the absence of close family ties, rather than, or in addition to, fear of rejection.

> I plan to tell nobody. This is a problem for me and my wife. (Ganda male, aged 29)

> I can't tell my father; how can I go about it. He would never understand. I don't tell him what happens to me. (Ganda female, aged 22)

Despite the concerns expressed by the persons with AIDS, however, family members who knew of the diagnosis did not express rejection of the patient. The only case in which a household member expressed a desire to separate the person with AIDS from the household involved a caretaker, who was an unrelated employer. The employer had been caring for an infected couple and their child and now stated the desire to be rid of the burden of caring for three sick persons.

> Now the problem is this. I want to get rid of them. These people are here because of me. I do not know how my husband takes it but I think he does not want to involve ourselves in any more expenses and other problems. We have cared for them for one year. If it were the boy alone with a woman then that is good – but three sick people is a great responsibility for the family. But the dilemma is letting them go, go to where? ... The reason for all of this is not because I do not want to help but because I fear to undertake more risks. And caring for three is not a joke. (Adult woman who is employer and caretaker for a couple and their child, all of whom have AIDS)

Historically, a common reason for rejection of persons with an infectious disease is fear of contagion and, in the case of HIV/AIDS worldwide, fears of casual contagion are common. In this sample, however, family members did not express fear of infection. Only four household members interviewed expressed concern about infection or inquired as to any possible risk of infection.

> Sometimes I wonder if whether mixing her cups with other cups will infect us. Do you think that we can be infected in such a way? (Adult female in household of Baganda female, aged 18)

With these exceptions, family members either made no statement about fear of infection or specifically denied being afraid of becoming infected by the patient.

> No, I do not think that it catches easily and it even doesn't seem to be any disease that I know. If it was one which catches fast we would all probably have it already. After all we share utensils with him, he sits in the same chair as us, a lot of personal contacts are made with him often. (Adult female in household of Ankole male, aged 35)

> We feared mostly because we knew she is going to die. But we did not fear her about infecting us. (Adult male in household of Baganda female, aged 24)

Instead of expressing rejection or fear of the patients, family members tended to emphasize the implications of AIDS, including fear of the loss of a loved one; the burden of care for the patient, and, perhaps, children who are left behind after the patient's death; and loss of future plans.

The two most common responses to the AIDS diagnosis from family and household members was a fear of the loss of a loved one (seven responses) and shock, disbelief and confusion over the diagnosis (six responses). To the families of the patients, the diagnosis of AIDS means that they will face the death of a loved one.

> I feared so much because I lost hope. I knew she was going to die. (Adult female in household of Baganda female, aged 28)

Another implication of the loss of the loved one is the burden of caring for children they have left behind.

> About when she is gone, I have not given it much thought although I know that I may remain with the responsibility of her daugher. (Mother of Baganda female, aged 22)

The presence of AIDS in the family affects the ability of the entire family to make plans for the future. In some cases this may be translated into a very personal loss, as represented by the woman who saw her husband's AIDS as a loss in the ability to bear children.

> To me the first and most important implication of his having AIDS was that I could not have the baby that I have so sought for all these years we have been together. All my plans of the future surrounded this baby that I thought we would have together. Suddenly all these plans were shattered. I have been consulting traditional doctors in order to help me conceive. When, however, they told me he had AIDS, I gave up all these efforts. I gave up all hope of bearing a child. (Wife of Ankole male, aged 26)

In summary, family concerns centred on issues of loss more than fear or concerns about either infection or the burden of caring for the patient, despite the concerns of some patients that their families would reject them. We cannot say, of course, how those families or family members who have not been informed of the diagnosis would respond if they had been told. It appears, however, that for the families where the diagnosis is known there is a disjunction between what individuals perceive will be the response of their families and the responses reported by the family members in this sample. This disjunction may result from the failure of either PWAs or their family members to speak truthfully regarding their feelings about AIDS. It may also stem, however, from experience with the response to AIDS of people outside of the household. As people acquire both more knowledge about AIDS and more experience with it, attitudes about PWAs also change. Patients may, in this case, be anticipating reactions based on observations of attitudes and events that have occurred previously, while family members are now responding on the basis of new knowledge and attitudes with regard to AIDS. Regardless, it is critical to examine the perceptions of both AIDS patients and their families with respect to the reception of a PWA within the neighbourhood.

WITHIN THE NEIGHBOURHOOD

Out of respect for confidentiality no individuals outside of the household were interviewed. Household members were asked what they perceived the response of the neighbours was or would be to the sick person and his or her family. Subjects often do not tell their neighbours that they have AIDS because they perceive that stigma will result. The stigma of AIDS results from its association with promiscuity and 'immoral' sexual behaviour. For a disease like AIDS, that stigma is felt not just by the patient themselves, but also by the family.

> We have not told anyone that he has AIDS for obvious reasons. AIDS is not a good thing to have you know the way people talk of you as having got it because of promiscuity. People even start avoiding you and you start feeling ashamed and embarrassed. So we haven't told anyone. Even our parents haven't been told because we don't like to worry them too much. (Wife of Baganda male, aged 38)

PWAs and their families often perceive that neighbours and other acquaintances, even if they have not been informed of the diagnosis of AIDS, have come to believe that a person has AIDS because of his or her physical appearance.

> Nobody except my family members have I told about it. After all, all outsiders think I have AIDS. (Kiga female, aged 26)

The lay model of AIDS ('slim') is one of continual decline in health, characterized by diarrhoea, fever and a rash. Individuals who seem to fit this model are often labelled as 'having slim'.

This labelling is perceived negatively by the person with AIDS and his or her family. Eleven subjects or their families report the subject is stared at and avoided when in public.

> At first people could miss steps while looking at me. Some even used to make comments when I am passing by. Some could call to others to come and see me pass by. (Ganda female, aged 24)

Two subjects commented that they find it unnerving and depressing when visitors who knew them before they got sick question them about the illness, while expressing shock at how bad they look.

> Back in the village ... the situation is difficult. Although the people there did not know for sure that I have AIDS having known me in better times when I was fat and my skin was smooth, they always exclaimed with dismay every time one of them saw me and they kept asking me what has happened to me. This got on my nerves and made my health even worse. (Ganda female, aged 55)

> Remember the day we travelled from the village. Everybody kept a distance. We were left alone on a seat in the bus. The bus was so

crowded but nobody could come near us. They could squeeze at each other away from us. Leaving a whole empty space around us. Leave alone travelling! Even here many come to see the sick but do not enter. They stand in the doorway and peep in the house as if something so dangerous is hiding in the house. Some people even refuse to greet the patient but just look straight at her and walk away mocking. They only come to see what an AIDS victim looks like. Some used to say that 'latest style of dressing' meaning that the patient decided to put on the style of thinness at her own choice. They could say this when all of us are hearing. (Adult female in the household of Baganda female, aged 28)

Because the stigma of AIDS is linked to the physical appearance of the patient, those patients who show some improvement are not thought to have AIDS. So, for example, a person who is treated for tuberculosis and gets better for a time is not thought to have AIDS, but 'just TB'.

At first when people thought that she has AIDS they were avoiding us, but when people see her improving they no longer stigmatize us. They believe they were mistaken at first. Because she is okay, the cough is not so much now. (Mother of Baganda female, aged 26)

Why, if she had it, has she taken so long to die? (Mother of Baganda female, aged 22)

Physical symptoms and progression of the condition, therefore, are key biological features of AIDS that carry extraordinary weight in influencing social and behavioural responses to the disease.

As long as the person remains reasonably healthy they may be able to maintain normal social intercourse. As symptoms develop, however, and their strength fails, the linkage of stigma to physical appearance may play a key role in encouraging withdrawal from social contacts. Not wishing to be seen and stared at results in individuals staying in the house and withdrawing from social activities, including going to church, the market, etc.

I keep in the house. Other people keep apart, away from me. This doesn't hurt me because I know it is their ignorance about the disease. (Ganda female, aged 24)

This isolation is felt by the family as well, particularly if visitors no longer come to the household.

Other people are isolating us. They have no longer come here. Since they saw our patient. We used to have many visitors. (Adult male in household of Baganda female, aged 24)

Responses such as closing a community toilet so the sick person cannot use it or banning use of a community water tap (examples cited by one family interviewed) affect household function and impede the patient's ability to continue to contribute to household tasks, such as fetching water. Even the activities of others in the household are affected.

> I used to sell ground-nuts here but people could refuse to buy because of having an AIDS patient. (Sister-in-law in household of Baganda female, aged 28)

Since neighbours were not interviewed, it cannot be ascertained whether the reaction of neighbours and acquaintances stems from fear of infection, stigma over 'immoral' behaviour, or other factors, but responses such as staring or rejection symbolize the stigmatization of AIDS to the person with AIDS and his or her family.

Not all the experiences with neighbours are negative, of course. Five of the subjects or their household members state that the neighbours have not responded badly.

> The neighbours have been understanding and sympathetic. They help us in any way and they don't discriminate against her in any way. They lend us their utensils and they too use ours without any sign of selectiveness or discrimination. (Adult female in household of Baganda female, aged 22)

Several reasons may exist for the lack of stigma in such cases. First, the 'appropriate' symptoms may not exist in these cases. Second, it may be simply that the relationship between neighbours and the family is closer, of longer standing, or otherwise less likely to be disrupted by the presence of AIDS in one of the families. Finally, it may be that these families themselves have experienced AIDS and are, therefore, more accepting of others with the disease. Unfortunately, we cannot determine which of these factors are most important at this time. It seems likely, however, that as the number of cases of AIDS continues to grow in Kampala, and throughout Uganda, more families will have experienced AIDS. Familiarity with the disease, including decreased fears of casual contagion, is likely to lessen stigma and increase openness and acceptance of persons with AIDS and their families.

The Direct Impact of AIDS on Family Functioning

HIV/AIDS, as a serious disease and illness, has direct impacts that affect family functioning. A primary impact is on the mobility of the patient and the economic welfare of the family. That AIDS has a negative impact on family and household economic well-being is expected. Clearly, loss of income due to disease and death presents a hardship to any family. The presence of an additional person in the household for a long period of time, especially one who doesn't contribute to household expenses, constitutes a significant burden. Add to this the medical costs if the person is sick, and the burden becomes even greater.

The most direct impact of AIDS on family economic well-being is through the inability of the patient to participate in income-generating work. Fourteen of the 24 individuals rely solely on household members' income for subsistence and medical care, as they are no longer able to work themselves. Both patients and their families feel the economic strain.

> My brothers buy food for me, they also pay for my room since I stopped working in 1988. The extra burden on my brothers is too much. (Baganda male, aged 29)

> I have many problems, I have two children in secondary school and I pay for their school fees. Yet my work was retarded by G's illness. She cannot go where she used to buy matooke . . . and I have also used my capital . . . to treat her. There is no one helping me. (Mother of a female Baganda, aged 26 years)

For families with limited resources and multiple demands, choices must be made. Families must decide which member warrants resources. For those families with more than one sick person this may result in the need to make a choice as to who will receive medicine and care. One woman explained:

> Now we have no money. We have used all the money on treatment of the children. We paid 4,000 shillings for laboratory tests and treatment for NK [the AIDS patient]. Now NM is also sick, even that boy did not go to school, he was feeling feverish. (Stepmother of Baganda female, aged 18 years)

> Daddy said that we did not have enough money to treat us both. (Stepsister of Baganda female, aged 18 years)

In a situation that forces choices regarding receipt of care, it is little wonder that some patients will be afraid to inform their families that they have AIDS. No person in the study reported active withdrawal of support, but, as is clear from the quote just given, some families are making choices regarding access to health care within the family. In other cases, as illustrated above, other things, such as school fees, are sacrificed to care for an HIV/AIDS patient.

Another aspects of AIDS that threatens economic well-being is the impact of the illness on mobility. As discussed above, mobility is a characteristic of this population and one determinant of mobility is economic opportunity and need. This mobility may occur at different levels. For example, as stated in the quote above, people may be unable to go to the location where they buy matooke to sell in their neighbourhood. Alternatively, mobility may be restricted on a larger scale, preventing relocation to where employment or better employment is available. Alternatively, the need for money may prohibit a return to the home village.

> If I am to go home, I have the problem of money. I do not go for my family alone but for the whole village and all the people are my people.

> So I cannot go to them when I am unable to attend to them and some of
> their needs. The war has made everything worse. Secondly, travel is a
> sign of work. Why should I travel when I am going to do nothing. If I had
> money I would move but I have no money. (Teso male, ages 28 years)

In a social system characterized by movement from location to location based on economic need, anything that jeopardizes the ability to move will endanger economic well-being. As an HIV infected individual progresses to AIDS and his or her strength decreases, mobility will be reduced and economic opportunity diminished.

Finally, reduced mobility also impacts on family assistance by decreasing the degree to which assistance can be shared across the dispersed network of kin. That is, in the absence of debilitating disease a person might move from household to household while in need of care, thus utilizing a network of relationships. If such movement is not possible one household may bear a disproportionate burden of care.

> Well of course he adds a substantial amount to the family's daily
> expenditure. You see in town, we have to buy everything from food, salt
> even up to water so one extra person adds a substantial bit to the
> household's expenditure. (Adult female in the household of an Ankole
> man, aged 35 years)

> My husband who is the one who provided the money for rent was
> nowhere to be seen and I couldn't pay rent so I was evicted from the
> house. Then I fell sick and much as I tried, I found that I couldn't look after
> myself so I had to come here ... as you realize this is not the most
> convenient place. The family here is quite big, things are expensive as
> you know and transport back is the same so it's definitely conditions that
> have forced me to live here. (Baganda female, aged 36 years)

In addition, choice of residence may be determined by access to health care.

> That village is unfortunately very far from Kampala and also from any
> health facilities. I don't hope to ever go back and live there. (Baganda
> female, aged 54 years)

> Now if I shift to my sister in Masaka, I will find a problem to get money to
> come and attend to regular clinics. (Baganda female, aged 28 years)

> I have to stay in the city to attend to treatment ... If I go home I am going
> to die. (Teso male, aged 28 years)

It should be noted, in this regard, that the majority of the patients in this study were receiving free care and medicine at St Francis Hospital AIDS clinic, Nsambya. Many, however, stated that they were unable to attend clinic on a regular basis because of the cost of transport to the hospital. Of course, families not able to access the clinic at either St Francis or Mulago Hospitals, or other charitable health care services, would have to pay for medical care, adding to the economic burden of AIDS.

Family Structure and Functioning in the Face of AIDS

McGrath (1991) argues that the impact of epidemic disease is increased by social responses that disrupt normal social group functions, such as economic activities. Because of the key role played by the family in social group functions, an examination of the impact of AIDS on family structure and functioning is appropriate. The data presented above indicate that several aspects of family structure and functioning are fundamentally affected by the presence of a person with AIDS within the family. These areas are: household composition, economic decisions, social interaction and access to health care.

Urban households in this population are typically characterized by a high degree of fluidity in composition. Family members move in and out of households depending on personal inclination, economic opportunity and family obligations. As noted above, AIDS truncates this normal pattern of mobility as the person becomes too weak to move or does not wish to travel away from available health care. The inability to care for oneself may result in adult children moving into their parents' home, young children being sent to relatives for care, or sick parents and siblings moving in with able-bodied adult family members.

> When I left that man [husband] I came with my children and I have been with him all the time. When I fell sick I came with them here. But the house has been too small. I had to get where to put this boy. He is a boy of 15 years who cannot stay with us in this congested house. There was a good friend of ours who accepted to keep him for nights. But thank God finally I managed to make the boy go back to his father. (Banganda female, aged 28 years)

> They [her children] are with their paternal aunts and relatives. (Baganda female, aged 36 years)

> With all these problems, I had to give away some children to the people who requested them. They have to do something to survive. (Baganda female, aged 45 years)

> When I fell sick, I had to go to my sister who is now caring for me. (Baganda female, aged 28 years)

In other words, the impact of AIDS on household composition is to alter the choices regarding where to stay and for how long, and to encourage traditional patterns of 'fostering'; that is, sending children to live with other kin.

The truncation of mobility also affects economic decision-making within the household. As described above, the presence of an additional family member who cannot provide economic assistance to the household becomes a burden and as the disease progresses, this burden grows. For those patients who can still work, the unpredictability of their future income impacts on the ability to make plans. Those who are forced to give up good jobs with good incomes will be faced with a lower standard of living.

The important influence of social networks and social support on health has been demonstrated (e.g. Berkman, 1985). As described above, persons with AIDS appear to be making decisions about who to inform of their diagnosis based on their perception of the reaction to AIDS within the community. In this context the issue of stigma and public perceptions of AIDS' aetiology becomes important in understanding family responses to the disease. The perception of stigma associated with HIV/AIDS encourages families to keep the diagnosis quiet.

As families try to shoulder the burden of care for an AIDS patient, their resources, both social and economic, become strained. To the extent that normal patterns of social interaction and economic exchange are affected by the care of the patient within the household, there is grave danger that household units will be unable to manage the care of persons with AIDS. If this happens and families become overwhelmed with the needs of caring for those with AIDS, then access to health care may be threatened for all family members.

At the present time, little can be done for AIDS patients other than providing treatment of basic symptoms and physical comfort to the extent possible. The vast majority of this care takes place within the home. If families cannot handle this burden on their own, they will have only a few alternatives. One is to seek assistance from the health care system, which is already taxed beyond its ability to respond. Another is to stop providing assistance to some family members. The impact of AIDS on health in Kampala, therefore, has the potential to extend well beyond HIV-infected individuals.

A primary determinant of social disruption resulting from epidemic disease is the loss of individuals with prime roles in the social system. AIDS is a particularly devastating disease in this respect because those most likely to become infected and die are also those who are most likely to have a prime role in the society. For families the loss of these productive members is particularly serious. The potential for a failure of the ability of the family to accommodate AIDS patients will continue to exist if the economic strain resulting from loss of productive family members is not addressed. Therefore, action must be taken to prevent social disintegration through extensive disruption of family function.

Although these data suggest that Ugandan families are attempting to deal with the AIDS crisis within the household, some unassisted by or isolated from the neighbours, it should be noted that these interviews were completed in 1989. Since that time the number of cases of AIDS in Kampala has continued to increase. A trend towards more acceptance to openness about the presence of AIDS appears under way as more and more families recognize the common bond of disease.

CONCLUSIONS

In summary, PWAs selectively inform family members of the diagnosis out of fear of stigma and rejection. The reaction of the family members who knew of the

AIDS diagnosis, however, was shock and concern about the future loss of a loved one, rather than rejection. Both PWAs and their families expressed a perception of isolation and rejection from others within their neighbourhood. This resulted not from direct knowledge of the diagnosis, but from the suspicion of diagnosis based upon physical appearance and symptoms. In addition, AIDS affects the economic well-being of the family by decreasing the ability to work and adding to the financial needs of the family. This results from reduced mobility that prevents regular employment as well as economically advantageous movement of family members between households.

Overall, the impact of AIDS on family function affects household composition, economic decisions, social interaction and access to health care. It is difficult to predict the final outcome of the epidemic on the family as an institution in Uganda. In Uganda mounting economic problems, despite structural adjustment efforts, are rendering more families poor. As a result, it is increasingly the case that the family having a member with AIDS is hard pressed to meet the needs of the person with AIDS alone or within the confines of the household.

Therefore, although material assistance, such as food, bedding, medicine and school fees, is needed to make up for lost income, more than money is needed to overcome the burden of AIDS on families. There must be a change in the climate of fear that prevents persons with AIDS from telling their families or other members of their social network of the diagnosis. Families must be able to continue to care for AIDS patients without having to choose that person over another family member needing assistance. Importantly, there must be ways that families can adapt to the loss of mobility that prevents normal patterns of family interaction in the dispersed kin network.

These data point to an urgent need for government, in collaboration with national and international non-governmental organizations, to develop assistance programmes for families to ensure that the family will continue to be the mainstay of members with AIDS.

REFERENCES

Ankrah, E. M. (1991) The impact of AIDS on the social, economic, health and welfare systems. AIDS: preserving the family of mankind, in: G. B. Rossi, E. Beth-Giraldo, L. Chieco-Bianchi, F. Dianzani, G. Giraldo and P. Verani (eds) *Science Challenging AIDS*, pp. 175–187 (Basel, Karger).

Ankrah, E. M., McGrath, J. W., Schumann, D. A., Nkumbi, S. and Lubega, M. (1989) The impact of AIDS on family structure and function in Uganda, presented at the meetings of the American Anthropological Association, November 1989.

Ankrah, E. M., McGrath, J. W., Schumann, D. A., Nkumbi, S. and Lubega, M. (1991) The impact of AIDS on urban families: an assessment of needs, presented at the VIth International Conference on AIDS in Africa, December 1991.

Berkman, L. (1985) The relationship of social networks and social support to morbidity and mortality, in: S. Cohen and S. L. Syme (eds) *Social Supports and Heath*, pp. 241–262 (New York, Academic Press).

Eberstein, I. W., Serow, W. J. and Ahmad, O. B. (1988) AIDS: consequences for families and fertility, in: A. F. Fleming, M. Carballo, D. W. FitzSimons, M. R. Bailey and J. Mann (eds) *The Global Impact of AIDS*, pp. 175–182 (New York, Alan R. Liss).

Fallers, L. A. (1964) *The King's Men: Leadership and Status in Buganda on the Eve of Independence* (East African Institute of Social Research, Oxford University Press).

Fallers, M. C. (1960) *The Eastern Lacustrine Bantu* (London, International African Institute).

Hunter, S. (1990) Orphans as a window on the AIDS epidemic in sub-Saharan Africa: initial results and implications of a study in Uganda, *Social Science and Medicine*, 31, pp. 681–690.

Janzen, J. M. (1978) *The Quest for Therapy in Lower Zaire* (Berkeley, University of California Press).

Kaijuka, E. M., Kaija, E. Z. A., Cross, A. R. and Loaiza, E. (1989) *Uganda Demographic and Health Survey, 1988/1989* (Entebbe, Uganda, Ministry of Health).

Kalibala, L. and Kaleeba, N. (1989) AIDS and community-based care in Uganda: the AIDS Support Organization, TASO, *AIDS Care*, 1, pp. 173–174.

Kilbride, P. L. and Kilbride, J. C. (1990) *Changing Family Life in East Africa: Women and Children at Risk* (University Park, Pennsylvania State University Press).

Levine, C. (1990) AIDS and changing concepts of family, *Milbank Quarterly*, 68, pp. 33–58.

Levine, R. A. (1970) Personality and change, in: J. Paden and E. Soja (eds) *The African Experience*, pp. 276–303 (Evanston, Northwestern University Press).

Lloyd, G. A. (1988) HIV-infection, AIDS, and family disruption, in: A. F. Fleming, M. Carballo, D. W. FitzSimons, M. R. Bailey and J. Mann (eds) *The Global Impact of AIDS*, pp. 183–190 (New York, Alan R. Liss, Inc.).

Macklin, E. M. (1989) *AIDS and Families: Report of the AIDS Task Force Groves Conference on Marriage and Family* (New York, Haworth).

Mandeville, E. (1975) The formality of marriage: a Kampala case study, *Journal of Anthropological Research*, 31, pp. 183–195.

Mandeville, E. (1979) Poverty, work and the financing of single women in Kampala, *Africa*, 49, pp. 42–52.

McGrath, J. W. (1991) Biological impact of social disruption resulting from epidemic disease, *American Journal of Physical Anthropology*, 84, pp. 407–419.

McGrath, J. W., Ankrah, E. M., Schumann, D. A., Lubega, M. and Nkumbi, S. (1991) The psychological impact of AIDS in urban families, presented at the VII International Conference on AIDS, June 1991.

Muller, O. and Abbas, N. (1990) The impact of AIDS mortality on children's education in Kampala (Uganda), *AIDS Care*, 2, pp. 77–80.

Nahemow, N. (1979) Residence, kinship, and social isolation among the aged Baganda, *Journal of Marriage and the Family*, 41, pp. 171–183.

Neel, J. V., Centerwall, W. R., Chagnon, N. A. and Casey, H. L. (1970) Notes on the effect of measles and measles vaccine in a virgin-soil population of South American Indians, *American Journal of Epidemiology*, 91, pp. 418–429.

Nelkin, D. and Gilman, S. (1988) Placing blame for devastating disease stress, *Social Research*, 55, pp. 361–378.

Obbo, C. (1980) *African Women: Their Struggle for Economic Independence* (London, Zed Press).

Okediji, P. A. (1975) A psychosocial analysis of the extended family. The African case, *African Urban Notes*, Series B, I, 3, pp. 93–99.

Parkin, D. J. (1966) Types of urban African marriage in Kampala, Africa, 36, pp. 269–285.

Perlman, M. L. (1970) The traditional systems of stratification among the Ganda and the Nyoro of Uganda, in: A. Tuden and L. Plotnikov (eds) *Social Stratification in Africa*, pp. 125-161 (New York, Macmillan).

Piot, P., Plummer, F. A., Mhalu, F. S., Lamboray, J.-L., Chin, J. and Mann, J. M. (1988) AIDS: an international perspective, *Science*, 239, pp. 573–579.

Preble, E. (1990) Impact of HIV/AIDS epidemic in sub-Saharan Africa: initial results and implications of a study in Uganda, *Social Science and Medicine*, 31, pp. 671–680.

Richards, A. I. (1966) *The Changing Structure of a Ganda Village* (Nairobi, East African Publishing House).

Serwadda, D., Mugerwa, R., Sewankambo, N. K., Lwebaga, A., Carswell, J. W., Kirya, G. B., Bayley, A. C., Downing, R. G., Tedder, R. S., Clayden, A. S., Weiss, R. A. and Dalgleish, A. G. (1985) Slim disease: a new disease in Uganda and its association with HTLV-III infection, *Lancet*, 19 October, pp. 849–852.

Southall, A. W. and Gutkind, P. C. W. (1957) *Townsmen in the Making: Kampala and Its Suburbs* (Kampala, Uganda, East African Institute of Social Research).

Southwold, M. (1965) The Ganda of Uganda, in: J. L. Gibbs (ed.) *Peoples of Africa*, pp. 41–78 (New York, Holt, Rinehart and Winston).

UNICEF (1990) *Children and AIDS: An Impending Calamity. The Growing Impact of HIV Infection on Women and Family Life in the Developing World* (New York, United Nations).

World Health Organization (1991) Acquired Immunodeficiency Syndrome (AIDS), *Weekly Epidemiological Record*, 66, p. 73.

SOCIAL
SUPPORT

FIVE

Social Support and HIV: A Review

Gill Green

INTRODUCTION

This paper reviews current research about social support and HIV. Following a brief discussion of theoretical problems inherent in studies about social support, general concepts emerging from the literature on social support and health, and social support and chronic illness are identified, and the extent to which these may be relevant to understanding HIV are considered. Current studies that specifically focus upon HIV and social support are then examined to identify which areas have been covered and which require more attention. Major findings from these and other HIV studies which address an aspect of social support are summarized and, finally, future developments are suggested. In order to make this review as comprehensive as possible, both published works and unpublished conference proceedings are included. The latter are indicated with an asterisk (*) where cited in the text.

THEORETICAL CONSIDERATIONS

Social support is an 'omnibus term' referring to a 'meta-construct' (Vaux et al., 1986) relating to different aspects of social relationships, including (a) the existence, quantity and type of interpersonal relationships (network structure of social interaction), (b) the functional context of these relationships (emotional, psychological, tangible or informational support) and (c) the perceived quality of this support (McAllister and Fisher, 1978; Barrera et al., 1981; Norbeck et al., 1981; Wellman, 1981; Barrera and Ainlay, 1983; Sandler and Barrera, 1984; Gottleib, 1985; House and Kahn, 1985; Weinert, 1987; Ormel et al., 1989; Stewart, 1989; Van Sonderen and Ormel, 1989). The number of definitions is endless; in this paper the term 'social support' is used in its broadest sense to cover all the above aspects.

The lack of consensus about how social support should be conceptualized is reflected in its measurement (Green, 1992). There are no standard, well-validated 'off-the-shelf' scales (Orth-Gomer and Unden, 1987; O'Reilly, 1988; Bowling, 1991). Typically each study devises its own measure depending on the focus of the research. Consequently, there are almost as many methodologies and instruments for collecting data about social support as there are theoretical or empirical discussions of the concept (Veiel, 1990). McGough (1990) has examined available measures in order systematically to assess social support needs of people with HIV.

A further theoretical problem is the socio-economic and cultural variation in the role of social support; support structures vary according to gender (Gove, 1975; Broadhead *et al.*, 1983), social class (Young and Willmott, 1957; Oakley and Rajan, 1991), household type (Bott, 1972; Wallman, 1984) and race (Hayes and Mindel, 1973; Wallman, 1984; Ostrow *et al.*, 1991). This has implications for studies of social support among people with HIV, since the population is so heterogeneous. Socio-cultural differences among people with HIV may be sufficiently large to make many of the measures used to collect data from one group inappropriate for other groups, e.g. childcare tends to be an issue affecting women rather than men, and it is unlikely that drug users in deprived areas of Edinburgh or single parents living in a shanty town in Kampala regularly go to dinner parties or have a need for someone to water their houseplants when they are out of town (two questions asked to measure social support among gay men in the United States: Martin and Dean, 1988). Social differences in the population may also be reflected in the association between social support and health (Schwarzer and Leppin, 1988). A recent study, for example (which is included in Table 5.1), reports racial differences in the relationship between social support and adaptation among black and white gay men with HIV (Ostrow *et al.*, 1991). A further problem is that a significant proportion of the HIV-positive population is institutionalized (e.g. in hospitals, hospices, rehabilitation centres or prisons) and, therefore, has quite different support requirements and opportunities compared to those living in the community. Finally, the social support requirements of people with HIV vary according to the stage of the illness: those who are asymptomatic may value someone to go out with more highly than the physical care required by someone with an opportunistic infection.

The lack of consensus about social support, the theoretical poverty of social support studies and the near impossibility of applying similar criteria to different populations may suggest that this concept is of little heuristic value in the study of health in general or HIV in particular. However, empirical data from studies of social support and health, as well as common-sense 'lay' explanations of well-being, indicate otherwise. Although few studies have demonstrated a causal relationship between social support and health, there is now ample evidence that various aspects of social support and health are positively associated: good social support either promotes healthiness or offers some protection from illness (Broadhead *et al.*, 1983). Put more crudely, social support seems linked to health although no one is quite sure how. This notion is supported by 'lay' explanations

Study	Sample	HIV status	Social support measure	Principal finding(s)*
Donlou et al. (1985) (pilot)	21 homosexual/bisexual men: 17 with AIDS; 4 with ARC attending an outpatient clinic at UCLA medical centre in Los Angeles	Diagnosis of AIDS or ARC	Resources and Social Support Questionnaire	Marked mood disturbance is not significantly correlated with total social support. Subjects report diminished social interactions since the onset of their illness and profound illness-related psychological stress
Zich and Temoshok (1987)	103 gay or bisexual men: 50 with AIDS; 53 with ARC attending an outpatient clinic at a general hospital and a private medical clinic in San Francisco	Diagnosis of AIDS or ARC received 2–8 weeks previously	Self-report rating of how desirable, available, often and useful are items covering emotional support, problem solving, indirect personal influence and environmental action	For persons with AIDS only increased physical distress is associated with perceiving less availability of support. For persons with AIDS and persons with ARC, the more available social support is perceived to be, the less hopelessness and depression
Wolcott et al. (1986)	50 homosexual/bisexual men attending an outpatient clinic at UCLA medical centre in Los Angeles	Diagnosis of AIDS received up to 3 months previously	Self-report rating importance and satisfaction with general support, and multiple factors of social network and resources	Social support satisfaction is significantly correlated with previously reported levels of psychologic distress and subjective (but not objective) measures of health status
Namir et al. (1987)	50 homosexual/bisexual men attending an outpatient clinic at UCLA medical centre in Los Angeles	Diagnosis of AIDS received up to 3 months previously	Self-report rating importance and satisfaction with general support, and multiple factors of social network and resources	Satisfaction with total support is strongly associated with an active-positive coping strategy
Namir et al. (1989a)	50 homosexual/bisexual men attending an outpatient clinic at UCLA medical centre in Los Angeles	Diagnosis of AIDS received up to 3 months previously	Self-report rating importance and satisfaction with general support, and multiple factors of social network and resources	Satisfaction with support and instrumental and emotional support is associated with good psychological and physical adaptation. Worse physical condition is related to less instrumental support but not to size of network or satisfaction with support
Namir et al. (1989b)	–	–	Review article	
Hart et al. (1990)	502 homosexual/bisexual men recruited from a range of community sources in London, Manchester, Oxford and Northampton	Not stated	Availability of friends and others in whom they could confide and seek practical help	The sample demonstrated high levels of willingness to disclose sexuality to others, sociability and social integration and access to practical help at times of temporary incapacity
Ostrow et al. (1991)	40 homosexual/bisexual men attending an HIV outpatient clinic in Detroit: 20 black men; 20 white men	HIV positive	Self-report rating of perceived material and emotional support, self-affirmation, and objective and subjective social integration and conflict	There is a positive association between social support and mental health for white gay men and a negative association for black gay men which is related to fundamental differences in the structure and composition of their social networks.

*All findings reported here are statistically significant $0.05 < P < 0.0001$ except where stated otherwise.

whereby one comes through bad times 'with a little help from your friends' while isolation leaves you 'lonely and blue'. Social support, for all its conceptual problems, is potentially too important to ignore in studies about health in general or HIV in particular. The relevance of findings from studies about social support and health for understanding HIV is, therefore, discussed below.

SOCIAL SUPPORT, HEALTH AND HIV

There are a few studies which show a direct association between social support and physical health (see Madge and Marmot, 1987, for a succinct summary): good social integration has been linked to reduced mortality (Berkman and Syme, 1979) and longevity (Olsen *et al.*, 1991). A positive link between good social support and lower mortality has possible implications for the rate of disease progression among people with HIV. Do those with good support survive longer?

Little is yet understood about the processes by which social support may affect physical health and whether or not an association reflects a direct causal relationship, although the concept of a neuroendocrine response to stress, which was introduced in the 1940s (Selye, 1946), has seen some interesting developments in the past decade in the field of psychoneuroimmunology (Solomon, 1987; Solomon *et al.*, 1987). Studies with both humans and animals provide evidence that behaviour and psychosocial factors can have profound influences on the functioning of the immune system, e.g. stress is a risk factor in the development of the herpes virus (Kiecolt-Glaser and Glaser, 1988), and psychological stress has been associated with increased susceptibility to the common cold (Cohen *et al.*, 1991). It has been suggested that absence of social support renders a person vulnerable to the effects of adverse life events and thus indirectly to decrements in immune function (Kaplan, 1991). Solomon (1987) hypothesizes that stress and psychosocial factors can influence the replication of HIV and the progression of AIDS, and Antoni *et al.* (1991) suggest that specific HIV stressors such as receiving a positive diagnosis may trigger an array of psychological and neuroendocrine events that impair cellular immune functioning. A programme of psychosocial stress management (including social support sensitization strategies) and aerobic exercise seems to have had modest success in retarding immune deterioration and disease progression in HIV-positive individuals (Antoni *et al.*, 1990, 1991), although aerobic exercise was also observed to have a beneficial immunological effect on subjects who tested HIV negative (LaPerriere *et al.*, 1990).

In general, social support is more readily shown to be associated with psychological well-being (Turner, 1981, 1983; Procidano and Heller, 1983; Sarason *et al.*, 1983; Sandler and Barrera, 1984; Cohen and Wills, 1985). The direction of causality of the association between social resources and psychological well-being and physical health status is poorly understood, and is a significant methodological problem to overcome, even in longitudinal studies (Madge and Marmot, 1987). Does good social support promote psychological well-being, which in turn promotes good health, or does good health ease psychological adaptation, which in turn attracts a wider support network? It is also unclear at which stage of disease (onset, progression or recovery) support is likely to be most influential (Cohen, 1988). These debates are relevant to the role of social support and the ability to cope among people with HIV.

There is an extensive literature on the role of social support at different stages of dying and variations in levels of social support according to the chronicity of illness, pain, type and location of symptoms, and the type of illness (e.g. Glaser and Strauss, 1968; Anderson and Bury, 1988; Corbin and Strauss, 1988). Studies examining the role of social support in the management of long-term chronic and/ or terminal illness have generally found a positive association between support and psychological resources which help the sufferer to cope with illness and promote recovery (Wortman and Dunkel-Schetter, 1979; DiMatteo and Hays, 1981; Wortman, 1984; Madge and Marmot, 1987).

There is evidence that diagnosis of a chronic illness may erode existing support (Peters-Golden, 1982; Bloom and Spiegel, 1984), and that those with poorer prognoses may receive less support (Wortman, 1984). The tendency for one's support network to attentuate when one is diagnosed with a chronic or terminal illness seems particularly pertinent to those diagnosed HIV-positive, owing to what has been called the 'double stigma' (Kowalewski, 1988) associated with HIV. HIV is socially defined as infecting already marginalized groups; hence the stigma attached to HIV is layered upon pre-existing stigma (based upon homophobia and negative feelings towards drug users; Herek and Glunt, 1988). There are numerous reports of discrimination and negative societal reactions against people with an HIV diagnosis, e.g. refusal of medical and dental treatment, loss of employment, travel restrictions, denial of insurance, social isolation, eviction from housing, rejection by family and avoidance by associates. In a study of gay HIV-positive men in London, 29% had received at least one negative reaction (King, 1989). Two studies of stigmatized groups 'at risk' for HIV, gay men (Kowalewski, 1988) and severe haemophiliacs (Schneider et al., 1991*), have observed that people belonging to these groups maintain social distance from gay men and haemophiliacs who are HIV-positive. The social unacceptability of an HIV diagnosis is reported to be one of the major concerns of people with HIV (Miller, 1988; Longo et al., 1990), and may lead to self-imposed familial estrangement, decreased socialization or withdrawal (Longo et al., 1990). An HIV diagnosis is commonly associated with depression, suicidal ideas, guilt and fears of social isolation (McKeganey, 1990; Platt, 1992), and symptomatic HIV disease is associated with an increase in psychiatric morbidity (Catalan, 1990). At the very least, coming to terms with an HIV diagnosis involves changes in outlook and relationships (Miller, 1987), and may involve the construction of a new identity (Sandstrom, 1990). It is, therefore, not surprising that social support was identified by a group of HIV-positive individuals as being crucial for coping (Mandel, 1986).

Other factors also make people with HIV particularly vulnerable, thus increasing their need for social support. First, the uncertainty associated with any chronic illness is particularly marked with HIV owing to its recent discovery, the high mortality rate, its effect upon multiple organs and systems of the body and the subsequent variety in the clinical course of infection, the debilitating effects of the latter stages of the illness, the unknown side-effects of treatment drugs and the episodic medical crises associated with the disease (Weitz, 1989). Second, it is a sexually transmitted disease which has profound implications for current and future sexual relationships and sexual and reproductive behaviour. Many people with HIV have sexual problems (Donlou et al., 1985; Catalan, 1990; Catalan et al., 1990*), become celibate and/or feel denied or restricted in their access to long-term sexual partnerships. Third, 'felt stigma' may lead to feelings of shame, low self-esteem and guilt about past behaviour (Siegel and Krauss, 1991), causing people with HIV to succumb to society's moral pressures to dictate their future behaviour. In Sweden, for example, those diagnosed HIV positive are required to sign a contract saying that they will inform all sexual partners of their HIV status (Mansson, 1990). Fourth, the population affected may already be relatively socially isolated. Severe haemophiliacs often suffer acute and chronic pain, which may influence their social life (Wilkie et al., 1990). Many gay men do not have strong links with a family network (Wolcott et al., 1986) and one-third of gay men interviewed in England and Wales were living alone (Hart et al., 1990). The lifestyle of many drug-users is often described as 'chaotic' and this may restrict their opportunities for establishing a strong support network.

In recognition of the various support requirements of many people with HIV infection, the need for counselling has been identified and incorporated into many of the services offered to people with HIV (Gold et al., 1986; Green, 1989; Sonnex et al., 1989). Many people with HIV are offered psychological intervention to help to come to terms with their diagnosis, improve the quality of their life and assist at times of crisis (Namir, 1986) or to give information (Lauer-Listhaus and Watterson, 1988). The need for support groups was identified early-on in the epidemic (Christ and Wiener, 1985; Mail and Matheny, 1989): 'buddies' were introduced to lend emotional support; many statutory and voluntary groups have been formed to provide emotional and practical assistance; and a number of self-help groups have been organized (particularly among the gay community).

CURRENT STUDIES OF SOCIAL SUPPORT AND HIV

Whereas a number of supportive services such as counsellors, buddies and home helps have been set up to help people with HIV, there is as yet only a small literature on the role of social support in the management of HIV disease. Table 5.1 lists all the published articles in English and Table 5.2 lists abstracts from the sixth and seventh international conferences on AIDS which examine an aspect of social support or social network in relation to the well-being of people who are HIV positive, or to behaviours of groups designated 'at risk' for HIV. Both tables are organized chronologically although all material from any one study is grouped together. The published papers were identified through Medline using 'social support' and 'AIDS' or 'HIV' as key words, and the abstracts were identified by the classification 'social support' and 'psychosocial'. Neither table is an exhaustive list, in that only work in which social support and/or network is a central focus has been included. Findings from other studies which consider social support among many other variables are, however, discussed in the following section ('Major findings'). Since this review focuses on the role of social support for people infected with HIV rather than social network analysis of HIV transmission, mathematical or socio-geographic studies linking social network to the spread of HIV (such as Wallace, 1991) are not included.

As the number of studies are relatively few in number, those included in Tables 5.1 and 5.2 are discussed concurrently. Clearly, the papers in peer-reviewed journals listed in Table 5.1, have been subjected to greater scrutiny by referees than the conference abstracts in Table 5.2, many of which include material of a very provisional nature. The studies in Table 5.1 should, therefore, be given more weight. In order to aid the reader in this respect, conference abstracts are identified in the text by an asterisk.

Table 5.1 gives some indication of how and which components of social support were measured in each study. These details are not included in Table 5.2 due to the brevity of conference abstracts. Each of the four studies which have generated published papers has conceptualized and measured social support quite differently, a fact which clearly illustrates the lack of consensus noted above. All have a sample of exclusively homosexual/bisexual men who are, in the main, white and middle class (with the exception of Ostrow *et al.*, 1991). This bias is less apparent in the studies listed in Table 5.2, which include two studies with samples of drug users (Frey *et al.*, 1990*, Nabila *et al.*, 1991*), one of haemophiliacs (Schneider *et al.*, 1991*), one of women (Nabila *et al.*, 1991*) and two studies with a mixed sample in terms of gender and transmission category (Eich *et al.*, 1990*, 1991*, Stoll *et al.*, 1991*). The majority of studies, and all but one of those which have already resulted in published articles, are based in North America, and only one is based in the Third World. There is, thus, a strong bias in the current literature (particularly in the published work) towards white, gay, North American males. Results from such studies may not be applicable to people with HIV who are drug users, black, working class, from the Third World or women, as social support requirements for drug users, who tend to have multiple social deprivations, or for women, who have quite distinct social roles to men, are likely to differ from those of gay men. Drug users or people living in the Third World, for example, may value material help more highly than the emotional support deemed so crucial to gay men with HIV.

In Table 5.1, all the studies (except Hart *et al.*, 1990) have an exclusively HIV-positive sample, as do all but three of those in Table 5.2 which focus upon 'at risk' groups. Of those in Table 5.1 with an exclusively HIV-positive sample, all control for disease progression and there is a strong bias towards those at a symptomatic stage of the illness; all except Ostrow *et al.* (1991) have samples of people with an AIDS or ARC diagnosis. Of those in Table 5.2 only two studies (Eich *et al.*, 1990*, 1991*; Persson *et al.*, 1991*) have asymptomatic samples and these both include subjects classified at CDC-stage II and III (at stage III subjects are showing

Table 5.2 Unpublished studies about social support and HIV (abstracts from Sixth and Seventh International Conferences on AIDS)

Study	Sample	HIV status	Principal finding(s)
Eich et al. (1990)*	70 HIV patients attending an outpatient clinic in Zurich: 50% homo/bisexual men, 25% heterosexual men, 25% women (majority of heterosexual drug users)	HIV positive: CDC stage II and III	The problems of the sample differ according to their specific socio-cultural context, e.g. drug users with HIV are threatened with social isolation whereas gay men have better social support systems
Eich et al. (1991)*	As above but sample increased to 114	HIV positive: CDC stage II and III	The sample may be clustered according to types of social relationships and socio-demographic data. Being 'old' as well as having a supportive social network correlates positively with a good sense of psychological well-being
Frey et al. (1990)* (pilot)	148 drug users in treatment, 96 drug users not in treatment in Philadelphia	Not stated	In-treatment drug users exhibit fewer high risk drug and sexual behaviours and have larger networks who they have more contact with, are more satisfied with and more influenced by than are drug users not in treatment.
Grace et al. (1990)*	225 male military patients in Washington, DC	HIV positive	Psychosocial support is related to depression primarily in the domain of self-esteem.
Turner et al. (1990)*	518 gay men drawn from census tracts with the highest incidence of AIDS in San Francisco	Some with HIV symptoms	The number of HIV symptoms and depression are both independently related to reductions in support satisfaction over a two-year period.
Daniel et al. (1991)*	16 male patients in Tel Aviv with one principal sexual partner	Symptomatic HIV positive	HIV positive men receive more support from heterosexual than homosexual HIV-negative partners.
McGrath et al. (1991)*	22 urban families in Kampala, Uganda	Families of subjects diagnosed with AIDS	Perception of stigma results in the withdrawal of HIV-positive individuals from activities outside the household.
Nabila et al. (1991)*	109 women in New York City on a methadone maintenance programme	Not stated	Good social support is associated with feeling comfortable discussing safer sex with sexual partners.
Persson et al. (1991)*	47 homosexual men attending a clinic at Malmo, Sweden	HIV positive CDC stage II or II	There is an association between weak social support and low levels of of CD4 lymphocytes.
Reisbeck et al. (1991)*	46 homosexual men in south Germany (not stated where recruited)	HIV positive	The gay community is a major social support and coping mechanism for people with HIV.
Schneider et al. (1991)*	52 haemophiliacs with severe haemophilia A in Munich (not stated where recruited)	30 HIV positive 22 HIV-negative interviewed shortly after test notification	HIV-positive haemophiliacs turn more to families and treatment centre for support whereas HIV-negative haemophiliacs tend to use non-medical social networks and avoid confronting HIV-positive individuals.
Stoll et al. (1991)*	54 HIV-positive subjects in Elangen Nurenberg of whom about 1/3 homosexual men, 1/3 heterosexual man and 1/3 women (majority of heterosexuals ex-drug users)	HIV positive, but not in terminal stage	Sufficient emotional support and a sense of belonging significantly decreases psychic distress and is very important for coping.

marked signs of progression). This no doubt reflects the difficulty in gaining access to people who are HIV-positive owing to issues of confidentiality, and the greater ease of recruiting those at later stages of the illness as they are more likely to be attending hospital clinics to receive treatment. Of all the studies of HIV-positive individuals in Tables 5.1 and 5.2 which state where the sample was recruited, all come from treatment settings (mostly hospital out-patient clinics). This may have implications for the relevance of the findings to the HIV-positive population as a whole. Frey *et al.* (1990*), for example, found that the social networks of drug users in treatment were larger, more often seen, more satisfactory and more influential than those not in treatment, and Alcabes *et al.* (1992) reported that drug users not in treatment were more likely to be male, younger and black than those currently in treatment. The over-representation of those at a symptomatic stage may provide an overly gloomy picture, given the tendency (noted among people with cancer) for support networks to attenuate as one becomes iller. Alternatively, it may provide an over-optimistic picture as many more voluntary and statutory services have been provided for those at later stages of the illness. Whatever the case, the support needs of people at different stages of the illness are likely to vary.

None of the studies in Table 5.1 and only one study in Table 5.2 (Schneider *et al.*, 1991*) has a control cohort of HIV-negative subjects. Given that HIV has to date infected predominantly already stigmatized groups, this is a potentially serious omission. The social support networks of the samples being monitored may reflect the social relationships of gay men or drug users, rather than of people with HIV. In order to understand more fully the effect of HIV upon social networks, matching HIV-positive samples with HIV-negative control groups from similar transmission categories is required.

Few studies in Tables 5.1 or 5.2 consider negative aspects of support (with the exception of Ostrow *et al.*, 1991), although this aspect may influence subjects' satisfaction with the support they receive. Patients may, for example, receive much support for medical staff during hospital visits but may acutely dislike the constant reminder of seropositivity or illnesses that such interactions inevitably entail.

The majority of studies in Table 5.1 are longitudinal (only Donlou *et al.*, 1985, and Hart *et al.*, 1990, are cross-sectional) and all rely heavily upon quantitative data; in the main the social support measures are self-completed by the respondent and those that are administered by an interviewer tend to have limited response categories. The longitudinal nature of the studies will enable change over time to be monitored, but the focus upon statistical associations may provide little information about the sociological processes which underlie or generate such associations. In contrast, many of the studies in Table 5.2 are cross-sectional and use a combined quantitative and qualitative approach. This provides useful information upon how HIV-positive individuals interact and use their social networks, but will not provide data about changes in social support in the course of HIV disease.

MAJOR FINDINGS

The majority of studies focus upon the association between social support and psychological well-being or coping. As yet, no published research definitively correlates the rate of progression of HIV disease with social support. With regard to longevity and social support, Reillo (1990*) reports that death within 12 months of an AIDS diagnosis was more likely to occur among those with no social support. Solomon *et al.* (1987) hypothesize from a pilot study that long-surviving individuals with AIDS (3–5 years) have more social support in the form of problem-solving assistance than those with short survival times after the diagnosis of AIDS, and Caumartin *et al.* (1991)* report that survival times is extended by involvement in the gay community. An association has also been found between a weak social support network and low levels of CD4-lymphocytes (Persson *et al.*, 1991*). Turner *et al.* (1990)*, found that the number of HIV symptoms was related to reductions in support satisfaction over a two-year period, while symptom development has been shown to be associated with less social support (Solano *et al.*, 1991*). It is unclear from these findings whether good social support promotes longevity or whether those who progress more quickly find support diminishing as a result of reduced social interaction or friends' fearful avoidance of them.

Some studies have found an association between self-reported physical health and some aspects of social support. Namir *et al.* (1989a) report a significant association between health measures and instrumental support (but not any other type of support); worse self-reported physical state was associated with the perception of less instrumental support. Zich and Temoshok (1987) found that the perceived availability of social support correlated strongly and negatively with reported number of physical symptoms for persons with AIDS (but not among persons with ARC). This could reflect those who are sicker either witnessing the attenuation of their network, or having a greater need for support as they become more disabled. There is, however, a strong suggestion that correlations between perceived social support and self-reported physical health may well be related to psychological state (Zich and Temoshok, 1987). Those who are depressed may well perceive both their health and social support negatively. The MACS study on a cohort of gay men unaware of their HIV status, for example, found that self-reported HIV-related symptoms (but not HIV status) were associated with more psychological symptoms (Ostrow *et al.*, 1989). Wolcott *et al.* (1986) report that those with *subjectively* higher levels of illness concerns had lower levels of satisfaction with their support, and Namir *et al.* (1989a) report that those who were satisfied with their support perceived their global health more positively. As yet, however, no significant correlation has been found between measures of psychological or social support and *objective* measures of health status.

There is evidence that psychological state (ability to cope, depression or mood disturbance) is correlated with satisfaction with, or perceived availability of, social support (Donlou *et al.*, 1985; Wolcott *et al.*, 1986; Zich and Temoshok, 1987; Ostrow *et al.*, 1989; Fleischman *et al.*, 1990*; Grace *et al.*, 1990*; Turner *et al.*,

1990*; Murphy *et al.*, 1991*; Stoll *et al.*, 1991*), and that those satisfied with their support have a greater ability to cope (Namir *et al.*, 1987). Wolcott *et al.* (1986) found satisfaction with support to be more highly correlated with psychological and subjective health status variables than with the number of people available to help. In general, those with a greater number of psychological symptoms are less satisfied with their support and perceive less support to be available. The direction of this association is unclear. Do those who are depressed either receive less or perceive their support to be less or are those with less support more vulnerable to depression? While the association between psychological well-being and social support is generally positive, this is not the case with all types of support or for all social groups. There are some indications of a negative association between mood disturbance and instrumental support (Namir *et al.*, 1989a), social support and mental well-being among black gay men (Ostrow *et al.*, 1991), and self-esteem and support for professional carers (Donlou *et al.*, 1985).

Of all the types of support measured, emotionally sustaining types of help tend to be rated by people with HIV disease as the most desirable, even though they are not significantly correlated to physical or psychological well-being (Namir *et al.*, 1989a; Wolcott *et al.*, 1986; Zich and Temoshok, 1987). This could reflect the high socio-economic status of the samples in these studies and may not be applicable to all those with HIV disease. It has also been suggested that perceived adequacy of support may be more important than the actual availability of support. Lennon *et al.* (1990) report that this was the key aspect of support in relation to levels of grief among bereaved gay men.

Support networks and the role of social support among those with or 'at risk' for HIV disease vary according to socio-economic and cultural circumstance, and stage of illness. A study comparing support across different socio-economic and transmission groups found gay men to have better support than the others in the sample who are predominantly drug users (Eich *et al.*, 1990*), and that a combination of greater age and a supportive social network was correlated with a good sense of psychological well-being, whereas a combination of youth and no support correlated with depression (Eich *et al.*, 1991*). Gay men in North America in general report quite good support and adequately sized networks although there is a tendency for them to have a degree of distance from their family, and fewer family members in their network (Donlou *et al.*, 1985; Wolcott *et al.*, 1986; Namir *et al.*, 1989a). In the UK, a sample of predominantly 'out' gay men report high levels of sociability and social integration (Hart *et al.*, 1990). Reliance on and support from partners and family seems to vary according to 'transmission category'. Individuals with AIDS in Kampala withdraw from activities outside the household, and increasingly rely on support from other family members (McGrath *et al.*, 1991), HIV-positive haemophiliacs in Munich turn more to their families for support than HIV-negative controls (Schneider *et al.*, 1991*), whereas gay men in southern Germany tend to receive most support from the gay community (Reisbeck *et al.*, 1991*). Daniel *et al.* (1991)* report that heterosexual HIV-positive men receive more support from their partners than HIV-positive gay men.

Ostrow *et al.* (1991) show that the relationship between social support and mental health among black and white gay men with HIV is quite different. White respondents are more likely to have a network identified with the white gay community whereas black respondents tend to be more reliant on family who are more likely (than the gay community) to hold stigmatizing attitudes towards homosexual behaviour and HIV infection, and therefore to be less able to provide adequate social support in mental health or behavioural domains. The differential relationship between mental health and social support may, therefore, be explained by fundamental differences in the structure and composition of social support networks. Differences in social networks according to social characteristics or sexual orientation may thus have important consequences for the relationship between social support and health.

A few studies have examined the relationship between social support and risk behaviour among 'at risk' groups, and generally have not found an association. Emmons *et al.* (1986) did not find a significant relationship between a measure of gay network affiliation and any behavioural outcome. Nor was any association found between social support and safer sexual and drug-using practices among 29 black drug users (Frey *et al.*, 1990*), the black gay men in Ostrow's (1991) study, or among gay men in Denmark (Brendstrup and Schmidt, 1990), Chicago (Joseph *et al.*, 1987) or New York (Siegel *et al.*, 1989). Indeed, this latter study reports that perception of good emotional support is positively and significantly associated with persistent participation in risky sex among gay men in New York. Among the white men in Ostrow's sample, however, there was a positive association between good social support and low risk-taking, and Nabila *et al.* (1991)* found that female drug users were more likely to feel comfortable discussing safer sex with sexual partners if they had good social support.

LOOKING FORWARD

There is evidence of a link between social support and the psychological well-being of people with HIV, but much information is still required about which particular aspects of social support and health are associated, and how this changes over time according to the stage of HIV disease. As a whole, many of the current studies from the United States are attempting to 'unpack' the diverse elements of social support in some detail, and many of these studies are longitudinal, thus enabling changes over time to be monitored. They tend, however, to place heavy reliance upon quantitative data; there is a need for more qualitative studies to put flesh upon skeletal statistical associations.

Current studies with large numbers of subjects tend to recruit from clinic settings, which often cater almost exclusively for a single transmission group, many of whom are at a symptomatic stage of the disease, and by definition all clients are 'in treatment'. The extent to which findings may be applicable to the HIV-infected population as a whole is questionable. The few existing studies with mixed samples (i.e. more than one transmission category) show important differences according to the social, cultural and sexual characteristics of the subjects, and the stage they have reached in their HIV career. This points towards a need for more information about such differences: more studies focused on those groups which have to date received less attention (women, drug users, those from the Third World, those not receiving treatment and 'asymptomatics'), and more studies which have a 'mixed' sample. A 'mixed' sample has the drawback of requiring much larger numbers in order to 'tease out' statistical associations, which is a very serious practical consideration given the limited size of the current HIV population and the difficulties in gaining access to interview them. Thus, it is likely that research of a truly mixed sample representative of the HIV population as a whole would require an in-depth study of a relatively small sample.

With regard to social support by social position, there is a substantial gap between the general social support literature, in which social parameters such as gender, class and race are basic differentiators, and much of the HIV literature, which emphasizes differences by transmission category. What is required is more information about the extent to which differences by transmission category are in fact social differences 'in disguise'. For example, the majority of 'out' gay men are broadly speaking 'middle class' and most injecting drug users are 'working class'. The finding that gay men are more dependent on their friends and less on their families for social support than drug users may, therefore, reflect the particular social class composition of each group rather than differences in sexual orientation or drug use.

There is also a need for more case–control studies as people who are HIV-positive are not representative of the general population. In Western countries, the HIV-positive population tends to be relatively young and largely male, and includes a high proportion of gay men, drug users and haemophiliacs. The social support networks of gay men, drug users and haemophiliacs may be quite different from those of the general population whether or not they are HIV-positive. Thus, the full impact of HIV on sufferers' social networks can only be gauged by comparing them to control subjects (from similar age, sex and transmission categories) who are HIV negative.

As HIV research is in its infancy, many of the general concepts noted in the literature have not been explored. There is clearly still much that is unknown about the relationship between social support and HIV, although the studies reported to date, taken together with the literature about social support and chronic illness, suggest that this is a fruitful avenue for further investigation. In particular, more studies which take account of the full diversity of the HIV-positive population, and the many different requirements and opportunities of the sub-groups within it, would facilitate appropriate supportive interventions being made for all.

REFERENCES

Alcabes, P., Vlahov, D. and Anthony, J. C. (1992) Correlates of human immunodeficiency virus infection in intravenous drug users: are treatment-program samples misleading? *British Journal of Addiction*, 87, pp. 47–54.

Anderson, R. and Bury, M. (1988) *Living with Chronic Illness: The Experience of Patients and Their Families* (London, Unwin Hyman).

Antoni, M. H., Schneiderman, N., Fletcher, M. A., Goldstein, D. A., Ironson, G. and LaPerriere, A. (1990) Psychoneuroimmunology and HIV-I, *Journal of Consulting and Clinical Psychology*, 58, pp. 38–49.

Antoni, M. H., LaPerriere, A., Schneiderman, N. and Fletcher, M. A. (1991) Stress and immunity in individuals at risk for AIDS, *Stress Medicine*, 7, pp. 35–44.

Barrera, M. and Ainlay, S. L. (1983) The structure of social support: a conceptual and empirical analysis, *Journal of Community Psychology*, 11, pp. 133–143.

Barrera, M., Sandler, I. and Ramsay, T. B. (1981) Preliminary development of a scale of social support on college students, *American Journal of Community Psychology*, 9, pp. 435–447.

Berkman, L. F. and Syme, S. L. (1979) Social networks, host resistance and mortality: a nine-year follow up study of Alameda County residents, *American Journal of Epidemiology*, 109, pp. 186–204.

Bloom, J. R. and Spiegel, D. (1984) The relationship of two dimensions of social support to the psychological well-being and social functioning of women with advanced breast cancer, *Social Science and Medicine*, 19, pp. 831–837.

Bott, E. (1972) *Families and Social Networks*, 2nd edn (London, Tavistock).

Bowling, A. (1991) *Measuring Health: A Review of Quality of Life Measurement Scales* (Milton Keynes, Open University Press).

Brendstrup, E. and Schmidt, K. (1990) Homosexual and bisexual men's coping with the AIDS epidemic: qualitative interviews with 10 non-HIV tested homosexual and bisexual men, *Social Science and Medicine*, 60, pp. 713–720.

Broadhead, W. E., Kaplan, B. H., Jones, S. A., Wagner, E. H., Shoenbach, V. J., Grimson, R., Heyden, S., Tibblin, G. and Gehlbach, S. (1983) The epidemiologic evidence for a relationship between social support and health, *American Journal of Epidemiology*, 1 (7), pp. 521–537.

Catalan, J. (1990) Psychiatric manifestations of HIV disease, *Baillière's Clinical Gastroenterology*, 4, pp. 547–562.

Catalan, J., Klimes, I., Bond, A., Garrod, A., Day, A., Hodges, S. and Rizza, C. (1990) Psychosocial status of HIV infected men with haemophilia. Controlled investigation. Abstract SB370 from the VIth International Conference on AIDS in San Francisco.

Caumartin, S., Joseph, J. G. and Chmiel, J. (1991) Premorbid psychosocial factors associated with differential survival time in AIDS patients. Abstract MC3105 from the VIIth International Conference on AIDS in Florence.

Christ, G. H. and Wiener, L. S. (1985) Psychosocial issues in AIDS, in: T. DeVita, S. Hellman and S. A. Rosenberg (eds) *AIDS: Etiology, Diagnosis, Treatment and Prevention*, pp. 275–297 (Philadelphia, J. B. Lippincott).

Cohen, S. (1988) Psychosocial models of the role of social support in the etiology of physical disease, *Health Psychology*, 7, pp. 269–297.

Cohen, S., Tyrrell, A. J. and Smith, A. P. (1991) Psychological stress and susceptibility to the common cold, *New England Journal of Medicine*, 29 August, pp. 606–612.

Cohen, S. and Wills, T. A. (1985), Stress, social support and the buffering hypothesis, *Psychological Bulletin*, 98, pp. 310–357.

Corbin, J. M. and Strauss, A. (1988) *Unending Work and Care: Managing Chronic Illness at Home* (San Francisco, Jossey-Bass).

Daniel, T., Lupo, P., Vardinon, N., Yust, I. and Burke, M. (1991) Variations in support for HIV-seropositive patients by sexual partner. Abstract WD4201 from VIIth International Conference on AIDS in Florence.

DiMatteo, M. R. and Hays, R. (1981) Social support and serious illness, in: B. H. Gottlieb (ed.) *Social Networks and Social Support*, pp. 117–148 (Beverly Hills, Calif., Sage Publications).

Donlou, J. N., Wolcott, D. L., Gottlieb, M. S. and Landverk, J. (1985) Psychosocial aspects of AIDS and AIDS-related complex: as pilot study, *Journal of Psychosocial Oncology*, 3, pp. 39–55.

Eich, D., Dobler-Mikola, A. and Luthy, R. (1990) Is quality of life associated with a specific risk behaviour in HIV-positive individuals? Abstract SB376 from the VIth International Conference on AIDS in San Francisco.

Eich, D., Dobler-Mikola, A. and Luthy, R. (1991) Psychosocial well-being in asymptomatic HIV-positive individuals is associated with age and social networks. Abstract WB2395 from the VIIth International Conference on AIDS in Florence.

Emmons, E. A., Joseph, J. G., Kessler, R. C., Wortman, C. B., Montgomery, S. B. and Ostrow, D. G. (1986) Psychosocial predictions of reported behaviour change in homosexual men at risk for AIDS, *Health Education Quarterly*, 13, pp. 331–345.

Fleischman, J., Piette, J. and Mor, V. (1990) Correlates of depressive symptomatology among people with AIDS. Abstract SB391 from the VIth International Conference on AIDS in San Francisco.

Frey, F. W., Metzger, D., Woody, G. E. and Trusiani, P. (1990) Social network characteristics and AIDS risk factors among intravenous drug users in Philadelphia. Abstract from the VIth International Conference on AIDS in San Francisco.

Glaser, B. and Strauss, A. (1968) *Time for Dying* (Chicago, Aldine).

Gold, M., Seymour, N. and Sahl, J. (1986) Counselling HIV seropositives, in: L. McKusick (ed.) *What to Do about AIDS: Physicians and Mental Health Professionals Discuss the Issues*, pp. 103–110 (Berkeley, University of California Press).

Gottlieb, B. H. (1985) Social networks and social support: an overview of research, practice and policy implications, *Health Education Quarterly*, 12, pp. 5–22.

Gove, W. R. (1975) Sex, marital status and mortality, *American Journal of Sociology*, 79, pp. 45–67.

Grace, W. C., Rundell, J. R. and Oster, C. N. (1990) Types of social support and their relationships to depressive symptoms in HIV positive men. Abstract SB379 from the VIth International Conference on AIDS in San Francisco.

Green, G. (1992) A review of the literature on social support and health with special reference to HIV, *MRC Medical Sociology Unit Working Paper No. 34*.

Green, J. (1989) Counselling for HIV infection and AIDS: the past and the future, *AIDS Care*, 1, pp. 5–10.

Hart, G., Fitzpatrick, R., McLean, J., Dawson, J. and Boulton, M. (1990) Gay men, social support and HIV disease: a study of social integration in the gay community, *AIDS Care*, 2, pp. 163–170.

Hayes, W. and Mindel, C. (1973) Extended kinship relations in black and white families, *Journal of Marriage and Family*, 35, pp. 51–57.

Herek, G. M. and Glunt, E. K. (1988) An epidemic of stigma: public reaction to AIDS, *American Psychologist*, 43, pp. 886–891.

House, J. S. and Kahn, R. L., with assistance of McLeod, J. D. and Williams, D. (1985) Measures and concepts of social support, in: S. Cohen and S. Syme (eds) *Social Support and Health*, pp. 83–108 (Orlando, Fla., Academic Press).

Joseph, J. G., Montgomery, S. B., Emmons, C. A., Kirscht, J. P., Kessler, R. C., Ostrow, D. G., Wortman, C. B., O'Brien, K., Eller, M. and Eshleman, S. (1987) Perceived risk of AIDS: assessing the behavioural and psychosocial consequences in a cohort of gay men, *Journal of Applied Social Psychology*, 17, pp. 231–250.

Kaplan, H. B. (1991) Social psychology of the immune system: a conceptual framework and review of the literature, *Social Science and Medicine*, 33, pp. 909–923.

Kiecolt-Glaser, J. K. K. and Glaser, R. (1988) Psychological influences on immunity: implications for AIDS, *American Psychologist*, 43, pp. 892–898.

King, M. B. (1989) Prejudice and AIDS: the view and experiences of people with HIV infection, *AIDS Care*, 1, pp. 137–143.

Kowalewski, M. R. (1988) Double stigma and boundary maintenance: how gay men deal with AIDS, *Journal of Contemporary Ethnography*, 17, pp. 211–228.

LaPerriere, A., Schneiderman, N., Antoni, M. H. and Fletcher, M. A. (1990) Aerobic exercise training and psychoneuroimmunology in AIDS research, in: L. Temoshok and A. Baum (eds) *Psychosocial Perspectives on AIDS*, pp. 259–286 (Hillsdale, NJ, Lawrence Erlbaum).

Lauer-Listerhaus, B. and Watterson, J. (1988) A psychoeducational group for HIV-positive patients on a psychiatric service, *Hospital and Community Psychiatry*, 39, pp. 776–777.

Lennon, M. C., Martin, J. L. and Dean, L. (1990) The influence of social support on AIDS-related grief reaction among gay men, *Social Science and Medicine*, 31, pp. 477–484.

Longo, M. B., Spross, J. A. and Locke, A. M. (1990) Identifying major concerns of persons with acquired immunodeficiency syndrome: a replication, *Clinical Nurse Specialist*, pp. 21–26.

McAllister, L. and Fisher, C. S. (1978) A procedure for surveying personal networks, *Sociological Methods and Research*, 7, pp. 131–148.

McGough, K. N. (1990) Assessing social support for people with AIDS, *Oncological Nursing Forum*, 17, pp. 31–35.

McGrath, J. W., Ankrah, E. M., Schumann, D. A., Lubega, M. and Nkumbi, S. (1991) The psychosocial impact of AIDS in Ugandan families. Abstract MD4261 from the VIIth International Conference on AIDS in Florence.

McKeganey, N. (1990) Being positive: drug injectors' experiences of HIV infection, *British Journal of Addiction*, 88, pp. 1113–1124.

Madge, N. and Marmot, M. (1987) Psychosocial factors and health, *Quarterly Journal of Social Affairs*, 3, pp. 81–134.

Mail, P. D. and Matheny, S. C. (1989) Social service for people with AIDS: needs and approaches, *AIDS*, 3 (suppl. 1), pp. S273–S277.

Mandel, J. S. (1986) Psychosocial challenges of AIDS and ARC: clinical and research observations, in: L. McKusick (ed.) *What to Do about AIDS: Physicians and Mental Health Professionals Discuss the Issues*, pp. 75–86 (Berkeley, University of California Press).

Mansson, S. A. (1990) Psycho-social aspects of HIV testing – the Swedish case, *AIDS Care*, 2, pp. 5–16.

Martin, J. L. and Dean, L. L. (1988) The impact of AIDS on gay men: a research instrument, unpublished questionnaire, Columbia University, New York.

Miller, D. (1987) *Living with AIDS and HIV* (Basingstoke, Macmillan).

Miller, D. (1988) HIV and social psychiatry, *British Medical Bulletin*, 44, pp. 130–148.

Murphy, D. A., Kelly, J. A., Brasfield, T., Koob, J. and Bahr, R. (1991) Predictors of depression among persons with HIV infection. Abstract WD4276 from the VIIth International Conference on AIDS in Florence.

Nabila, E. B., Gilbert, L. and Schilling, R. F. (1991) Social support networks and sexual risk taking in female IV drug users. Abstract WD4026 from the VIIth International Conference on AIDS in Florence.

Namir, S. (1986) Treatment issues concerning persons with AIDS, in: L. McKusick (ed.) *What to Do about AIDS: Physicians and Mental Health Professionals Discuss the Issues*, pp. 87–94 (Berkeley, University of California Press.)

Namir, S., Wolcott, D. L., Fawzy, F. I. and Alumbaugh, M. J. (1987) Coping with AIDS: psychological and health implications, *Journal of Applied Social Psychology*, 17, pp. 309–328.

Namir, S., Alumbaugh, M. J., Fawzy, F. I. and Wolcott, D. L. (1989a) The relationship of social support to physical and psychological aspects of AIDS, *Psychology and Health*, 3, pp. 77–86.

Namir, S., Wolcott, D. L. and Fawzy, F. I. (1989b) Social support and HIV spectrum disease: clinical research perspectives, *Psychiatric Medicine*, 7, pp. 97–105.

Norbeck, J. S., Lindsey, A. M. and Carrieri, V. L. (1981) The development of an instrument to measure social support, *Nursing Research*, 30, pp. 264–269.

Oakley, A. and Rajan, L. (1991) Social class and social support: the same for different?, *Sociology*, 25, pp. 31–59.

Olsen, R. B., Olsen, J., Gunner-Svensson, F. and Waldstrom, B. (1991) Social networks and longevity: a 14 year follow-up study among elderly in Denmark, *Social Science and Medicine*, 33, pp. 1189–1195.

O'Reilly, P. (1988) Methodological issues in social support and social network research, *Social Science and Medicine*, 26, pp. 863–873.

Ormel, J., Van Tilberg, T. G. and Van Sonderen, F. L. P. (1989) Personal network delineation and social support: a comparison of four delineation methods. Paper presented at the European Conference on Social Network Analysis, June 1989, Groningen, The Netherlands.

Orth-Gomer, K. and Unden, A.-L. (1987) The measurement of social support in population surveys, *Social Science and Medicine*, 24, pp. 83–94.

Ostrow, D. G., Monjan, A., Joseph, J., Vanraden, M., Fox, R., Kingsley. L., Dudley, J. and Phair, J. (1989) HIV-related symptoms and psychological functioning in a cohort of homosexual men, *American Journal of Psychiatry*, 146, pp. 737–742.

Ostrow, D. G., Whitaker, R. E. D., Frasier, K., Cohen, C., Wan, J., Frank, C. and Fisher, E. (1991) Racial differences in social support and mental health in men with HIV infection: a pilot study, *AIDS Care*, 3, pp. 55–63.

Persson, L., Ostergren, B. S. and Moestrup, T. (1991) Social network social support and the amount of CD-4 lymphocytes in a representative urban population of asymptomatic HIV seropositive homo- and bisexual men. Abstract MC3176 from the VIIth International Conference on AIDS in Florence.

Peters-Golden, H. (1982) Breast cancer: varied perceptions of social support in the illness experience, *Social Science and Medicine*, 16, pp. 483–491.

Platt, S. (1992) Suicidal ideation and behaviour in human immuno-deficiency virus (HIV) disease, *Epidemiologia e Psichiatria Sociale*, 1, pp. 11–13.

Procidano, M. E. and Heller, K. (1983) Measures of perceived social support from friends and from family: three validation studies, *American Journal of Community Psychology*, 1, pp. 1–24.

Reillo, M. (1990) Psychosocial factors associated with prognosis in AIDS. Abstract SB372 at the VIth International Conference on AIDS in San Francisco.

Reisbeck, G., Hutner, G., Oliveri, G., Seidl, O. and Ermann, M. (1991) Social support networks of HIV-infected homosexuals. Abstract WD4212 from the VIIth International Conference on AIDS in Florence.

Sandler, I. N. and Barrera, M. (1984) Toward a multimethod approach to assessing the effects of social support, *American Journal of Community Psychology*, 12, pp. 32–52.

Sandstrom, K. L. (1990) Confronting deadly disease: the drama of identity construction among gay men with AIDS, *Journal of Contemporary Ethnography*, 19, pp. 271–294.

Sarason, I. G., Levine, H. M., Basham, R. B. and Sarason, B. R. (1983) Assessing social support: the social support questionnaire, *Journal of Personality and Social Psychology*, 44, pp. 127–139.

Schneider, M. M., Seidl, O., Ermann, M., Rommel, F. and Schramon, W. (1991) Use of social network among HIV-infected and non-infected haemophiliacs. Abstract WB2399 from the VIIth International Conference on AIDS in Florence.

Schwarzer, R. and Leppin, A. (1988) Social support and health: a meta-analysis, *Psychology and Health*, 2, pp. 1–15.

Selye, H. (1946) The general adaptation syndrome and the diseases of adaptation, *Journal of Clinical Endocrinology*, 6, pp. 117–230.

Siegel, K. and Krauss, B. J. (1991) Living with HIV infection: adaptive tasks of seropositive gay men, *Journal of Health and Social Behavior*, 32, pp. 17–32.

Siegel, K., Mesagno, F. P., Chen, J. Y. and Christ, G. (1989) Factors distinguishing homosexuals practising risky and safer sex, *Social Science and Medicine*, 28, pp. 561–569.

Solano, L., Costa, M., Salvati, S., Coda, R., Aiuti, F., Mezzaroma, I. and Bertini, M. (1991) Psychosocial factors and symptomatic development in HIV positives. Abstract MC3107 from the VIIth International Conference on AIDS in Florence.

Solomon, G. F. (1987) Psychoneuroimmunologic approaches to research on AIDS, *Annals of the New York Academy of Sciences*, 496, pp. 628–636.

Solomon, G. K., Temoshok, L., O'Leary, A. and Zich, J. (1987) An intensive psychoimmunologic study of long-surviving persons with AIDS, *Annals of the New York Academy of Sciences*, 496, pp. 647–655.

Sonnex, C., Petherick, A., Hart, G. J. and Adler, M. W. (1989) An appraisal of HIV antibody test counselling of injecting drug users, *AIDS Care*, 1, pp. 307–311.

Stewart, M. J. (1989) Social support instruments created by nurse investigators, *Nursing Research*, 38, pp. 268–275.

Stoll, P., Leiberich, P., Porsch, U., Engeter, M., Olbrich, E., Narrer, T. and Kalden, J. R. (1991) Social support as assistance for effective coping in HIV-positives. Abstract WB2385 from the VIIth International Conference on AIDS in Florence.

Turner, R. J. (1981) Social support as a contingency in psychological well-being, *Journal of Health and Social Behavior*, 22, pp. 357–367.

Turner, R. J. (1983) Direct, indirect and moderating effects of social support upon psychological distress and associated conditions, in: H. B. Kaplan (ed.) *Psychosocial Stress: Trends in Theory and Research*, pp. 105–155 (New York, Academic Press).

Turner, H. A., Hays, R. B. and Coates, T. J. (1990) Determinants of social support among gay men. Abstract SB380 from the VIth International Conference on AIDS in San Francisco.

Van Sonderen, E. and Ormel, J. (1989) The relationship between social network characteristics and social support. Paper presented at the European Conference on Social Network Analysis, June 1989, Groningen, The Netherlands.

Vaux, A., Phillips, J., Holly, L., Thomson, B., Williams, D. and Stewart, D. (1986) The social support appraisals scale (SS-A): studies of reliability and validity, *American Journal of Community Psychology*, 14, pp. 195–219.

Veiel, H. O. F. (1990) The Mannheim interview on social support: reliability and validity data from three samples, *Social Psychiatry and Psychiatric Epidemiology*, 25, pp. 250–259.

Wallace, R. (1991) Social disintegration and the spread of AIDS: thresholds for propagation along 'sociogeographic' networks, *Social Science and Medicine*, 33, pp. 1155–1162.

Wallman, S. (1984) *Eight London Households* (London, Tavistock Publications).

Weinert, C. (1987) A social support measure: PRQ85, *Nursing Research*, pp. 273–277.

Weitz, R. (1989) Uncertainty and the lives of persons with AIDS, *Journal of Health and Social Behavior*, 30, pp. 270–281.

Wellman, B. (1981) Applying network analysis to the study of support: in: B. H. Gottlieb (ed.) *Social Networks and Social Support*, pp. 171–200 (Beverly Hills, Calif., Sage Publications).

Wilkie, P. A., Markova, I., Naji, S. A. and Forbes, C. D. (1990) Daily living problems of people with haemophilia and HIV infection: implications for counselling, *International Journal of Rehabilitation Research*, 13, pp. 15–25.

Wolcott, D. L., Namir, S., Fawzy, F. I., Gottlieb, M. S. and Mitsuyasu, R. T. (1986) Illness concerns, attitudes towards homosexuality, and social support in gay men with AIDS, *General Hospital Psychiatry*, 8, pp. 395–403.

Wortman, C. B. (1984) Social support and the cancer patient: conceptual and methodological issues, *Cancer*, 53 (supplement), pp. 2339–2359.

Wortman, C. B. and Dunkel-Schetter (1979) Interpersonal relationships and cancer: a theoretical analysis, *Journal of Social Issues*, 35, pp. 120–155.

Young, M. and Willmott, P. (1957) *Family and Kinship in East London* (London, Routledge & Kegan Paul).

Zich, J. and Temoshok, L. (1987) Perceptions of social support in men with AIDS and ARC: relationships with distress and hardiness, *Journal of Applied Social Psychology*, 17, pp. 193–215.

SIX

Coping with the Threat of AIDS: The Role of Social Support

Jane Leserman, Diana O. Perkins and Dwight L. Evans

Infection with HIV raises a wide spectrum of concerns and fears among infected individuals. Even before symptoms occur, those infected with HIV have concerns about future economic security; sexuality and disease transmission; rejection from family, friends, and lovers; and eventual ill health and death. Previous research has focused on psychiatric alterations associated with HIV-positive status, most notably depression and anxiety (Atkinson *et al.*, 1988; Kessler *et al.*, 1988; Ostrow *et al.*, 1989; Dew *et al.*, 1990; Perry *et al.*, 1990). The present study focused on how asymptomatic HIV-positive homosexual men cope with the threat of AIDS. Among seropositive men, we (a) examined the relationship of coping to dysphoria and self-esteem in order to determine the positive or negative aspects of various coping strategies and (b) explored how social support and race are related to coping. We also studied the coping strategies (e.g. fighting spirit, helplessness, denial) used by HIV-positive men and compared these strategies with those of seronegative comparison subjects.

Much has been written about the role of coping in buffering the psychological impact of stress and possibly altering the progression of disease (e.g. cancer, AIDS). In cancer patients, Greer *et al.* (1979) found that fighting spirit and denial were associated with a better prognosis than was helplessness or stoicism. Regardless of whether coping has a direct role in HIV disease outcome, it may have an important role in preventing depression as the threat of AIDS becomes a reality for those who were previously asymptomatic. The following questions remain: (a) which coping strategies indicate the most healthy adaptive pattern?; and (b) what role does social support play in eliciting adaptive coping styles?

Coping generally refers to 'the cognitive and behavioural efforts to manage specific external and/or internal demands appraised as taxing or exceeding the resources of the individual' (Folkman and Lazarus, 1988). To our knowledge, however, there has been no agreement on or exhaustive list of cognitive and behavioural efforts or strategies that people use to deal with threats. Although it has been assumed that active strategies are good and that passive strategies are bad, only a few studies have delineated the mental health correlates of a variety of coping styles in people with HIV infection. Among homosexual men coping with HIV-related illness, two studies (Namir *et al.*, 1987; Wolf *et al.*, 1991) showed that active-behavioural coping was associated with enhanced mood and self-esteem and that avoidance coping (denial) was related to greater total mood disturbance and lower self-esteem. One study (Dew *et al.*, 1990) showed no significant association between active or avoidant coping and psychological distress. In cancer patients, passive and suppressive coping strategies were related to emotional distress, whereas active coping styles (e.g. confronting problems, sharing concerns) were associated with less dysphoria (Weisman, 1989). Our determination of adaptive or healthy coping strategies has been based on the relationship of the coping measures to depression, tension, anger and self-esteem.

Given that more active coping strategies indicate better adaptation, what is the evidence that social support may lead to more adaptive coping styles? Among HIV-infected homosexual men, social support was shown to correlate positively with active coping and negatively with avoidance (Namir *et al.*, 1987; Wolf *et al.*, 1991). Other studies of HIV-infected men have shown a clear relationship of social support to less mood disturbance (Donlou *et al.*, 1985; Zich and Temoshok, 1987; Namir *et al.*, 1989; Dew *et al.*, 1990; Rabkin *et al.*, 1990), less helplessness (Zich and Temoshok, 1987), and greater self-esteem (Donlou *et al.*, 1985). In addition, social support has been linked to less anxiety and depression in a variety of community samples (Turner, 1981; Flannery and Wieman, 1989).

In the present study we extended the work of others by looking at the relationship of seven specific coping styles to several measures of dysphoria, self-esteem and social support. We hypothesized that coping by maintaining a fighting spirit, planning, personal growth and seeking social support would be related to positive affect and self-esteem, whereas denial and helpless coping would be associated with negative affect and self-esteem. Furthermore, we hypothesized that social support, as measured by a variety of indicators (e.g. support satisfaction, participation in the AIDS community), would be associated with more fighting spirit, planning, personal growth, seeking social support and religious coping, and with less helplessness and denial. In addition to these hypotheses, we explored possible race differences in social support and coping. Furthermore, to describe the seropositive men, we compared their coping strategies to those of seronegative comparison subjects, since the threat of AIDS is inherently more immediate for those infected with HIV.

METHODS

Subjects

We studied 105 homosexual volunteers: 52 asymptomatic HIV-positive men and a comparison group of 53 HIV-negative men. This group is part of the Coping in Health and Illness Project, a large, multidisciplinary, longitudinal study. The study was approved by our institutional committee for the protection of human rights, and all subjects provided written informed consent. Subjects were recruited from North Carolina county health departments and through homosexual organizations, advertisements and word of mouth.

The men were between the ages of 18 and 50 years and were required to have at least a tenth-grade education or a general equivalency diploma and to have spoken English as their primary language before the age of 12. All HIV-positive subjects were asymptomatic, without AIDS or AIDS-related complex (e.g. night sweats, herpes zoster, oral candidiasis, hairy leukoplakia, shingles, unexplained fever or diarrhoea, and unexplained weight loss or fatigue in the presence of other symptoms) according to the Centers for Disease Control criteria. All subjects were further screened to exclude any individual with important medical illness, a recent operation or a history of intravenous drug use as a risk factor for HIV exposure. These screening criteria were included for the neuropsychological and psycho-immune aspects of the larger study.

Procedure

Over two nights and days at an inpatient research centre, the subjects underwent psychiatric, physical, neurological and neuropsychological examinations and several blood samples. On the first evening, before any testing, each subject completed a packet of self-report questions about coping.

Measures

Coping was assessed by means of the Coping in Health and Illness Project questionnaire with a modification of the COPE (Carver *et al.*, 1989). The subjects were asked to indicate on a four-point scale ('not at all' to 'very much') how they 'generally cope with, or handle the threat of getting AIDS'. The subjects indicated their coping responses to items included in five of the 14 scales of the COPE: (1) planning (e.g. 'I try to come up with a strategy about what to do'), (2) positive reinterpretation and personal growth (e.g. 'I try to see it in a different light, to make it seem more positive, (3) seeking emotional social support (e.g. 'I try to get emotional support from friends or relatives'), (4) denial (e.g. 'I pretend that it hasn't really happened'), and (5) turning to religion (e.g. 'I seek God's help'). In addition, we added items to create two additional scales, helpless coping and fighting spirit. Items for these two coping measures were modified versions of items from Greer and Watson's coping questionnaire for cancer patients (Greer and Watson, 1987). To create indexes of helpless coping and fighting spirit, we ran a principal factor analysis with quartimax rotation for each index; quartimax was used because we wanted to find the factor structure of a set of items. Initially, 11 fighting spirit items and nine helpless coping items were analysed (for both the 52 HIV-positive and the 53 HIV-negative homosexual men). Items loading (greater than 0.38) on the primary factor were retained, yielding nine fighting spirit items and eight helpless coping items. Cronbachs alphas for both the HIV-positive and HIV-negative men were checked to ensure reliability of the scales for both groups. The item scores were summed and divided by the number of items to create all coping indexes, which ranged from 1 to 4. Table 6.1 shows the intercorrelations among coping indexes and the substantial Cronbach's reliability coefficients on the diagonal of the matrix (ranging from 0.77 to 0.93).

Table 6.1 Intercorrelations of scores on coping scales for 52 HIV-positive homosexual men

Coping scale	Correlation (r)*						
	Helpless coping	Denial	Fighting spirit	Personal growth	Planning	Seeking social support	Turning to religion
Helpless coping	0.77	0.48†	−0.32‡	−0.25	−0.35†	−0.20	−0.02
Denial		0.82	−0.00	0.06	−0.13	−0.11	0.18
Fighting spirit			0.80	0.65†	0.60†	0.34‡	0.34‡
Personal growth				0.83	0.42†	0.56†	0.41†
Planning					0.88	0.41†	0.11
Seeking social support						0.82	0.15
Turning to religion							0.93

*Cronbach's alpha shown on diagonal. †$P<0.01$, two-tailed; d.f. = 50. ‡$P<0.05$, two-tailed; d.f. = 50.

Depression and dysphoric mood for the past week were assessed with the self-report Carroll Rating Scale for Depression (Carroll *et al.*, 1981), the Profile of Mood States (POMS) (McNair *et al.*, 1981) and the interview-based Hamilton Rating Scale for Depression (Hamilton, 1960). Consensus psychiatric diagnoses were made by reviewing a structured diagnostic interview (modified Structured Clinical Interview for DSM-III-R) (Spitzer *et al.*, 1989; Perkins *et al.*, 1990) at a diagnostic conference. The Rosenberg Self-Esteem Scale (Pearlin *et al.*, 1981), a ten-item evaluation of the subject's self-esteem, was also administered.

We assessed social support in several ways. The Sarason Brief Support Questionnaire (Sarason *et al.*, 1987) assessed the degree of satisfaction with people the subject counted on for social support or help (Cronbach's alpha = 0.86). Social conflict was measured with a seven-item inventory used in the Multicenter AIDS Cohort Study (unpublished 1989 paper by K. O'Brien *et al.*) in its coping and change survey. The social conflict scale (Cronbach's alpha = 0.87) addresses the degree of conflict the individual has experienced in the past month with the people in his personal life (e.g. 'Have you felt irritated or resentful towards people in your personal life?'). We also developed a six-item scale to measure participation in the AIDS community (e.g. belonging to AIDS support groups and organizations, socializing with HIV-positive people) (Cronbach's alpha = 0.75).

Statistical Methods

To describe the coping strategies of the study group, we first compared the seropositive and seronegative subjects on the seven coping variables by using multivariate analysis of variance (MANOVA). Significant results from MANOVA (Wilks's lambda, $F = 3.79$, d.f. = 7, 97, $P = 0.001$) allowed us to perform separate analyses of covariance on the coping measures, with serostatus as the independent variable and education and race as covariates (Table 6.2). Education and race were controlled, since these variables were correlated significantly with both serostatus and coping. The assumption of parallel regression of the covariates was met. The probability values in Tables 6.2 are two-tailed.

Table 6.2 Scores on coping scales for HIV-positive and HIV-negative homosexual men

| | Score* | | | | | |
| | HIV-positive men ($n = 52$) | | HIV-negative men ($n = 53$) | | ANOVA† | |
Coping scale	Mean	s.d.	Mean	s.d.	F	P
Helpless coping	1.56	0.46	1.35	0.45	5.17	0.03
Denial	1.57	0.61	1.27	0.61	5.96	0.02
Fighting spirit	3.40	0.55	3.15	0.55	5.20	0.02
Personal growth	3.09	0.73	2.96	0.73	0.78	0.38
Planning	3.07	0.80	2.86	0.80	1.64	0.20
Seeking social support	2.86	0.80	2.91	0.81	0.08	0.78
Turning to religion	2.64	1.02	2.37	1.01	1.76	0.19

*Adjusted mean scores are from analysis of covariance with race and education controlled. Range of possible scores is 1 to 4.
†Two-tailed P values; d.f. = 1, 101.

The remaining analyses were performed only for the HIV-positive subjects. Pearson product-moment correlation (with two-tailed significance tests) was used to show the interrelationships among the coping measures (Table 6.1). Principal factor analysis with varimax rotation was used to confirm the pattern of correlation among the coping indexes (with 0.38 as the cut-off for inclusion in a factor). Cronbach's alpha for each coping index indicates the reliability or internal consistency of each measure.

To examine the relationship between coping and measures of dysphoria, we performed multiple regression analyses with the dysphoria measures as the dependent variables and the coping variables run separately as independent variables, holding constant age, education, race and months since the subject learned he was HIV positive. These background variables were chosen because they were significantly related to some of the coping measures. They were controlled to rule out the possibility of spurious findings. Only race altered the relationships of some coping measures to dysphoria (regression coefficient change of 20% or more). Therefore, Table 6.3 shows the partial correlations of coping with depression, tension, anger and self-esteem, with race controlled. All tests are one-tailed.

Table 6.3 Partial correlations between scores on coping and dysphoria scales for 52 HIV-positive homosexual men*

Coping scale	Partial correlation with dysphoria scale (race controlled) (r)					
	Carroll depression scale	Hamilton depression scale	Profile of mood states			Rosenberg self-esteem scale
			Depression	Tension	Anger	
Helpless coping	0.47†	0.39†	0.37†	0.28‡	0.12	−0.40†
Denial	0.26‡	0.28‡	0.28‡	0.30‡	0.41†	−0.10
Fighting spirit	−0.33†	−0.28‡	−0.25‡	−0.24‡	−0.13	0.51†
Personal growth	−0.29‡	−0.26‡	0.00	−0.15	0.08	0.33†
Planning	−0.05	−0.02	−0.04	−0.06	−0.11	0.28‡
Seeking social support	−0.16	−0.11	0.07	−0.02	−0.14	0.18
Turning to religion	0.05	0.12	0.18	−0.09	0.00	−0.07

*Because of missing data, $n = 49$ for the Hamilton scale and $n = 58$ for the POMS indexes. In the statistical analyses, d.f. = 49 (Carroll and Rosenberg scales), d.f. = 46 (Hamilton scale) or d.f. = 48 (POMS).
†$P<0.01$, one-tailed test. ‡$P<0.05$, one-tailed test.

We were next interested in testing the relationship of coping to social support variables; support satisfaction, participation in AIDS groups and social conflict. Since only race (and not age, education or time since the subject learned he was seropositive) was related to social support and coping variables, we determined partial correlations between support and coping variables, holding race constant. Since a few of the zero-order relationships were diminished when we controlled for race, the results of the partial correlation analysis are shown in Table 6.4. All tests are one-tailed because of the testing of directional hypotheses. We will also report the zero-order correlation coefficients (two-tailed) for the correlations of race with the coping and social support variables, as well as partial correlations of race and coping when social support is held constant.

RESULTS

The HIV-positive subjects had a mean age of 30.0 years (s.d. 6.7) and an average education of 14.4 years (s.d. 2.5), and 76.9% ($n = 40$) were white. The HIV-negative subjects had a mean age of 30.9 years (s.d. 6.9) and an average education of 15.9 years (s.d. 2.4), and 90.6% ($n = 48$) were white. Since we were interested in race effects on psychosocial variables, we compared the background

Table 6.4 Partial correlations between scores on coping scales and social support measures for 51 HIV-positive homosexual men

| Coping scale | Partial correlation with support measure (race controlled) | | | |
| | Satisfaction with support* | | Participation in AIDS groups† | |
	r	P‡	r	P‡
Helpless coping	−0.34	0.008	−0.13	0.19
Denial	−0.02	0.45	−0.02	0.43
Fighting spirit	0.35	0.006	0.11	0.22
Personal growth	0.46	0.0004	0.32	0.01
Planning	0.06	0.35	0.08	0.30
Seeking social support	0.52	0.0001	0.33	0.01
Turning to religion	0.36	0.005	0.14	0.16

*Score on Sarason brief social support questionnaire.
†Rating on six-item measure.
‡One-tailed test; d.f. = 48.

characteristics of the black and white seropositive subjects. Although the differences were not significant, the blacks had less education (mean 13.3 years, s.d. 1.9) than the whites (mean 14.7, s.d. 2.6) ($t = 1.74$, d.f. = 50, $P = 0.09$) and the blacks were younger (mean age 27.8 years, s.d. 3.9) than the whites (mean 30.7, s.d. 7.2) ($t = 1.8$, d.f. = 34, $P = 0.08$). Only two (16.7%) of the blacks met the DSM–III–R criteria for lifetime drug dependence or drug abuse, compared to 19 (47.5%) of the whites ($\chi^2 = 3.65$, d.f. = 1, $P = 0.06$).

Table 6.2 shows the means (adjusted for race and education) and standard deviations for the ratings of coping measures for the seropositive and seronegative subjects. Most subjects endorsed fighting spirit, personal growth, planning and seeking social support and rejected helpless coping and denial. The seropositive subjects generally coped with the threat of AIDS with more fighting spirit, yet also more denial and helplessness, than did the seronegative comparison subjects.

Table 6.1 shows the pattern of intercorrelation among the coping measures in the HIV-positive subjects. Factor analyses of these scales confirmed the two-factor pattern of correlation shown in Table 6.1 (two factors with eigenvalues above 1). The first factor (explaining 69% of the variance in the matrix) included fighting spirit, personal growth, active planning, seeking emotional social support and, to a lesser extent, religious coping. These five indexes might represent more active or positive coping strategies. The second factor (explaining 31% of the variance in the matrix) included helpless coping and denial. Thus, subjects who felt helpless when confronting the threat of AIDS also tended to deny this threat ($r = 0.48$, d.f. = 50, $P = 0.0004$). Denial and helplessness may represent more passive or negative coping responses.

Our next question was whether particular coping strategies were related to positive or negative affect (dysphoria) or to self-esteem. Overall the seropositive subjects scored relatively low on our depression measures (Hamilton Rating Scale for Depression: mean 4.69, s.d. 4.79; Carroll Rating Scale for Depression: mean 9.13, s.d. 6.76). Only five (9.6%) met the DSM–III–R criteria for a current major depression, although fully 21 (40.4%) had had major depression during their lifetimes. Table 6.3 shows the partial correlations of coping with depression, tension, anger and self-esteem when race was controlled (race was the only covariate that altered the relationships of coping to dysphoria and self-esteem). The homosexual men who felt helpless about the threat of AIDS were significantly more depressed and tense and had lower self-esteem. Denial was also consistently associated with dysphoric states, particularly angry moods. The subjects with fighting spirit tended to be less depressed on all measures and had much higher self-esteem. Reacting to the AIDS threat by seeing it as an opportunity for personal growth was also significantly associated with less depression and with more self-esteem. Having plans to cope with the threat of AIDS was unrelated to all dysphoria measures, although it was related to better self-esteem. Finally, coping by seeking social support or by turning to religion was not significantly correlated with the dysphoria measures or with self-esteem.

Before analysing the relationship between social support and coping, we were interested in whether there were race differences on the coping and social support measures. Blacks were more likely than whites to endorse the coping strategies of helplessness ($r = 0.29$, d.f. $= 50$, $P = 0.04$), denial ($r = 0.33$, d.f. $= 50$, $P = 0.02$), and turning to religion ($r = 0.32$, d.f. $= 50$, $P = 0.02$) and were less likely to seek emotional support ($r = -0.42$, d.f. $= 50$, $P = 0.002$) to cope with AIDS. These race differences were not explained by age, education or time since the subject learned of his serostatus. The races did not differ on the other coping indexes. Blacks' greater dissatisfaction with existing social support networks ($r = -0.28$, d.f. $= 50$, $P = 0.05$) largely explained their greater feelings of helplessness (partial $r = 0.13$, d.f. $= 49$, $P = 0.36$) and somewhat explained their lower tendency to seek emotional support (partial $r = -0.29$, d.f. $= 49$, $P = 0.04$).

Table 6.4 shows the relationship between social support measures and coping strategies when race was held constant. Satisfaction with support contributed to significantly less helpless coping, more fighting spirit, more personal growth, greater likelihood of seeking social support to deal with AIDS, and more turning to religion to help. Furthermore, participation in the AIDS community was associated with significantly more personal growth and a significantly greater tendency to seek emotional support as a way of coping with AIDS. Conflict in social relationships was unrelated to coping except that the subjects with more conflict were significantly less likely to seek social support when threatened by AIDS (partial $r = -0.33$, d.f. $= 49$, $P = 0.02$).

Planning was unrelated to any social support variable except coping by using social support ($r = 0.41$, d.f. $= 50$, $P = 0.002$). Using denial was also not correlated with any social support variable. Denial, was, however, related to anger, depression, helpless coping, and being black. In a regression model predicting denial, we found that being black ($\beta = 0.26$, $t = 2.21$, d.f. $= 47$, $P = 0.03$), being angry ($\beta = 0.35$, $t = 3.02$, d.f. $= 47$, $P = 0.004$) and feeling helpless about dealing with AIDS ($\beta = 0.38$, $t = 3.20$, d.f. $= 47$, $P = 0.003$) explained 39% of the variance in denial.

DISCUSSION

A major finding of this study was that homosexual HIV-positive men can be characterized as coping with the threat of AIDS by adopting a fighting spirit, reframing stress to maximize personal growth, planning a course of action, and seeking social support. To a large extent, our study subjects scored low on denial and helplessness, and most did not have noteworthy depressive symptoms or current major depression. The low values on denial and helplessness may be due to the subjects' adaptive coping strategies, their asymptomatic status, the nature of subjects who volunteer for an HIV study and/or the undesirability of admitting to helplessness. The high scores for fighting spirit and the low helplessness scores are consistent with findings from other research studies (Rabkin *et al.*, 1990; Wolf *et al.*, 1991). Interestingly, the HIV-positive subjects scored higher on fighting spirit, helplessness and denial than did the HIV-negative men. Given that the threat of AIDS is more real and immediate to HIV-positive men, they may more actively mobilize all coping strategies.

We examined the relationship of coping strategies to each other and to measures of dysphoria and self-esteem to determine which coping strategies are associated with more healthy adaptation to HIV infection. Fighting spirit, personal growth, active planning, seeking emotional support and, to a lesser extent, religious coping appeared to represent similar active or positive coping responses. Denial and helplessness appeared to represent passive and pessimistic coping strategies. As one might expect, helplessness was related to dysphoria and lowered self-esteem, whereas fighting spirit and positive growth tended to be correlated with favourable affect and better self-esteem. These findings support the use of strategies that are emphasized in stress management programmes, such as fighting spirit and reframing stress through positive reinterpretation and personal growth. Those who cope with the threat of AIDS by more planning, seeking social support or turning to religion appear not to be better or worse off with regard to dysphoric mood.

The relative merit or harm of denial (pretending HIV infection has not happened) is less apparent in the available literature. Whereas Greer *et al.* (1979) found that denial had positive survival value in breast cancer patients, studies in the psychological literature have tended to be less clear about the mental health implications of denial. In our group of HIV-positive homosexual men, it appears that underlying the denial of HIV-positive status were depression, feelings of helplessness, and anger. These findings are consistent with other studies of HIV-infected men (Namir *et al*, 1987; Wolf *et al.*, 1991). Possibly, the HIV-positive individuals who feel overwhelmed by the threat of AIDS express this by more denial, depression, anger and helplessness.

Finally, we were interested in whether social support is related to particular coping strategies. To a large extent, we found that being satisfied with one's social support networks and participating in the AIDS community were related to more healthy coping strategies (e.g. more fighting spirit, more personal growth, less helplessness). These findings are consistent with previous research (Namir *et al.*, 1987; Wolf *et al.*, 1991). Given the cross-sectional design of the present study, however, we cannot determine whether having strong social support leads to enhanced ability to cope with the threat of AIDS or whether those who cope effectively with stress are then better able to elicit social support. These relationships will be studied in our longitudinal follow-up of these subjects. It seems more likely that social support buffers some of the difficulties associated with the threat of AIDS and helps subjects maintain a positive and empowering approach to this disease. Socializing with other HIV-positive men and participating in AIDS support groups, the buddy programme and AIDS organizations may be other ways to help those with HIV infection to adapt and perhaps grow from this experience. For homosexual men, who may receive less support from their families, these other sources of support may be critical. Establishing strong social support networks before the onset of HIV-related symptoms may help to buffer the mental health consequences of this devastating illness.

The black subjects in our study tended to cope by means of more helplessness, denial and turning to religion, and by less seeking of social support. To some extent, this was because of less satisfaction with their social support networks. It seems that HIV-positive blacks, because they bear the stigma and isolation of race, homosexuality and HIV infection, should be particularly targeted for social support interventions.

In conclusion, our findings suggest that: (1) these subjects primarily coped with the threat of AIDS by adopting a fighting spirit, reframing stress to maximize personal growth, planning a course of action and seeking social support; (2) more helpless coping, less fighting spirit and less personal growth were related to dysphoria and poor self-esteem; (3) denial was related to more depression, anger and helpless coping; (4) satisfaction with one's social support networks and participating in the AIDS community were related to more healthy coping strategies; and (5) black subjects experienced more denial, more helplessness and less social support. These results suggest that health professionals treating HIV-positive patients should promote a fighting spirit and help patients reframe this health crisis as an opportunity for personal growth and challenge. Patients who are coping by denial (pretending that HIV infection has not happened) may really be expressing helplessness, anger or depression, and thus may need psychological or psychiatric services. As noted previously (Evans and Perkins, 1990), patient evaluations should include assessment of available family, friend, and other social support networks. Most important, professionals should encourage patients to use their existing sources of positive social support and should help patients, particularly black patients, to find new supports in the community.

REFERENCES

Atkinson, J. H., Grant, I., Kennedy, C. J., Richman, D. D., Spector, S. A. and McCutchan, J. A. (1988) Prevalence of psychiatric disorders among men infected with human immunodeficiency virus, *Archives of General Psychiatry*, 45, pp. 859–864.

Carroll, B. J., Feinberg, M., Smouse, P. E., Rawson, S. G. and Greden, J. F. (1981) The Carroll rating scale for depression, I: development, reliability and validation, *British Journal of Psychiatry*, 138, pp. 194–200.

Carver, C. S., Scheier, M. F. and Weintraub, J. K. (1989) Assessing coping strategies: a theoretically based approach, *Journal of Personality and Social Psychology*, 56, pp. 267–283.

Dew, M. A., Ragni, M. V. and Nimorwicz, P. (1990) Infection with human immunodeficiency virus and vulnerability to psychiatric distress: a study of men with haemophilia, *Archives of General Psychiatry*, 47, pp. 737–744.

Donlou, J. N., Wolcott, D. L., Gottlieb, M. S. and Landsverk, J. (1985) Psychosocial aspects of AIDS and AIDS-related complex: a pilot study, *Journal of Psychosocial Oncology*, 3, pp. 39–54.

Evans, D. L. and Perkins, D. O. (1990) The clinical psychiatry of AIDS, *Current Opinion in Psychiatry*, 3, pp. 96–102.

Flannery, R. B. and Wieman, D. (1989) Social support, life stress, and psychological distress: an empirical assessment, *Journal of Clinical Psychology*, 45, pp. 867–872.

Folkman, S. and Lazarus, R. S. (1988) Manual for the ways of coping questionnaire: research edition (Palo Alto, Calif., Consulting Psychologists Press).

Greer, S., Morris, T. and Pettingale, K. W. (1979) Psychological response to breast cancer: effect on outcome, *Lancet*, ii, pp. 785–787.

Greer, S. and Watson, M. (1987) Mental adjustment to cancer: its measurement and prognostic importance, *Cancer Surveys*, 6, pp. 439–453.

Hamilton, M. (1960) A rating scale for depression, *Journal of Neurology and Neurosurgical Psychiatry*, 23, pp. 56–62.

Kessler, R. C., O'Brien, K., Joseph, J. G., Ostrow, D. G., Phair, J. P., Chmiel, J. S., Wortman, C. B. and Emmons, C. A. (1988) Effects of HIV infection, perceived health and clinical status on a cohort at risk for AIDS, *Social Science and Medicine*, 27, pp. 569–578.

McNair, D. M., Lorr, M. and Droppleman, L. F. (1981) *Profile of Mood States* (San Diego, Educational and Industrial Testing Service).

Namir, S., Alumbaugh, M. J., Fawzy, F. I. and Wolcott, D. L. (1989) The relationship of social support to physical and psychological aspects of AIDS, *Psychology and Health*, 3, pp. 77–86.

Namir, S., Wolcott, D. L., Fawzy, F. I. and Alumbaugh, M. J. (1987) Coping with AIDS: psychological and health implications, *Journal of Applied Social Psychology*, 17, pp. 309–328.

Ostrow, D. G., Monjan, A., Joseph, J., Van Raden, M., Fox R., Kingsley, L., Dudley, J. and Phair, J. (1989) HIV-related symptoms and psychological functioning in a cohort of homosexual men, *American Journal of Psychiatry*, 146, pp. 737–742.

Pearlin, L. I., Menaghan, E. G., Leiberman, M. A. and Mullan, J. T. (1981) The stress process, *Journal of Health and Social Behavior*, 22, pp. 337–356.

Perkins, D. O., Dickison, J. A. and Evans, D. L. (1990) SCID-RDC: DSM–III–R and RDC integrated interview, in *New Research Programme and Abstracts*, 143rd Annual Meeting of the American Psychiatric Association, Washington, DC.

Perry, S., Jacobsberg, L. B., Fishman, B., Frances, A., Bobo, J. and Jacobsberg, B. K. (1990) Psychiatric diagnosis before serological testing for the human immunodeficiency virus, *American Journal of Psychiatry*, 147, pp. 89–93.

Rabkin, J. G. Williams, J. B. W., Neugebauer, R., Remien, R. H. and Goetz, R. (1990) Maintenance of hope in HIV-spectrum homosexual men, *American Journal of Psychiatry*, 147, pp. 1322–1326.

Sarason, I. G., Sarason, B. R., Shearin, E. N. and Pierce, G. R. (1987) A brief measure of social support: practical and theoretical implications, *Journal of Social and Personal Relationships*, 4, pp. 497–510.

Spitzer, R., Williams, J. B. W., Gibbon, M. and First, M. B. (1989) *Instruction Manual for the Structured Clinical Interview for DSM–III–R (SCID)* (New York, New York State Psychiatric Institute, Biometrics Research).

Turner, R. J. (1981) Social support as a contingency in psychological well-being, *Journal of Health and Social Behavior*, 22, pp. 357–367.

Weisman, A. D. (1989) Vulnerability and the psychological disturbances of cancer patients, *Psychosomatics*, 30, pp. 80–85.

Wolf, T. M., Balson, P. M., Morse, E. V., Simon, P. M., Gaumer, R. H. Dralle, P. W. and Williams, M. H. (1991) Relationship of coping style to affective state and perceived support in asymptomatic and symptomatic HIV-infected persons: implications for clinical management, *Journal of Clinical Psychiatry*, 52, pp. 171–173.

Zich, J. and Temoshok, L. (1987) Perceptions of social support in men with AIDS and ARC: relationships with distress and hardiness, *Journal of Applied Social Psychology*, 17, pp. 193–215.

SEVEN

Gay Men, Social Support and HIV Disease: A Study of Social Integration in the Gay Community

Graham Hart, Ray Fitzpatrick, John McLean, Jill Dawson
and Mary Boulton

INTRODUCTION

In the UK, homosexual and bisexual men constitute 80–85% of people with AIDS (PWAs) and about half of all HIV-1 antibody reports are of men with homosexual and bisexual behaviour as their primary risk factors for exposure to HIV infection (PHLS, 1989). Despite evidence of a levelling off in the incidence of HIV in this population (PHLS Working Group, 1989; Loveday et al., 1989) as a result of changes in risk behaviour (Evans et al., 1989; Johnson and Gill, 1989), homosexual and bisexual men will continue to represent a large proportion of the people requiring formal and informal HIV-related health care and social support in the foreseeable future. Yet while the clinical management of HIV disease has seen rapid development, the social dimensions of care have so far received little attention, except in so far as this involves the counselling of people with HIV disease (Carballo and Miller, 1989).

In 1986 the then Secretary of State for Health, Norman Fowler, visited San Francisco and praised the model of community care for people with AIDS developed in that city by the gay community; he also suggested that this was a suitable model for AIDS services in the United Kingdom. This model has been described in a paper by Peter Arno (1986), in which he emphasizes that many of the non-profit agencies which arose in response to the AIDS epidemic relied in great part on the efforts of a mass of volunteers donating their time and energy to the needs of PWAs. In the UK the term 'community care' embraces a range of interventions, from the highly organized statutory and non-statutory services to informal, unpaid care provided by family members and others (Bulmer, 1987). In this paper we therefore address the issue of the extent to which gay men in the UK may have access to the latter – informal resources, rather than services provided by non-statutory agencies or AIDS charities, which could be mobilized to provide support at times of illness. It will be suggested that, even with high levels of social integration as measured by openness to others regarding sexuality, leisure time spent with other gay men and knowledge of, and willingness to provide help to, people with HIV-related disorders, the routine and long-term provision of practical support to gay men with chronic disease cannot be borne to any great degree at an individual level by members of the gay community.

Data presented here derive from a large study of gay men in England which was primarily concerned with the effects of HIV and AIDS on sexual behaviour. We have reported elsewhere on some of the key behavioural findings of this research (Fitzpatrick *et al.*, 1989a, b, c), and so discussion here will be limited to the study population's social integration and access to informal care networks.

METHODS AND SAMPLE

Most studies of gay and bisexual men in the UK are clinically based; few have attempted to recruit from non-clinical settings. The criterion for inclusion in this study was any man who had had sex with another man within the last five years. We recruited our sample (*n* = 502) from a variety of predominantly community sources: 283 (56%) were identified through gay clubs, pubs and gay organizations; 96 (19%) came from 'snowball' sampling, that is respondents who have been referred by people already interviewed; and 123 (25%) came from genito-urinary medicine clinics. London provided 227 (45%) of the sample; however, 144 (29%) were recruited in Manchester, 65 (13%) in Oxford and 31 (6%) in Northampton. A further 32 (7%) came from towns, cities and rural areas near to the four main centres of the study. These locations were selected mainly to determine whether there were differences between men recruited in London and those from other centres; as there have been no studies of the distribution of homosexual men in the UK, it was not possible to select a 'representative' sample of gay men. The mean age of the sample was 31.6 (s.d. 10.4), with a range from 16 to 67.

Data was collected by two research officers (JM, JD) using interviews which included demographic information, sexual orientation and recent sexual behaviour, attitudes to and use of condoms and safer sex, attitudes to the HIV antibody test, health beliefs and behaviours and level of social integration as measured by disclosure of social orientation, sociability, social support, domestic arrangements and access to practical help.

Statistical analysis was undertaken using the chi-square test for significance.

RESULTS

Disclosure of Sexual Orientation

Seventy-eight per cent (372) of the men described their sexual orientation to us as gay, with a further 43 (9%) describing it as homosexual and 51 (10%) as bisexual. A further 16 (3%) preferred no designation or unique terms not included in the checklist, such as 'transsexual'. When asked whether they used these terms when talking to others about themselves, 454 (90%) maintained that they did so. Of those with heterosexual friends ($n = 494$) and work colleagues ($n = 483$), 439 (89%) said that close friends were aware of their sexual orientation, 398 (78%) that other friends were aware of this and 345 (71%) said that colleagues knew of their sexuality. Those who used the terms homosexual, gay or bisexual were significantly more likely ($P<0.001$) to have disclosed their sexuality to heterosexual friends, other friends, work colleagues and their employers.

The parents of the men in this sample were also aware of their sons' sexual orientation. Seventy per cent of those whose mother was alive and presently or previously in contact (308 of 440) knew that the respondent was gay. The fathers of 62% of the men (245 of 398) were aware of their sons' sexual orientation. The term frequently used to describe a person's willingness to disclose homosexual sexual orientation is 'out of the closet'; the majority of our sample can therefore be described as an 'out' population of gay men. There were no significant differences in 'outness' between men recruited in different parts of the country.

Sociability

The men were asked a series of questions relating to their social networks; this included how often they went out with friends socially. Seventy-seven per cent (386) maintained that they went out socially, either several days a week (66%) or every day (11%), 78 (15%) that they went out socially once a week, and only 38 (8%) said that they would go out socially two or three times a month or less. This is always, or often, with a group of friends (291 of 502; 58%) rather than always or often alone (121; 24%).

In general, the friends of the men in this sample were also gay; 66% ($n = 336$) maintained that a half or more of their friends were gay men. Seventy-five per cent (378) said that a half or more of their social life was spent with other gay men, and for 175 (35%) proximity to the 'gay scene' (i.e. gay pubs, clubs and organizations) had been a consideration in their decision to live in their present location. Men living in cities, towns or other areas outside of London were significantly less likely, however, to have chosen their present location because of its proximity to the gay scene ($P<0.0001$).

Social Support

In order to gain some measure of the extent to which the men in the sample were part of, or had access to, a network of social support, a number of questions were asked relating to the availability of friends and others in whom men could confide and from whom practical help might be sought. For example, 347 (69%) of the men felt that they belonged to a close circle of friends and that they were part of a group who kept in close contact with each other. However, many more (474; 94%) said that there were people among their circle of friends to whom they found it helpful to talk. Indeed, 82% of this group (387 of 474) spoke to such friends once a week or more and for some of these daily contact was the norm (105 of 387). Again, a large proportion of the men (462 of 502; 92%) maintained that they had at least one person with whom they could share their most private feelings and in whom they could confide on a regular basis. This was usually a male friend (293 of 462; 63%) or partner (241; 52%), although family members (176; 38%) and female friends 148 (32%) also fulfilled this function. Access to social support did not vary by centre of recruitment.

Domestic Arrangements and Practical Help

To establish the nature of the men's domestic situation and their access to practical help at times of temporary incapacity, questions were asked regarding their living arrangements and the availability of people locally to whom they could turn for help when ill.

Over one-third of the sample lived alone (180; 36%). Of those who did not live alone (322; 64%), 89 (28%) lived with a male partner, and this group constituted 18% of the total study population. Others lived with one other male friend (56; 17%) in a mixed-sex (63; 20%) or an exclusively male (46; 14%) household, or with parents (52; 16%) or wife or female partner (15; 5%).

As domestic situation *per se* does not necessarily determine access to informal care, the men were asked whether there were people in their neighbourhood ('nearby') to whom they could turn for practical help if, for example, they were ill and required shopping to be done or needed help around the house. The majority of the sample 463 (92%) said that they did have access to such a person. In this group this was most frequently a friend (230; 50%), although others had a partner (112; 24%) or parent or other relative (82; 18%) on whom they could rely. Finally, 39 of 463 in this position (8%) said they could turn to a neighbour for practical help during illness.

HIV, AIDS and Other Gay Men

In Table 7.1 we report on the extent to which men in the sample either know or have known people with HIV infection, people with symptomatic HIV disease or people with AIDS, or have been involved in the practical help or support of people with AIDS. We also investigated the relationship between these variables and whether the respondent was recruited from, or interviewed in, London, Oxford, Northampton or Manchester.

It is clear from the final column of Table 7.1 that although the majority of men in the study know or have known at least one person who is HIV antibody positive, and between 42 and 46% have known a person or persons with HIV symptomatic disease, AIDS and somebody who has died of AIDS, only 25% have actually been involved in helping somebody with AIDS. In addition, there are differences between the men in the sample according to their area of recruitment and interview on all but the last of these questions. The greatest difference is between men recruited in London as compared to Oxford ($P<0.0001$) in relation to knowing

Table 7.1 Knowledge and support of people with HIV infection, HIV disease and AIDS according to area of recruitment

	London n = 227 (%)	Oxford n = 65 (%)	Northampton n = 31 (%)	Manchester n = 144 (%)	Other n = 32 (%)	Total n = 499 (%)
Known person(s) ab+	161* (17%)	26 (40%)	16 (52%)	93* (65%)	19 (59%)	315) (63%)
Known person(s) ab+ and ill	122** (54%)	18 (28%)	12 (39%)	66** (46%)	14 (44%)	232 (46%)
Known person(s) with AIDS	115*** (51%)	14 (21%)	11 (35%)	57*** (40%)	13 (40%)	210 (42%)
Known person(s) to have died of AIDS	128* (56%)	13 (20%)	9 (29%)	49* (34%)	14 (44%)	213 (43%)
Provided practical help and support to person(s) with AIDS	66 (29%)	7 (11%)	9 (29%)	36 (25%)	5 (16%)	123 (25%)

*$P<0.0001$; **$P<0.001$; ***$P<0.0005$.

somebody with HIV disease, from asymptomatic infection through to AIDS.

Looking at these data in a different way, however, it is clear that the most consistent differences are to be found between the large cities of London and Manchester and the smaller towns of Oxford and Northampton. If we exclude the men recruited from outside these four towns, then 68% of respondents interviewed in London and Manchester knew someone who was HIV antibody positive, as compared to 44% of those recruited in Oxford and Northampton ($P<0.0001$). Similarly, 61% of men recruited from London and Manchester knew someone with HIV disease as compared to 31% of those from Oxford and Northampton ($P<0.001$). Men from the large cities were more likely to know someone with AIDS (46%) than those from the smaller towns (26%) ($P<0.0005$), and to have known someone who has died from AIDS (48% versus 28%) ($P<0.0001$). Only in relation to helping someone in a practical way in relation to AIDS does this not apply; there were no significant differences between the towns and cities. Finally, 85 men in the total sample (17%) had a close friend, lover or former lover who had died of AIDS. These men were significantly more likely to have provided practical help or support to a person with AIDS than others in the study population (76% versus 24%; $P<0.0001$).

DISCUSSION

Men with homosexual and bisexual behaviour as their primary risk factor for HIV infection will continue to constitute the largest risk specific group of people with AIDS in the UK in the foreseeable future. Yet there have been no published reports to date of the requirements of this population in relation to the statutory and non-statutory health and social services, nor of the more informal resources to which they may have access within the gay community. Our aim has been to investigate elements of the latter – the social integration of this community and the informal support available to its members.

It is clear that our population of homosexual and bisexual men had friends, colleagues and families who, for the most part, were aware of their sexual orientation. Indeed, this knowledge was not fortuitous; the men in the sample were likely to have informed most of these people of their sexuality. We would like to stress, therefore, that our findings in relation to social support, access to informal care, knowledge of people with HIV infection and disease and help given to people living with AIDS is limited to a group of men who are, in common parlance, firmly 'out of the closet'. By definition, we did not generally recruit men who were isolated from other gay men and unable to confide in, or discuss issues of sex and sexuality with, others. We are not in a position to claim that this is a representative population of gay men; in the absence of data collected systematically on the sexually active population of the UK as a whole, no claims to representativeness are possible. This group was, however, recruited from a variety of sources and from different areas of the UK; the need to sample widely in this population has been discussed elsewhere (Hart, 1989).

We found that the men had active social lives and that much of their leisure time was spent with other gay men. All but 6% of the men interviewed had people with whom they found it helpful to talk, and all but 8% maintained that they had at least one person in whom they could confide on a regular basis. This situation may be contrasted with negative media images of isolation and deviance in this group (Watney, 1987).

Our interest in the sample's domestic arrangements was related to one aspect of informal care, namely the extent to which the carers of people with chronic illness frequently are related to, and live with, the sick person (Bulmer, 1987). Although describing a predominantly healthy gay population, whose living arrangements might change were serious illness to occur, we found that while 31% lived with partners or relatives, over two-thirds of the sample were not in households where a partner or relative was present. It is not possible to determine whether this has consequences in terms of gaining access to long-term help and support in dealing with serious illness, but it does demonstrate that partners or relatives are not immediately at hand to provide such care.

Yet the majority of the men in the sample did feel that there were people to whom they could turn in times of illness for help with shopping or around the house. This finding should, however, be treated with caution. One question was limited to small-scale needs at specific times and by no means represents the full social service needs of a person with AIDS (Mail and Metheny, 1989), or indeed of the more demanding personal and physical needs of a person with chronic illness (Bulmer, 1987). It has been demonstrated elsewhere that relationships *outside* the family are less easily maintained by the chronically ill, even when ambulatory (Fitzpatrick *et al.*, 1988), and so it cannot be assumed that the social relationships and integration described earlier would necessarily be sustained at times of serious illness. Further research is necessary to determine the extent to which non-family members, such as friends, are willing to undertake tasks such as shopping and cleaning for the chronically ill.

A quarter of the men had contributed to the practical help or support of a person with AIDS, which does demonstrate one aspect of the extent to which AIDS has had an impact on the gay community. Generally, the men interviewed in the large cities of London and Manchester were significantly more likely to know people at every stage of HIV infection than those recruited from Oxford or Northampton, indicating that the extent to which this disease has impinged upon communities may be determined by urban concentration, rather than by geography. Men who had a close friend, lover or former lover who had died of AIDS were more likely to have been involved in AIDS-related practical help or support than other men, and this indicates that close and intimate, rather than diffuse or more distant, relations may be necessary for help to be provided; resort to a 'gay community' in general is insufficient to fulfil adequately the informal care needs of its members at times of long-term serious illness. We need to investigate further possible variations within and between gay communities in order to determine the type and level of service provision required in different parts of the country.

The support of the Secretary of State for Health in 1986 for community care in San Francisco is understandable if one considers that the cost of this is borne in great part by local (as opposed to national) government, and that it relies upon the mobilization of mass volunteer labour by a highly cohesive community committed to its own people; in addition, all of this occurs in a geographically discrete area. Community care in the UK in relation to other illness relies to a large extent on unpaid, informal carers, often women, who provide daily support to relatives (Bulmer, 1987). In this paper, we have reported on a population which is distributed unevenly throughout the country and which cannot assume the presence or availability of partners or relatives at times of serious illness. Men who are not as willing as our sample to disclose sexual identity may be even less likely to expect or receive such support, as it is not unknown for friends and relatives to reject those found to be living with HIV disease or AIDS.

It has been our aim to describe aspects of the social integration of a population of 'out' gay men and their access to support, both psychosocial and practical. The final range of this group's needs is yet to be addressed, but in providing a preliminary report on these issues, we hope that future detailed investigations of care requirements will now have available baseline data on a large population of healthy gay men, which will inform discussion of how these needs may properly be met.

REFERENCES

Arno, P. S. (1986) The non-profit sectors' response to the AIDS epidemic: community based services in San Francisco, *American Journal of Public Health*, 76, pp. 1325–1330.

Bulmer, M. (1987) *The Social Basis of Caring* (London, Allen & Unwin).

Carballo, M. and Miller, D. (1989) HIV counselling: problems and opportunities in defining the new agenda for the 1990s, *AIDS Care*, 1, pp. 117–123.

Evans, B. A., McLean, D. A., Dawson, S. G., Teece, S. A., Bond, R. A., MacRae, K. D. and Thorp, R. W. (1989) Trends in sexual behaviour and risk factors for HIV infection among homosexual men, 1984–1987, *British Medical Journal*, 298, pp. 215–218.

Fitzpatrick, R., Newman, S., Lamb, R. and Shipley, M. (1988) Social relationships and psychological well-being in rheumatoid arthritis, *Social Science and Medicine*, 27, pp. 399–403.

Fitzpatrick, R., Boulton, M., Hart, G., Dawson, J. and McLean, J. (1989a) High risk sexual behaviour and condom use in a sample of homosexual and bisexual men, *Health Trends*, 21, pp. 76–79.

Fitzpatrick, R., Dawson, J., McLean, J., Hart, G. and Boulton, M. (1989b) The life-styles and health behaviours of gay men, *Health Education Journal*, 48, pp. 131–133.

Fitzpatrick, R., Hart, G., Boulton, M., McLean, J. and Dawson, J. (1989c) Heterosexual sexual behaviour in a sample of homosexually active men, *Genitourinary Medicine*, 65, pp. 259–262.

Hart, G. (1989) AIDS, homosexual men and behaviour change, in: C. J. Martin and D. V. McQueen (eds) *Readings for a New Public Health* (Edinburgh University Press).

Johnson, A. M. and Gill, O. N. (1989) Evidence for recent changes in sexual behaviour in homosexual men in England and Wales, *Philosophical Transactions of the Royal Society, London*, B325, pp. 153–161.

Loveday, C., Pomeroy, L., Weller, I. V. D., Quirk, J., Hawkins, A., Smith, A., Williams, P., Tedder, R. S. and Adler, M. W. (1989) Human immunodeficiency viruses in patients attending a sexually transmitted disease clinic in London, 1982–7, *British Medical Journal*, 298, pp. 419–421.

Mail, P. D. and Matheny, S. C. (1989) Social services for people with AIDS: needs and approaches, *AIDS*, 3 (Suppl. 1), pp. S273–S277.

PHLS (1989) *AIDS/HIV Quarterly Surveillance Tables: Data to end September 1989* (London, Public Health Laboratory Service).

PHLS Working Group (1989) Prevalence of HIV antibody in high and low risk groups in England, *British Medical Journal*, 298, pp. 422–423.

Watney, S. (1987) *Policing Desire* (London, Comedia).

EIGHT

The Role of Informal Carers in Supporting Gay Men Who Have HIV-Related Illness: What Do They Do and What Are Their Needs?

Kathy McCann and Emma Wadsworth

INTRODUCTION

Health care for people with HIV infection and AIDS, like care for people with a number of other health problems, would, it is argued, benefit from a shift from the present hospital based care to community based care (National AIDS Trust, 1989; HMSO, 1987). Such a move is seen as important in order to rationalize the use of acute services and create a sensible balance between care in the community and in hospitals (Adler, 1987; Smits, 1989; Bebbington and Warren, 1989), and because it is the preferred option of the person with HIV-related illness, as home is the place where most people would want to be (National AIDS Trust, 1989).

Though community care is made up of a number of elements, including statutory and commercial services, voluntary organizations and informal care (Bulmer, 1987), it has been argued that the term is simply a euphemism for informal care, the main element being care by the family and particularly by female relatives (Parker, 1985; Graham, 1984; Finch, 1987; Levin *et al.*, 1983). Furthermore, the role of statutory services in the community has increasingly come to be support for the family in its caring (Parker, 1985; Wenger, 1984), such that non-statutory and informal unpaid care systems are relied upon to provide main support (Bulmer, 1987; Green, 1989; Ashley-Miller, 1990). Indeed, the White Paper, *Caring for People: Community Care in the Next Decade and Beyond*, acknowledged the importance of the family and informal carers in sustaining community care when it stated: 'the government acknowledge that the great bulk of community care is provided by family, friends and neighbours' (HMSO Cmnd 849, para. 1.9, 1989).

Community care thus relies on the availability of people to do the caring, and the range of support undertaken informally and the period over which this occurs are important in understanding the nature of care in the community and the balance between statutory and informal care, and in identifying the gaps which might exist. The White Paper went on to say it was essential, when designing packages of care for dependants, that consideration should be given to the needs of carers. To do this policy makers need to take into account what carers describe as being necessary for them.

This paper describes the contribution which informal carers made to people with HIV infection and AIDs (PWA) in terms of practical and emotional support and looks at the relationship between having an informal carer and access to statutory services. It also examines the ways in which carers themselves felt they were left unsupported.

BACKGROUND AND METHODS

Information about informal carers presented here formed part of a wider study in which gay men with HIV infection, and both lay and professional carers, were asked about their experience of an attitude towards a variety of health, social and voluntary care services. Respondents to the study were recruited through the genito-urinary medicine and immunology clinics and the designated wards of a London teaching hospital between November 1988 and June 1989. Eighty per cent of all gay men who attended the hospital during this period completed a form expressing interest in the study. Structured personal interviews, covering all aspects of care as well as social circumstances, took place with 265 individuals; 86% of those who completed the form (McCann, 1991). The whole range of HIV disease was represented, from HIV-positive and asymptomatic to AIDS; 66% of the men interviewed in the first part of the study were working, the majority full-time. Just under half (47%) were professionals or had intermediate occupations (social classes I or II). Forty-five per cent owned their own accommodation and 40% lived alone.

Informal carers were contacted through respondents to the first part of the study. During the initial interview, PWA respondents were asked a series of questions about any help and support they had received and if they could or would nominate someone who had given them 'help or care' on an informal basis; 55% did so. The majority of PWAs nominated one carer (76%), 22% nominated two and 2% three. One hundred and twenty-five informal carers were interviewed, 71% of those nominated. Reasons why the carers were not interviewed included because they had died (1%), the people they were caring for had died (2%) or they refused despite the initial nomination (7%). Similar numbers could not be contacted or were left to contact us themselves and did not (19%). Not all those diagnosed with AIDS or AIDS-related complex (ARC) who had received help wished us to approach their carer. Twenty-three people who were diagnosed AIDS or ARC did not want us to contact their carer for interview, although most of these (*n* = 19) had received some help from friends or family.

As a whole there were no age or social class differences between those who did and those who did not nominate a carer. There were, however, clear differences in health as almost all the informal carers had been supporting someone who had been ill (92%). Thirty per cent of the people who had been given a diagnosis of AIDS or ARC did not nominate a carer, though almost all of these people (83%) said they had actually received help from someone, particularly practical help, but did not want us to approach their carer for interview. The present data thus represent the responses of two-thirds of the potential carers of the group of PWAs we interviewed, and this is very much an opportunistic sample.

RESULTS

Informal Carers: Who Are They?

The relevant carer was most commonly identified as a close friend (45%) or a partner (42%). Four per cent of PWAs nominated parents and a further 4% siblings, 2% a buddy (i.e. volunteer) and 3% other people. The majority of carers were male (77%): 62% were aged between 30 and 45 years. Of the others equal numbers were under 30 and over 45. Questions which were included as part of the General Household Survey (GHS) in 1985 provide information about a sample of carers from the general population (Green, 1989). Although the carers in this study form such a selected subsample of the population, comparisons were made with the GHS since no more appropriate data were available. These data indicate that those caring within the present study were younger, with the peak age for caring in the general population between 45–64. There was no gender difference in the national study among those caring within the same household though women were more likely to be caring for someone outside their own household. In this study, males predominated whether they were living in the same household or elsewhere.

Twenty-eight per cent of our carers had a specific health problem themselves, 5% saying they were in poor health. Over half (53%) of the people who mentioned a health problem said that it affected their ability to care. In the national study about half of the carers reported long-standing illness (Green, 1989).

When asked the question, 'Do you worry or have you ever worried/thought about being HIV positive yourself?', a third of carers (34%) said they did not worry about being positive. Where they did, approximately half (49%) reported that this was unrelated to the person they were supporting. One in ten carers were HIV positive themselves. A further fifth (22%) had had a test which proved to be negative. Virtually all those tested were male (90%).

Carers were marginally more likely to live separately from the person who had nominated them (54%) than to live with them. Of those living elsewhere only 6% were within five minutes walk and 37% spent at least three-quarters of an hour travelling, 5% saw the respondent every day and half between two and six times a week. Frequency of visiting was related to the time spent travelling, with those living more than half an hour away visiting significantly less often than those who lived nearer ($\chi^2 = 14.90$, d.f. $= 1$, $P<0.001$). Our group were more likely to be living with the person who they were helping than was true in the GHS sample

(46% compared to 29% nationally) (Green, 1989). Seventeen per cent of the carers had someone dependent upon them, besides the person in the sample who had nominated them as a carer; for five this was another person with HIV infection. Information from the General Household Survey showed that a third of carers had someone dependent on them though this was almost always dependent children (Green, 1989).

Over half (56%) the informal carers we interviewed considered that they 'bore the brunt' of the care, though one in nine said they shared it with another person and one in six felt someone else did the major part. Eleven per cent described the issue of caring as irrelevant because the persons predominantly cared for themselves, and 4% of people did not feel able to answer this question or objected to the term 'bearing the brunt'. In 15% of cases we interviewed more than one carer for the same PWA.

What Did Carers Do to Support People with HIV Infection?

Because of the variable nature of HIV infection and because some PWAs had more than one carer, the calls on individual carers themselves differed. Informal care here covers a huge variation in support within intimate relationships, from purely practical help to emotional support, or a combination of both. Taking those doing the main caring, a small proportion said they spent time doing practical tasks only (4%), while a quarter (26%) said they gave only emotional support. The majority (70%) did both. In terms of the practical help, under half (44%) said they had increased the time they had spent doing household tasks. This was particularly true of those living with the person who nominated them (57% compared to 33% of those who lived elsewhere).

When asked questions about practical help, half said they had assisted with various personal and household tasks (see Table 8.1).

Table 8.1 Personal and household tasks which the carers helped with

Tasks	%
Household	
Shopping	46
Cooking	32
Cleaning	35
Household repairs	18
Personal	
Getting in or out of bath/shower	14
Having a bath	12
Dressing	10
Going to toilet	3
Shaving	6
Feeding	3
Help at night	25
Other	14
n = (100%)	125*

*More than one response was possible

Other things which people reported included giving advice about health or welfare, psychological reassurance, help with heavy lifting, gardening or moving house, mobility (particularly getting up and down stairs or accompanying the person to hospital outpatient appointments). The average number of tasks was four, with 25 people reporting that help was needed with five or more. The most usual combination of tasks was shopping, cooking and cleaning, with help with getting in and out of the bath, dressing or household repairs as additions.

Almost half of those carrying out specific tasks said they had been doing so continuously for at least 14 days. In the case of cooking, cleaning and shopping exactly half had been helping continuously for six months or more. A quarter (24%) were helping at night, half of whom were also working outside the home. Unfortunately, we are unable to explore in detail the kind of help people gave overnight, but one in four said their assistance at night had taken place over a period of time, the majority of these (five out of seven) for at least six months. As might be expected, relatively fewer people reported that they carried out personal tasks such as bathing, shaving and help with going to the toilet, on a long-term basis; where they did, it was likely to be for periods of up to three months.

Apart from practical help in the home, the carers also gave assistance to their loved ones during stays in hospitals.

A third of carers who visited the persons while they were in hospital provided practical help while there, as this man explained:

> I live here [in the hospital] – I was staying when he was at his worst – 24 hours a day for three weeks. I'm in charge of his pills and everything, I bathe him and clean him and cook and massage him.

A further 5% felt they would have liked the opportunity to help while their partner or friend was in hospital. The majority (58%) said they did not want to (4% did not express a wish about this). Exactly half the carers had also accompanied the person to outpatients appointments at times, 23% always did so.

For many people, rather than helping with any of these particular physical tasks, their contribution was more general and perhaps less quantifiable as the following comments illustrate:

> I keep things ticking over.

> I have offered full mental and financial help.

> He's always relied on me for things to keep him together, e.g. I financially support him – I just do more.

Or it was predominantly emotional support:

> He needs more emotional support than anything.

> It was more emotional support. He knows I'm here.

> I've only given moral support, thank God – at least that means he is okay.

But it was sometimes a mixture of both:

> He can't make his bed completely and needs some help at home with cleaning but currently he can manage. He has psychological fluctuations rather than physical ones.

Eleven per cent of carers said the person carried out almost all practical tasks for themselves, as this one man explained:

> He has hardly needed any help really, he has only needed support.

Some people either found it hard to quantify what they did or did not feel their contribution was substantial:

> He's a friend who just happens to have HIV. End of story so far.

This was despite the person with HIV infection nominating them as their carer, though it could be that in identifying the person as a carer the PWA may be anticipating an increase in the help needed in the future, hoping that help might be forthcoming or even desiring to give the interviewer an answer to a question they had not yet thought about. Clearly a lack of recognition of their own role mitigates against their obtaining any support for themselves. It could illustrate a reluctance to accept a loved one as dependent and denote the grey areas where usual support within a relationship becomes something more.

One in eight people said they wished they could have given more help than they already did.

Presence of an Informal Carer and Use of Services

A log linear model was used to examine the relationship between the identification of an informal carer and use of statutory services, taking into acount the possibility that it might be confounded by illness. Independent of illness more people who identified an informal carer than those who did not, were in contact with a psychologist ($\chi^2 = 6.8$, d.f = 1, $P<0.01$) and more were in contact with the hospital community support team, responsible for liaison between patients, the hospital and community ($\chi^2 = 15.62$, d.f. = 1, $P<0.001$). Some differences also remained with the detailed work of the community liaison team. Where there was an informal carer the team was more likely to do home visits ($\chi^2 = 16.14$, d.f. = 1, $P<0.001$); but where no informal carer was identified the team was more likely to spend time talking to the person (88%) than when an informal carer was identified (76%), though this difference was not significant. Where the team was involved 42% of carers felt that the team supported the person with HIV infection only, 49% felt they supported both the person and themselves as carer. One in twenty felt that the team was useful to them as carers, rather than to the PWA. Finally, those with an informal carer ($\chi^2 = 4.42$, d.f. = 1, $P<0.05$) and those with a diagnosis of AIDS or AIDS-related complex ($\chi^2 = 4.45$, d.f. $= 1$, $P<0.05$) were, independently, more likely to have been admitted to hospital. For all the other relationships the person's diagnosis was the factor associated not whether or not they had an informal carer.

Only one person was not in contact with either a professional or an informal carer.

Unmet Need, Gaps in the Service and How to Fill These

I don't think carers get much support. I've noticed that with other friends. They're getting tired out, then ill themselves and it sounds whiney but sometimes you think no one is bothered.

Finally, we asked about the support carers had received for themselves and 15% of them said that on balance they had received insufficient emotional support and 13% insufficient practical help.

Altogether just under a third (30%) said they would have liked more help but had not obtained it. Fifteen per cent of these identified the social services as the possible source of this help, 21% the hospital, 24% volunteers and 40% others, mostly relatives and friends. While some people mentioned needing help with specific health problems, or things like sleep, hearing and literacy, other requirements were more general:

I would have liked someone here during the day doing odd things that he couldn't do, just to help out and occasionally in the evening so I could go out without feeling guilty.

[I would like] two or three hours' break a day.

The kinds of practical support that were identified included transport, particularly to the clinic, shopping, financial and legal help as well as help that would allow a continuation of paid employment. Improved communication between themselves and medical professionals was also seen as desirable.

Often what was needed was not physical but moral or emotional support, particularly counselling. Ten people mentioned this specifically and the following comments illustrate the substance of what people wanted:

We both would have liked good local reliable counselling on all aspects of being HIV positive, i.e. from the PWA's point of view and from my own including information regarding what help is available and someone to discuss his moods and say how dreadful I feel.

Counselling for him and for me, to cope with him and having a boyfriend who doesn't know what is going on.

Or mutual support:

I am sure there is a need for a support group.

Lovers, etc. have to stand around and wait. It's the same for cancer or any other illness, these people are left in limbo. There is a need for some sort of support organization.

As this man explained, what he required was less structured and was simply someone to talk to:

Physically no, a bit of moral support would come in useful.

I'd have liked someone to go and shout at.

In general, there was sometimes a disparity between people's recognition of a need for assistance and their willingness to ask for it. For example, though 15 people said they would have liked to have a home help, only five had asked for one. Four people said they would have liked a social worker, two support from the community liaison team, eight some kind of community nurse and 13 a psychologist. Only a minority had asked for help from any of these.

People gave various explanations for not obtaining help. Among these were: they did not know where to go; they were too busy or tired to obtain the help; or they had simply not asked. These comments illustrate some of the things that were said:

We haven't asked for it [help] but that doesn't mean we didn't need it.

I haven't come to the point where I need specific help to cope.

Others did not feel it appropriate to involve outsiders:

I wanted to do it all myself. If the opportunity had arisen for someone else to come in I'd have still rather be doing it myself.

He needs such personal, intimate help. It needs continual attention to a thousand little things all the time. I know by instinct.

Equally, the person with HIV infection may not have wanted to involve others:

I haven't approached anyone. He doesn't want to involve outsiders. I find it stressful.

He just didn't want publicity about being ill.

I've agonized about whether I'm making myself indispensable – he's quite resistant to letting others into his life.

Or professionals in particular:

I'd prefer if it wasn't professional help but help from others in a similar situation, i.e. partners of PWAs who can whinge together.

Where approaches for professional help had been made but were not fruitful, carers described this as simply that 'nothing had happened' and no one had pursued it. This is an area in which professionals' responsibility for referrals could be pursued more aggressively.

DISCUSSION

Data presented here provide information as to the possible role of the informal carer in helping someone with HIV infection and AIDS. Discussions about community care for HIV-related illness have indicated that the resource of informal care, which is taken for granted in other areas, may not be readily available here (Aggleton and Homans, 1987). Instead, because people are inhibited by the cultural associations of HIV-related illness, they may be unwilling to disclose information about their condition to people who, in other circumstances, might be expected to help (Miller, 1987). Indeed they may feel unable to discuss their HIV status and any illness even with the people closest to them for fear of being rejected or discriminated against (Aggleton et al., 1989; Hart et al., 1990). It would seem from the information provided in the present study that friends, partners and other relatives played a considerable part in supporting people with HIV infection and that there was also a huge range of things people did to help. However, the nature of informal care is, as one would expect, a continuum of different kinds of help and support. There is a grey area when everyday and accepted support present in a relationship becomes 'care'. Because the physical contributions people make are tangible, it is easy to concentrate on these when discussing informal care and to underestimate the emotional support people give, even though the physical tasks people perform may not be the most important feature of caregiving (Twigg et al., 1990). Moreover, because emotional support is part of an existing loving relationship it can be difficult to quantify for research and policy purposes. Here the emotional support people gave was substantial.

Only six people had been ill and not received some support from family and friends; all except one had received help from professionals. That carers were predominantly male represents an unusual gender distribution. Some people were not willing to accept that they were dependent in some way, or that they were providing for the needs of a loved one. Issues of reciprocity were relevant as were the special problems created when two people are both affected by HIV-related illness, as implied by this man:

> We joke about the photo finish.

Carers in our group were much more likely than carers in general to be caring for someone with the same complaint. This will obviously carry with it extra demands for the people involved. Those responsible for making care plans therefore need to take into account the fact that there may be circumstances where carers themselves may suffer ill health, may be supporting more than one person and alternate between offering support and needing it.

Informal carers appear to be important in the use of some statutory services, namely the psychologist and the community liaison team. This could imply a number of things: having a carer facilitates access to these professionals; or the effects of dependency or the demands of caring require the skills, particularly counselling or emotional support, that these professionals provide; or these are better supported people who are more easily able to access services. Admission to hospital was more likely when people had informal carers, which is contrary to what one might expect if the presence of lay carers in the community were to reduce demands on acute facilities. One possible explanation for this could be that informal carers give people more confidence to obtain care or make demands on the services when they need help. Another may be that the services themselves are sensitive to the stress placed upon the carer, and are willing to provide hospital admission as a relief to someone supporting an ill person at home. The fact that these were the only statistically significant associations is perhaps surprising. If statutory services supplement informal care, it might have been expected that more home helps would be involved where there was no informal carer, or indeed that there would be a social worker involved, or more frequent use of voluntary organizations. This suggests that the relationship between informal care and use of services is a complex one which warrants further research.

Informal carers were able to identify the areas where they felt unsupported or needed additional assistance. Emotional support was one such area, as was help with specific practical tasks and, finally, ways of maintaining work outside the home. Family and friends were mentioned as the people who carers would most like additional help from which does indicate the possibility that once they take on a supporting role those individuals are often left to get on with it without the routine support of others.

Though the White Paper on community care recognized that the needs of informal carers had to be considered when developing health and social services it was vague about how this might be achieved. A recent leaflet by the King's Fund Centre Carers' Unit outlined a ten-point plan for supporting carers in general. Targets included: recognition of their contribution and their own needs; opportunities for them to take a break; practical help including domestic help; someone to talk to about their own needs; income to cover costs of caring which does not preclude employment; and services designed through consultation with carers (King's Fund Centre Carers' Unit, 1989). From the reports of informal carers here, it would seem that this could be an appropriate starting point.

REFERENCES

Adler, M. (1987) Care for patients with HIV infection and AIDS, *British Medical Journal*, 195, pp. 27–30.

Aggleton, P. and Homans, H. (eds) (1987) *Social Aspects of AIDS* (London, Falmer Press).

Aggleton, P., Homans, H., Mojsa, J., Watson, S. and Watney, S. (1989) *Aids: Scientific and Social Issues: A Resource for Health Educators* (London, Churchill Livingstone).

Ashley-Miller (1990) Community care, *British Medical Journal*, 300, p. 487.

Bebbington, A. and Warren, P. (1989) What role for local authorities? *Insight*, 4 (11), pp. 12–14.

Bulmer, M. (1987) *The Social Basis of Community Care* (London, Allen & Unwin).

Finch, J. (1987) A question of choice, *Carelink*, Summer, pp. 4–5.

Graham, H. (1984) *Women, Health and the Family* (Brighton, Harvester Press).

Green, H. (1988) *Informal Carers*, OPCS Social Survey Division No. 15, suppl. A (London, OPCS).

Hart, G., Fitzpatrick, R., McLean, J., Dawson, J. and Boulton, M. (1990) Gay men, social support, and HIV disease: a study of social integration in the gay community, *AIDS Care*, 2 (2), pp. 163–170.

HMSO (1987) *Social Services Select Committee: Problems associated with AIDS*, Vol. 1, Recommendations and Vol. 11, Minutes of Evidence, 13th May, Session 86–87.

HMSO (1989) *Caring for People: Community Care in the Next Decade and Beyond*, Cmnd 849 (London, HMSO).

King's Fund Centre (1989) Carers' needs: a ten point plan for carers, *Community Care*, November. Supplement for carers for people.

Levin, E., Sinclair, I. and Gorbach, P. (1983) *The Supporters of the Confused Elderly at Home: Extract from the Main Report* (London, National Institute of Social Work Research Unit).

McCann, K. (1991) Methodological issues encountered in researching HIV-related health care for gay men (manuscript available from ISSMC, 14 South Hill Park, London NW3 2SP).

Miller, D. (1987) *Living with Aids* (London, Macmillan Education).

National AIDS Trust and King's Fund (1989) *AIDS: Can We Care Enough?* Report of conference for World AIDS Day, 1988.

Parker, G. (1985) *With Due Care and Attention: A Review of Research on Informal Care*, Family Policy Studies Centre, No. 2.

Smits, A. (1989) Home Support team. Data Sept. 1987–1988, District Health Authority report.

Twigg, J., Atkin, K. and Perring, C. (1990) *Carers and Services: A Review of Research* (London, HMSO).

Wenger, G. C. (1984) *The Supportive Network: Coping with Old Age*, National Institute, Social Studies Library, No. 46 (London, Allen & Unwin).

NINE

Significant Relationships and Social Supports of Injecting Drug Users and Their Implications for HIV/AIDS Services

Aaron Stowe, Michael W. Ross, Alex Wodak, Gillian V. Thomas
and Sigrid A. Larson

The issue of the systems in which HIV-related issues develop and which those at risk of infection inhabit (including family, medical workers and counsellors, and friends: Bor *et al.*, 1992) is central to their adaptation and adjustment. Bor *et al.* note that the 'family' may be the individual's most important social system, whether it is a biological (family of origin) or social (family of affiliation) entity. From a purely clinical perspective, systems theorists argue that the context of risk or disease has implications for the nature of the psychological problems that patients experience and how they may be dealt with.

Little is known about the family relationships and friendship networks of injecting drug users (IDUs), yet the vast literature on social support suggests these relationships may play a crucial role in a person's health and well-being. As a part of a pilot study we investigated the supportive resources which IDUs have in their day-to-day life, and those which they could rely on in times of crisis or stress. Since IDUs comprise the second largest group of HIV-infected people in Australia, we focus on how being HIV seropositive may mediate support from friends and family, and what services and agencies IDUs would seek if they needed help. Unlike most research which investigates social support our research is not experimental in design, as our aim is not to model the impact of social support on IDUs' health and well-being (physically, mentally or socially defined). The goal of this research is to explore the nature of the family relationships and friendship networks, and identify what social supports exist for this stigmatized group whose behaviour may lead to further marginalization if they were to become HIV infected.

Previous research has found strong relationships between social support and positive outcomes for health and well-being throughout the life-cycle. In an early review, Cobb (1976) reported that adequate social support protected people in crisis from a variety of pathological states; from birth to death, as a result of chronic diseases, depression and other illnesses. The influence of social support has been investigated in relation to mortality (Berkman and Syme, 1979), diseases such as cancer (for example, Broadhead and Kaplan, 1991) and rheumatoid arthritis (Goodenow *et al.*, 1990) and negative life stress (for example, Cohen and Hoberman, 1983). While there is an overall conclusion that social support and positive outcomes for health are related, in their comprehensive review of the literature Cohen and Syme (1985) state that the relationship is almost entirely correlational.

It is not known why social support is associated with health, but two hypotheses have been proposed to explain the relationship: the main or direct effect model and the buffering model. The direct effect model posits that social support enhances health and well-being irrespective of stess because large social networks provide people with regular positive experiences and a set of stable, socially rewarded roles in the community (Cohen and Wills, 1985). Cohen and Syme (1985) explain that the perception that others will provide aid in the event of a stressful situation has an overall positive effect on people's health and may elevate their self-esteem, stability and control over their environment. The impact on people's psychological states may also affect the health outcome by influencing the susceptibility to illness by its impact on the immune system or through the influence on behaviour and physiological responses.

In the buffering model resources provided by others have beneficial outcomes by protecting people from the pathogenic effects of stress (Cohen and Syme, 1985). Intervention by supports may redefine and reduce the potential harm posed by the occurrence and/or they may aid by confidence building so the event is not recognized as stressful. Cohen and Syme suggest that a second way the buffer model works is by the support directly intervening between the source of the stress, thereby reducing or eliminating the pathological outcome, or by influencing the responsible illness behaviours or physiological processes.

The presence of perception of social support on the psychological distress and physical well-being of homosexual and bisexual men has been investigated with regard to AIDS and HIV infection. In so far as homosexual men experience similar psychological distress to IDUs, as both groups face stigmatization in the community and similarly face exposure to HIV infection, the research highlights the need to examine the social supports of IDUs. Noh *et al.* (1990) reported that men who had close confidants experienced less emotional strain imposed by the threat of exposure to HIV. HIV-positive gay men who reported having social supports have been reported to experience less emotional distress (Blainey *et al.*, 1991), and to demonstrate active-behavioural coping (Wolf *et al.*, 1991) and lower levels of mood disturbance, greater global health perception and higher self-esteem (Wolcott *et al.*, 1986). For those men with AIDS increased physical distress has been associated with lower perceived social support and for men with both AIDS and ARC the more available social support was perceived to be, the less hopeless and depressed they felt (Zich and Temoshok, 1987).

The research into the health and well-being of homosexual and bisexual men in relation to HIV/AIDS clearly indicates the importance of social supports, not only to mediate the stress of having AIDS or being HIV infected, but also to confront the threat of infection. These are issues which also confront IDUs yet we do not know what resources (family, friends or formal services) IDUs can rely upon. Furthermore, apart from issues related to psychological health and AIDS and HIV infection, the importance of social support has been identified as a factor associated with risk reduction among IDUs (Abdul-Quader *et al.*, 1990; El-Bassel *et al.*, 1991).

However, the absence of data on social supports of IDUs has meant that researchers have little idea of the baseline or context of social support in this population, or of the best ways to measure it. Following Cohen and Wills (1985), who suggest that structural measures of support only indirectly index the availability of support, we used both structural and functional indices. The structural measurement assesses the existence of support and aspects of the respondent's social integration whereas the functional refers to the extent to which the family and friendship relationships provide specific aspects of support. We used a modified Interpersonal Support Evaluation List (ISEL: Cohen and Hoberman, 1983) which measures four functional categories of social support: esteem, informational, social companionship and instrumental support. The present study was designed both to provide some baseline data and to explore measurement of social support in IDUs.

METHODS

The sample of 100 IDUs was interviewed by two experienced interviewers during December 1991. The face-to-face interview, which was part of a pilot test of a new research instrument, took approximately 45 minutes to complete and responses were written on the questionnaire form by the interviewers.

Recruitment was by advertisements at treatment clinics, needle exchanges, word of mouth and personal contacts. Respondents were eligible to carry out the interview if they had injected within the last two years, and had to telephone to make an appointment ahead of the interview time. Interviews were carried out in an office next to a methadone clinic in the King's Cross–Darlinghurst area of Sydney with separate entry off the street. Respondents were paid A$20 for the anonymous interview. The research was endorsed by the relevant ethics committee.

Questions about who people could discuss a personal problem with were phrased, 'If you had a personal problem could you discuss this problem with any people you know and rely on them for help – emotionally or in other ways?' and, for family, 'people' was replaced by 'family members'. Respondents were asked to provide initials of each person to ensure that estimates of numbers were based on actual individuals rather than guessed, as well as whether the person knew of their injecting drug use, their relationship to the respondent, gender and own IDU status.

Modified ISEL Scale

The ISEL was revised by taking the four items from each of the four aspects of social support scales (belonging, self-esteem, tangible and appraisal), which appeared to be relevant to IDUs, and modifying them to make them appropriate to the IDU's situation where appropriate, by specifically referring to problems related to drug use or sexually transmissible infections. Items appear in Table 9.1. The scoring of the initial scale (probably true or probably false) was retained. Instructions were:

> Below is a list of statements which may or may not be true about you. For each statement could your circle PROBABLY TRUE (PT) if the statement is true about you or PROBABLY FALSE (PF) if the statement is not true about you. If the statement does not apply to you, try to decide *quickly* whether it is probably true or probably false. Please make sure you circle a response for every question.

In order to determine if the items clustered into the original dimensions of the ISEL, a factor analysis was carried out using principal components analysis followed by varimax rotation. Negatively worded items (half of the items) were first recoded so that all items were worded in the same direction (and thus loadings are unipolar in Table 9.1).

Table 9.1 Factor structure of the ISEL scale as modified for injecting drug users

Item	Loading
Factor 1: Tangibility of people and support scale	
I know someone who would give me old dishes if I moved into my own place.	0.73
People hang out in my place during the day or evening.	0.69
I know someone who I see or talk to regularly who I could talk to about problems I might have with drugs.	0.69
I know someone who I see or talk to regularly who I could talk to about sexually transmissible diseases (STDs) if I had one.	0.61
I know someone who would bring my meals to my room or place if I was sick.	0.60
I don't know anyone who would give me some old furniture if I moved into my own place.	−0.46
(24.9% of variance)	
Factor 2: Appraisal of friendship	
Lately, when I've been troubled, I keep things to myself.	0.71
I hang out with friends at their place a lot.	0.68
I have a group of friends who I meet with regularly or do things with regularly.	0.57
I don't know someone who I see or talk to regularly who I could talk to about sexual problems if I had any.	0.55
(9.9% of variance)	
Factor 3: Self-esteem	
Most people are more attractive than I am.	0.74
Most of my friends are more satisfied or happier with themselves than I am.	0.71
Most of my friends have more control over what happens to them than I do.	0.54
Most people who know me think highly of me.	−0.43
(9.2% of variance)	

Data analysis was carried out using SPSS[x]. Frequency tabulations of the social support measures were utilized, along with Spearman rank-difference correlation coefficients between social support measures.

RESULTS

The sample was comprised of 60 men and 40 women. Their age ranged from 16 to 45 years with a mean of 28 years (s.d.d. 7). The respondents were generally well educated with 42% completing years 11 or 12 at high school, 35% completing 10 years of education, and 42% completing a post-school qualification (39% trade or technical courses and 3% tertiary).

Table 9.2 indicates that the sample were largely not employed and some were in receipt of social security benefits for an extended period of time. The average period on social security was two years (23.5 months s.d.d. 31.7) with the median period 12 months.

Table 9.2 Employment status and social security history

	(%)	n
Employment status		
Not employed	80.0	80
Full-time	7	7
Part-time	2	2
Casual	8	8
Student	1	1
Home duties	1	1
Other	1	1
Social security benefit		
Unemployment	36.0	31
Sickness	48.8	42
Pension	15.1	13
Period on social security		
<3 months	20.9	18
3–6 months	17.5	15
7–12 months	15.2	13
1–2 years	23.4	20
3–6 years	12.8	11
>6 years	10.6	9

Most (78%) of the sample were Australian born, with 86% (19 of 22) of those born overseas coming from English-speaking countries: New Zealand, United Kingdom, Canada and the USA. The majority (68%) of respondents were single and 32% were married or living in a sexual relationship. Most (74%) respondents did not have children and of the 26 who did have children only 10 of these respondents were financially responsible for them. Forty-one respondents were currently in treatment with the most common treatment being methadone maintenance (20 respondents). Of the 41 respondents who had been in prison over one-third (15 of 41) had been released within the past 12 months. Three respondents reported being HIV infected.

Details of social support networks are illustrated in Table 9.3. It is apparent that for personal problems, friends constituted the major source of social support, with two-thirds reporting that partners and/or lovers did not exist or were not available. Where family was a source of social support, mother and siblings were most often noted. Counsellors and social workers were rarely mentioned. Table 9.4 illustrates the degree of openness and expected support from family and friends if respondents were HIV seropositive. There is an inverse relationship between openness with biological family and with friends, and a tendency to expect greater support from friends rather than family.

Table 9.3 Family and non-family social support networks

	n	(%)		*n*	(%)
Non-family			*Family*		
Total non-family			Total family		
Zero	9	9.0	Zero	51	51.0
1 to 2	45	45.0	1 to 2	33	33.0
3 to 5	35	35.0	3 to 5	16	16.0
>5	11	11.0	>5	0	0.0
Friends			Mother		
Zero	20	20.0	Yes	30	30.0
1 to 2	43	43.0	Father		
3 to 5	30	30.0	Yes	10	10.0
>5	7	7.0	Siblings		
Partners and lovers			Zero	64	64.0
Zero	66	66.0	1 to 2	32	32.0
1	30	30.0	3 to 5	4	4.0
>1	4	4.0	Other family		
Counsellors and social workers			Yes	5	5.0
Yes	6	6.0	*Family and non-family*		
			Total support network		
			Zero	6	6.0
			1 to 2	40	40.0
			3 to 5	28	28.0
			>5	26	26.0

Respondents were asked: 'If you had a personal problem could you discuss this problem with any people you know and rely on them for help – emotionally or in other ways?' and 'If you had a personal problem could you discuss this problem with your family and rely on them for help – emotionally or in other ways?'

Characteristics of the social support networks are illustrated in Table 9.5. Nearly half the respondents indicated that the majority of the people they 'hang around with' are also IDUs. A majority also indicated that all or most of the time in the past six months had been spent living with IDUs, and that almost all of these had been known for longer than six months. Table 9.6 illustrates places where help would be sought if respondents became infected with HIV and other services and agencies which were identified as helpful. The majority of respondents identified medical services.

Table 9.4 The degree of openness with friends and family, and expected support from friends and family if HIV positive*

	Friends (%)	Family (%)
Degree of openness		
Not at all open	3.0	29.0
A little open	0.0	9.0
Somewhat open	3.0	12.0
Quite a lot open	16.0	10.0
Totally open	59.0	21.0
Variable responses	9.0	11.0
Don't know/non-response	10.0	8.0
Expected support		
Totally rejecting	2.0	7.0
Somewhat rejecting	2.0	10.0
Neither rejecting nor supportive	3.0	5.0
Quite supportive	29.0	22.0
Totally supportive	34.0	13.0
Don't know	6.0	13.0
No response	4.0	5.0

Respondents were asked: 'Could you tell me how open you could be with these people and you know/your family, for example could you tell them if you were HIV positive?' and 'How would you expect your friends/family to react if you told them you were HIV positive?'
* $n = 100$.

Responses to the five-point scale which asked 'When you are having problems are you satisfied with the support you are getting from your friends?' were skewed towards satisfaction (24% very satisfied, 30% satisfied, 28% reasonable/OK). Knowledge of respondent's injecting drug use was limited to a modal number of 1–2 non-family members (46%; 3–5, 36%) with 21% of mothers, 6% of fathers and 29% of siblings being aware of it.

Correlations between the total score on the modified ISEL scale (sum of three subscales) and satisfaction with support from friends was -0.39 ($n = 85$, $P<0.001$), with number of close friends 0.52 ($n = 92$, $P<0.001$), with total number of non-family supports 0.63 ($n = 92$, $P = 0.001$), with total support (family, friends and others) 0.65 ($n = 92$, $P<0.001$). There was an insignificant correlation between satisfaction with support from friends and number of close friends (-0.10, $n = 91$, $P>0.10$). Openness with family and anticipated family reaction to HIV were correlated (0.53, $n = 78$, $P<0.001$) although openness with non-family and friends was not (0.15, $n = 82$, $P<0.05$).

The results of the factor analysis of the modified ISEL scale appear in Table 9.1. Five factors with eigenvalues >1 were extracted, but included factors with less than three items with loadings >0.3, so rotations of a lesser number of factors were carried out. The rotation of three factors (accounting for 44% of total variance)

Table 9.5 Characteristics of the friendship networks

	n	(%)
Proportion of people 'hang around with' who are IDUs		
None	7	7.0
Less than half	28	28.0
About half	17	17.0
Greater than half	31	31.0
All	17	17.0
Time in the past 6 months living with IDUs		
All the time	44	44.0
Most of the time	8	8.0
Half of the time	13	13.0
Some of the time	18	18.0
No time	17	17.0
*Percentage of close friends known for more than 6 months**		
None	1	1.1
1–50	7	7.5
51–75	7	7.5
76–99	10	10.8
100	69	73.4

Respondents were asked: 'How many of the people you hang around with now inject drugs?', 'How much of the last six months have you been living with anyone who injects drugs?' and 'How many of your close friends have you known for more than six months?'
*n = 94 as six respondents did not have any close friends.

Table 9.6 Places where help would be sought if HIV positive and other services and agencies identified as helpful if HIV positive (n = 100)

Services and agencies where help would be sought	
General practitioners	35
Specialist medical centres	25
Drug treatment centres	15
Counsellor or social worker	15
HIV support groups	12
Other services	11
Hospitals	10
Other services and agencies known as helpful	
Specialist HIV medical centres	22
HIV support groups	16
Drug treatment centres	14
Counsellor or social worker	10
Community-based AIDS organizations	12
Hospitals	11
Other services	8

Respondents were asked: 'Who or where would you go for help if you were HIV positive?' and 'What other services do you know about that would be helpful to you if you were HIV positive?' Respondents would often identify more than one source of help within a category. However, the percentages indicate that a particular source of help was nominated, not how many times.

provided the most interpretable solution. The three factors were readily interpretable and consisted of dimension of tangibility of people and support, appraisal of friendship and self-esteem. The self-esteem scale was the only scale which was identical to the full unmodified ISEL scale. Two items ('I don't get invited to things with other people' and 'I don't know anyone who would loan me their car for a couple of hours') loaded below 0.4. They were discarded from the scale and are not illustrated in Table 9.6. Many respondents were unable to answer the latter item as they were unable to drive. Alpha coefficients for the three scales were, respectively, 0.72, 0.59 and 0.57.

DISCUSSION

These data should be interpreted with several caveats in mind. First, they are based on a sample of unknown representatives, but which from its derivation and demographics, and the fact that there was payment for the interview, appears orientated to more drug-dependent IDUs. Second, these data are based on respondents who in some cases appeared to be mildly intoxicated (although not to the point of being unable to complete the interview: if this appeared the case, respondents had the interview terminated and were invited to make a further appointment for interview). Third, there were no appropriate scales for measurement of social support in IDUs, and this study had to attempt to adapt instruments and questions from other studies to this task; reliability and validity for several of our measures are thus not available. In the case of the modified ISEL, the negative direction of the wording of half of the questions interspersed with positive wording apparently confused some respondents. Fourth, the meaning of the term 'close friend' may have differed between respondents, although the precaution of getting them to give initials or first name of the friends and family members meant that these were estimated on the basis of recall of actual individuals rather than guesstimates. It was apparent to the interviewers (GVT and SAL) that some respondents tended to name almost everyone they knew (often the younger respondents), while others were more considered in their listings. Furthermore, the interviewers noted that the concept of emotional support appeared alien to many respondents and there was a vagueness about needs and the concept of 'going for help' in general in this population.

These points made, it is apparent that there are few if any previous useful data on social support in this population and that this lack may have arisen in part from the perception of IDUs as neither deserving of support nor being prepared to utilize it. Nevertheless, the broad literature on the influence of social support on mental and physical illness makes investigation of this group worth while, particularly in view of the suggestion in some of the literature that self-esteem and self-efficacy may influence HIV risk behaviours. A further factor that makes this group important from a research perspective is the suggestion that stigmatized status may magnify the effects of life events (Ross, 1990).

These data confirm that IDUs have social support networks and that friends appear more important than biological family in providing support. Where family is involved in support, mothers and some siblings are the family members who are most likely to provide it, and to know of the respondent's drug use. However, less than a third listed mother or at least one sibling as knowing, which combined with the fact that half of the sample of IDUs in a previous study (Ross *et al.*, 1992a, b) reported moving to Sydney from elsewhere in the state or from interstate suggests that available family support is poor. Indeed, the preference for non-family support mirrors the role of the adopted subcultural family as providing more support than the biological family in homosexual men. This is supported by the greater degree of anticipated openness about HIV if infected and the greater expected support from friends rather than family. The sample reported a broad range of the proportion of the people they 'hung around with' who were IDUs, but the majority had spent the past six months living with other IDUs, again confirming the status of other IDUs as a surrogate family in terms of availability of support.

Nevertheless, where family were likely to be supportive if the respondent became HIV-seropositive, the correlation with the modified ISEL was of the same magnitude, suggesting that provided there was availability, some family members were as useful as friends in the perceived position of support. The ISEL score was significantly and positively correlated with numbers of friends, total non-family supports and family supports. However, it was moderately *negatively* correlated with satisfaction of support from friends, and uncorrelated with satisfaction of support from close friends, suggesting that tangibility and appraisal of friendship may not be related to the quality of it or to the number of friends.

The ISEL as modified for use with IDUs suggests that rather than the four factors as found with college students in the United States, IDUs see support in terms of its tangibility of people and support, and in terms of an appraisal of having friends, as well as a self-esteem measure. There was a moderate correlation between these three scales. It would appear that it has some concurrent validity in terms of its intercorrelations with other rating-scale measures of social support and could form a useful basis for measurement of social support in IDUs in other contexts.

It is interesting, when looking at the services and agencies where help would be sought if respondents became HIV seropositive, that these were conceptualized predominantly in terms of medical services. Where these were specialized drug or HIV clinics, it would be expected that they would be able to provide appropriate referral to social support or counselling. However, this may not be the case with many general practitioners as they are generally reluctant to deal with IDUs (Roche *et al.*, 1991).

This paper presents data on the social supports of IDUs in Sydney. While the sample is one with a high proportion of unemployed respondents, and control data are not available for non-IDUs, it is apparent that they have some social supports, but that they are more likely to be friends (often other IDUs) and less likely to be family. If they were to become HIV-seropositive, they were more likely to expect support from friends than family, although where the family was judged to be supportive, there was little difference in the magnitude of the correlation with the modified ISEL scale for family or friends. The ISEL scale modified for use with IDUs appears to have adequate reliability and concurrent validity for further use, and suggests that IDUs see social support in terms of tangibility of people and support, and appraisal of friendship, as well as being related to self-esteem. There is no necessary relationship between numbers of supports and satisfaction with such support, suggesting that quality and quantity are relatively independent or even inversely related.

The implications of these data for social support of HIV-infected IDUs are threefold. First, social support in this population is measurable and further research is needed. Second, friends are more likely to be a source of support than biological family and, if people are HIV infected, they are perceived as being more supportive than family. Third, support for HIV-infected people is predominantly conceptualized in terms of the medical model. However, there is clearly available social support for most IDUs, although its effects on adjustment to HIV, as well as the accuracy of these perceptions, needs to be investigated in IDUs infected with HIV as well as compared with that in comparable non-IDUs.

REFERENCES

Abdul-Quader, A.S., Tross, S., Friedman, S. R., Kouzi, A. C. and Des Jarlais, D. C. (1990) Street recruited intravenous drug users and sexual risk reduction in New York, *AIDS*, 4, pp. 1075–1079.

Berkman, L. F. and Syme, S. L. (1979) Social networks, host resistance, and mortality: a nine year follow-up study of Alameda County residents, *American Journal of Epidemiology*, 109, pp. 186–204.

Blainey, N. T., Goodkin, K., Morgan, R., Feaster, D., Millon, C., Szapoczinik, J. and Eisdorfer, C. (1991) A stress-moderator model of distress in early HIV-1 infection: concurrent analysis of life events and social support, *Journal of Psychomatic Medicine*, 35, pp. 297–305.

Bor, R., Miller, R. and Goldman, E. (1992) *Theory and Practice of HIV Counselling: A Systemic Approach* (London, Cassell).

Broadhead, W. E. and Kaplan, B. H. (1991) Social support and the cancer patient, *Cancer*, 67, pp. 794–799 (February Supplement).

Cobb, S. (1976) Social support as a moderator of life stress, *Psychosomatic Medicine*, 38, pp. 300–314.

Cohen, S. and Hoberman, H. M. (1983) Positive events and social supports as buffers of life change stress, *Journal of Applied Social Psychology*, 13, pp. 99–125.

Cohen, S. and Syme, S. L. (1985) Issues in the study and application of social support, in: S. Cohen, and S. L. Syme (eds) *Issues in the Study of Social Support*, pp. 3–22 (Sydney, Academic Press).

Cohen, S. and Wills, T. A. (1985) Stress, social support, and the buffering hypothesis, *Psychological Bulletin*, 98, pp. 310–357.

El-Bassel, N., Gilbert, L. and Schilling, R. (1991) Social support and sexual risk taking among female recovering IV drug users, *VII International Conference on AIDS*, Florence, 16–21 June 1991, Abstract W.D. 4026, Vol. 2.

Goodenow, C., Reisine, S. T. and Grady, K. E. (1990) Quality of social support and associated social and psychological functioning in women with rheumatoid arthritis, *Health Psychology*, 9, pp. 266–284.

Noh, S., Chandarana, P., Field, V. and Posthuma, B. (1990) AIDS epidemic, emotional strain, coping and psychological distress in homosexual men, *AIDS Education and Prevention*, 2, pp. 272–383.

Roche, A., Guray, C. and Saunders, J. (1991) General practitioners' experiences of patients with drug and alcohol problems, *British Journal of Addiction*, 86, pp. 263–275.

Ross, M. W. (1990) The relationship between life events and mental health in homosexual men, *Journal of Clinical Psychology*, 46, pp. 402–411.

Ross, M. W., Wodak, A. and Gold, J. (1992) Sexual behaviour in injecting drug users, *Journal of Psychology and Human Sexuality*, 5, pp. 89–104.

Ross, M. W., Wodak, A., Gold, J. and Miller, M. E. (1992) Differences across sexual orientation on HIV risk behaviours in injecting drug users, *AIDS Care*, 4, pp. 139–148.

Wolcott, D. L., Namir, S., Fawzy, F. I., Gottelieb, M. S. and Mitsuyasu, R. T. (1986) Illness concerns, attitudes towards homosexuality, and social support in gay men with AIDS, *General Hospital Psychiatry*, 8, pp. 395–403.

Wolf, T., Balson, M., Morse, E., Simon, P., Gaumer, R., Dralle, P. and Williams, M. (1991) Relationship of coping style for affective and perceived social support in asymptomatic and symptomatic HIV-infected persons: implications for clinical management, *Journal of Clinical Psychiatry*, 52, pp. 171–173.

Zich, J. and Temoshok, L. (1987) Perceptions of social support in men with AIDS and ARC: relationships with distress and hardiness, *Journal of Applied Social Psychology*, 17, pp. 193–215.

TEN

The Extended Family and Support for People with AIDS in a Rural Population in South West Uganda: A Safety Net with Holes?

Janet Seeley, Ellen Kajura, Cissy Bachengana, Martin Okongo, Uli Wagner and Daan Mulder

INTRODUCTION

It is commonly assumed that the extended family in Africa provides social and economic support for its members in times of need. The United Nations Regional Adviser on Social Welfare Policy and Training, Economic Commission for Africa explained in 1972 (Shawky, 1972, pp. 4–5):

> In rural Africa, the extended family and clan assume the responsibility for all services for their members, whether social or economic. People live in closely organised groups and willingly accept communal obligations for mutual support. . . . The sick, the aged and children are all cared for by the extended family.

The care of AIDS patients is seen as falling within the sphere of extended family care. Indeed, in a brief article in *WorldAIDS*, Ngugi (1990, p. 8) described the care given to one young man who died of AIDS at his parental home in Kenya. After cataloguing the care given to the patient by a range of people, she remarks 'In Kenya, as in many parts of Africa, we still enjoy the extended family kinship systems. On average, 10 people from the village, including distant family members, visited . . . daily.'

Panos (1990, p. 61) notes 'In the contexts of AIDS care and prevention, the extended family network found in many developing countries is a national strength.' But, as they go on to point out, as the AIDS burden grows it can also easily be over-exploited: 'Some doctors and social scientists in the south are concerned that reliance on the extended family is overplayed . . . they argue that for many people the extended family as a safety net can be no more than a myth.' It is this assertion which this paper sets out to explore, using data from rural Uganda.

BACKGROUND

Since 1990 an HIV/AIDS counselling component has been developed within the Medical Research Council (UK) Programme on AIDS in Uganda, a population-based research project on the dynamics of the HIV-1 transmission in a rural community (Seeley *et al.*, 1991).

The study area of the MRC Programme is a rural subcounty in Masaka District, two hours' drive southwest of Kampala. Most of the population are Baganda, living in dispersed settlements and small trading centres. They are banana and coffee cultivators. The descent system of the Baganda is patrilineal with virilocal marriage (where the woman moves to the man's home). It is not uncommon for women to move some distance from their natal home for the purpose of marriage. However, marriage is not always patrilocal: young men do not always stay close to their fathers and brothers when they set up their own households. Thus the extended family group is often dispersed over a number of villages or a wider area. The median household size in the area is five.

HIV-1 seroprevalence is 5% in the general population, or 8.3% in adults aged 13 years and older.

METHODS

During the period January–June 1991 a total of 195 clients received pre-test counselling; of these 147 returned for their results and post-test counselling. Of those, 30 HIV-positive clients (17 women, 13 men) requested home-based care because they were sick. All were included in this study. They were visited and assisted on a regular basis (at least once a fortnight) by a programme counsellor (a local person) and/or a medical officer. Data on the care received were gathered through observation and informal interviews recorded in counsellor and medical reports of visits and, in the case of death, from interviews with carers, relatives or neighbours.

RESULTS

The age distribution of the clients included in this study is shown in Table 10.1.

Table 10.1 Clients visited for home care

Age (years)	Men	Women
15–24	2	0
25–34	7	11
35–44	3	2
45–54	1	2
55+	0	2
Total	13	17

The age distribution is similar to that recorded for non-care-seeking post-test clients. The majority were aged 25–34 years. The oldest client was a 66-year-old woman, the youngest was a 22-year-old man. Table 10.2 summarizes who the principal carers and assistants of these patients were.

Table 10.2 Carers

Carers	Principal		Assistants		
	Males	Females	Males	Females	Total
Mother	2	8	2	1	13
Husband/wife	4	1	–	–	5
Sister	1	3	–	–	4
(Grand)children	1	3	–	–	4
Other relative	5	2	5	7	19
Counsellor	–	–	–	2	2
None	–	–	6	7	13

The word 'principal' does not imply anything about the quality of care: the named carer was the individual recognized as being responsible for the care of the patient by the household and by the counsellor/medical officer. None of the patients included in this study was living alone.

Mothers and 'other relatives', usually sisters, most commonly took on the role of principal carer, followed by wives (for the men). In 13 cases there was no assistance for the principal carer. In 15 cases the principal carer had assistance from close relatives, usually a woman. For the remaining two clients a female counsellor gave assistance by preparing food for the patient, cleaning the patient's surroundings and washing bed clothes.

During their visits the counsellors and medical staff identified reasons why the care given by carers often fell short in some way and were told a number of reasons why relatives did not give assistance to the principal carer. In 27 of the 30 cases there was evidence of limited care. Some of the main reasons are set out below.

Lack of food in the home, particularly food suitable for a patient, and/or lack of money to buy medications (both Western and treatments for indigenous healers) were mentioned in 12 cases.

For ten cases carers' other responsibilities, which included care of children, work responsibilities (usually in the case of mothers, wives or sisters, cultivating the land to get food for the household) and the care of other sick relatives, were mentioned. For three clients the sole carer, one case the husband and two cases the mother, was also ill.

Belief that the illnesses associated with AIDS were caused by witchcraft affected the care in four cases, since Western medicine is thought to be ineffective and indeed harmful for the treatment of such illnesses. Local indigenous healers were consulted in these four cases, although in three the practitioners had proved too expensive and the consultations were stopped.

Care was also limited, or denied, because of stigma. In three cases the patient was subjected to ridicule by relatives who blamed her (in all cases the patient was female) for her condition.

Other reasons given included lack of adult assistance in the home (three clients were cared for by children) and fear of treatment (some clients and their families believed that they would be given drugs to kill them). For three men, their wives had left the home when the men had become sick and their mothers or sisters had taken on their care. This may not have resulted in limited care.

Seventeen (12 women, 5 men) died during the six-month period of study. Of those who died, records of seven cases (6 women, 1 man) show that other relatives had been asked to help but had refused on the grounds of poverty or other family responsibilities.

Medical reports were available on eight of the 17 deaths. For three of these (2 women, 1 man) neglect was cited as contributing to the death. In one case this was because of poverty, in another the principal carer was too sick to provide care and in the third the family continued to blame the patient for her condition and provided only minimal care. However, in 16 of the 17 cases extended families did provide assistance for the funeral as is their customary obligation. The one case where they did not was that of a 28-year-old woman where her mother was in dispute with her father and relatives refused to come to the funeral.

To help us to understand the situation better we can look at four cases in more detail.

The first was a 35-year-old woman whose husband had died earlier in the year. She was living close to her elderly mother-in-law, who was too weak to help. She had seven children. The youngest two, aged six months and three years, were sick. Her son aged 16 and daughter aged 15 cared for their mother. On two occasions the eldest son went to fetch his maternal grandmother, who lived some distance away, when he believed his mother to be dying. On both occasions when this proved not to be the case, the grandmother returned to her own home because of her own family responsibilities. When the client did die the extended family gathered for the funeral, but returned to their homes after the funeral rites, leaving the 16-year-old boy as household head in charge of his six siblings.

The second was a 55-year-old woman, cared for by her husband, who was also sick. There was a 17-year-old relative living in the household but he was not involved in the woman's care. She died alone while her husband was in hospital.

The third was a 35-year-old woman who, when her husband had died, was brought with her baby daughter who was also sick from her marital home to her natal home for care. Her family blamed her for her sickness and left her alone at home during the day without anyone to take care of her, even though she was bedridden. The counsellor took on the role of carer, visiting the client daily to check on her condition. During the last weeks of her client's life a sister assisted the counsellor in preparing food and cleaning the room. Other family members remained reluctant to assist.

Finally, there was a 40-year-old man who was divorced, and lived with his three primary school children, who took care of him. He was landless and lived close to his elderly brother, who had a large family. They had not been helping and told the counsellor that they could give little assistance because of their own family responsibilities. The Programme counsellor made regular visits to check on the care given by the children to the client.

DISCUSSION

Our findings suggest that the care of AIDS patients in the community of study often falls on individuals with limited assistance from extended kin and neighbours. A similar situation is recorded by Ankrah *et al.* (1991) in their study of the impact of AIDS on the families of 24 people with AIDS in Kampala. They observe that as the number of AIDS cases grows 'A crisis in functioning to meet the basic needs of sick and well members will occur in more and more families, that cannot be addressed by the extended family.' However, despite limited resources some families do cope with the care of AIDS patients through their own efforts.

There are additional factors that need to be considered which may have influenced the care given in the 30 cases in our study, which were not referred to by the clients, their families or the counsellors involved.

First, a version of the 'Hawthorne effect' (a term coined when research participants' knowledge that they were being observed had a positive effect on their responses: Roethlisberger and Dickson, 1939) may have been taking place. It is possible that regular visits by a counsellor may cause a family to exaggerate their difficulties and perhaps rely more on the counsellor's participation in care than may have been the case if the counsellor had not been available. The fact that the counsellors were local people with an understanding of the family backgrounds of their clients and, consequently, were often able to see through attempts to fabricate 'need' went some way towards negating the effect of their presence on the family demands. Alternatively, being under observation a family may have given better care to the patient than if they had not been observed. One may assume that the presence of an observer in the household would have affected behaviour in some way.

Second, a not uncommon argument for limiting care is that the person will die anyway, so why waste money on drugs or food? This may have played a part in the decision-making process of the families concerned. Some terminally ill clients request their carers (and sometimes the visiting counsellor/medical assistant) not to try to keep them alive any longer, because they are tired of suffering. This was not documented for the cases in this study, but the possibility exists that these feelings played a part in the decision making about care.

Finally, there is a question over the role of the extended family in the care of members in traditional Baganda culture. Roscoe (1965, p. 12) in his idealized account of traditional life states:

> The Baganda were charitable and liberal; no one ever went hungry while the old customs were observed, because everyone was welcome to

go and sit down and share a meal with his equals. ... There were no orphans, because all the father's brothers were fathers to a child.

Iliffe (1987, p. 59) questions this view. In his discussion of the treatment of the poor in Buganda he notes that the Luganda oral literature 'was exceptionally rich in proverbs about poor men, emphasising their isolation as individuals: "A poor man is like a yam; he creeps alone".' He cites sources which describe such poor solitary individuals as being debtors, women widowed by violence, victims of famine, epileptics and 'especially leprosy sufferers, who were treated with a ruthlessness unusual in Africa'. Bennett and Mugalula-Mukibi (1967) in their analysis of people living alone in one Baganda community noted the presence of the old and sick among their number. It may be worth while to question the assumption that there has always been a tradition of the *extended* family caring for its members in Buganda.

This raises a more general issue: the definition of the family and the extended family. As Iliffe notes (1987, p. 7), when one talks of 'African families as universal providers of limitless generosity' one tends to forget that 'Africans lived in different kinds of families, from the Yoruba compound with scores of related residents to the elementary households of Buganda'. Jaenson *et al.* (1984, p. 165) in their study of four different communities in Uganda (Busoga, Kigezi, Baganda and Teso) noted that 'Not only do households vary considerably in size but also in internal organization both between and within areas.' This variation will influence the coping strategies of the members. We must also expect the variation in social organization to affect strategies adopted to cope with the care of AIDS patients. Iliffe (1987, p. 8) cautions that 'family structure was not an immutable ethnic characteristic but could change to meet changing needs'. Consequently, blanket statements about the role of the extended family in Africa as a safety net need to be questioned and assumptions that the extended family will be ready and able to assist sick members need to be treated with caution.

Coping with HIV infection, AIDS and subsequent death places a particularly heavy burden upon the caring capacity of the family. Barnett and Blaikie (1992, p. 87) observe that the impact of AIDS deaths on households is not like other disasters (drought, famine, war, etc.) because 'It is gradual and incremental and occurs over a period of at least five years.' AIDS would thus wear down the family resources over what may be a lengthy period of sickness. In addition, as observed among our counselling clients, it is the breadwinners of the family who are most at risk and who leave behind the dependent old and young when they die.

Our research findings suggest that although families with AIDS patients in the population under study often require material support, many families need moral and practical support, in the form of encouragement, reassurance and practical advice on how best to care, in order to provide adequate care for their sick members. As we have attempted to show, it is unrealistic to expect the extended family, in all situations, to provide these services and 'to cushion the impact of illness' (Claxton, 1973, p. 477).

REFERENCES

Ankrah, E. M., McGrath, J. W., Schumann, D., Nkumbi, S., Lubega, M. and Misanya, G. A. (1991) The impact of AIDS on urban families: an assessment of needs (Poster WA251), *VIth International Conference on AIDS in Africa*, 16–19 December 1991, Dakar, Senegal.

Barnett, T. and Blaikie, P. (1992) *AIDS in Africa: Its Present and Future Impact* (London, Belhaven Press).

Bennett, F. J. and Mugalula-Mukibi, A. (1967) An analysis of people living alone in a rural community in East Africa, *Social Science and Medicine*, 1, pp. 97–115.

Claxton, M. (1973) The sick person in Ugandan society, *Social Science and Medicine*, 4, pp. 471–478.

Iliffe, J. (1987) *The African Poor: A History* (Cambridge, Cambridge University Press).

Jaenson, C., Harmsworth, J., Kabwegyere, T. and Muzaale, P. (1984) *The Uganda Social and Institutional Profile*. Prepared for USAID, Uganda, by Experiment in International Living, Kampala, Uganda.

Ngugi, E. (1990) Caring: the cost to a community, *WorldAIDS*, March, p. 8.

Panos (1990) *Triple Jeopardy: Women and AIDS* (London, PANOS Institute).

Roethlisberger, F. J. and Dickson, W. J. (1939) *Management and the Worker* (Cambridge, Mass., Harvard University Press).

Roscoe, J. (1965) *The Baganda*, 2nd edn (London, Frank Cass).

Seeley, J., Wagner, U., Mulemwa, J., Kengeya-Kayondo, J. and Mulder, D. (1991) The development of a community-based HIV/AIDS counselling service in a rural area in Uganda, *AIDS Care*, 3, pp. 207–217.

Shawky, A. (1972) Social work education in Africa, *International Social Work*, 15, pp. 4–5.

CHILDREN

ELEVEN

Impact of HIV/AIDS on African Children

Elizabeth A. Preble

INTRODUCTION

With the end of the 1980s, the first decade of the human immunodeficiency virus/ acquired immunodeficiency syndrome (HIV/AIDS) pandemic has been completed. (In keeping with increasingly common usage, the term HIV/AIDS is used in this paper to describe the range of HIV-related illnesses, including what was formerly referred to as full-blown AIDS. Also, in Africa, many fatal cases of HIV-related illness do not fit the current clinical definition of AIDS.) The impact of the disease on adults in both developed and developing countries is now generally understood, and the process of defining and quantifying the clinical, epidemiological and demographic effects is well under way. Paediatric AIDS, however, has remained a more elusive disease, particularly in developing countries, because clinical and laboratory diagnosis is more difficult. AIDS case-reporting systems rarely include children and children lack a collective political voice to express the gravity of their situation.

For Central and East Africa, estimates of the major direct impact of HIV/AIDS-related illness on children, under-five mortality, as well as estimates of the major indirect impact, orphanhood, are urgently required, even if necessarily imprecise. Attention must be focused on the problems of HIV/AIDS in this vulnerable group and efforts to develop appropriate responses for HIV/AIDS prevention and for short- and long-term care must be intensified.

The estimates of HIV/AIDS-related under-five mortality and AIDS orphanhood are targeted for ten geographically contiguous countries in Central and East Africa (see Figure 11.1); Burundi, Central African Republic, Congo, Kenya, Malawi, Rwanda, Tanzania, Uganda, Zaire and Zambia. These countries were chosen because they are among those most severely affected by HIV/AIDS in the developing world (Center for International Research, 1989). They have, in 1990,

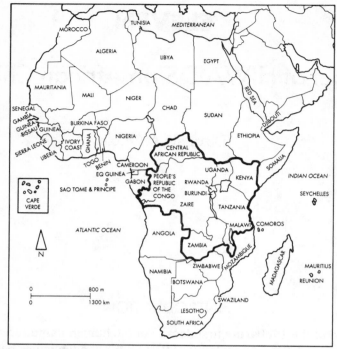

Figure 11.1 Africa

an estimated combined total population of 141 million and an annual total number of births of nearly seven million (United Nations Department of International Economic and Social Affairs, 1989).

The World Health Organization (WHO) estimates that at least one million women in Africa are already infected with HIV (Chin *et al.*, 1989). Owing to the long incubation period of this disease and the shortage of HIV testing facilities in Africa, the vast majority of these women are unaware that they are infected. While many deaths from HIV/AIDS have already occurred, the major impact of HIV infection and AIDS on children will occur in the 1990s as increasing numbers of HIV-positive women have children and as men and women who are HIV-infected in the 1980s and 1990s progress from infection to fatal cases of AIDS. Education, screening of blood supplies and other steps to prevent HIV infection in adults need to be urgently accelerated.

The impact of HIV/AIDS on child morbidity and mortality is devastating, as children progress to disease and death after HIV infection much faster than do adults. Since symptoms of HIV/AIDS resemble other common childhood diseases, most deaths from paediatric HIV/AIDS are not recognized as such.

AIDS orphans in Africa are emerging as another tragic manifestation of this worldwide pandemic. They are joining those now referred to by the United Nations Children's Fund as 'children in extremely difficult circumstances', including children endangered by armed conflict and other disasters, those exploited by child labour, street children and children who are victims of abuse and neglect (United Nations Children's Fund, 1989). While the phenomenon of AIDS orphans is also affecting Western cities like New York City (Norwood, 1989), the predominance of heterosexual transmission and the absolute numbers of parents infected with HIV give the problem considerably greater proportions in Africa.

The origin of this widespread orphanhood due to HIV/AIDS and the large numbers of children involved will render traditional systems of adoption and institutional care insufficient to meet increasing demands for long-term child care. Governments need urgently, therefore, to develop policies for these orphans, and to develop feasible and culturally acceptable models for child care that ensure, as far as possible, that children's basic needs are met.

DATA

Baseline Seroprevalence Data

Estimates of HIV seroprevalence among women of reproductive age form the foundation for this study's estimates of both HIV/AIDS-related under-five mortality (through vertical transmissions of HIV to the fetus) and HIV/AIDS-related orphanhood (as mothers progress from HIV infection to AIDS and death). Seroprevalence surveys in Africa have limitations (in sample size and selection, reliability of HIV laboratory tests and so forth). However, for the purposes of this study, seroprevalence data were thought to form a more reliable basis for projections than numbers of reported AIDS cases (which are significantly underreported in Africa) or computer simulation models of HIV transmission (which are dependent upon highly speculative assumptions about risks of infection through acts of unprotected intercourse, societal sexual patterns and so on).

HIV seroprevalence estimates for women aged 15–49 in urban and rural areas of each of the ten selected countries were derived from a published review of all available studies (Center for International Research, 1989). Rates were selected and applied independently for urban and rural areas since urban rates tend to be considerably higher than rural rates. Urban and rural findings were weighted accordingly. Data from studies which focused on high-risk groups of women (such as prostitutes) were not utilized. In the few urban or rural areas of countries where seroprevalence studies of women of reproductive age were not available, estimates of seroprevalence rates were derived from survey results from neighbouring countries with similar cultural and health patterns. These estimates are recognized to be highly speculative in some cases; however, where a range of options was available, the more conservative (and hence optimistic) assumptions were always selected. For the baseline 1988 seroprevalence rates, urban rates ranged from 4.0 to 22.9% with a median rate of 8.1%. Rural rates ranged from 1.0 to 9.4% with a median rate of 2.3%.

Seroprevalence studies from which these rates were selected were undertaken between 1985 and 1988, but were all attributed to 1988 to form the baseline data for this study (hence, the current and future rates are, in several cases, underestimated).

While consideration of age-specific HIV infection rates in women would have improved the precision of this model, they are unavailable for most of the ten countries included here.

From the 1988 baseline HIV seroprevalence data for urban and rural women aged 15–49, three models of increase of HIV infection were constructed: (a) a 'low HIV progression' model, which assumes HIV seroprevalence rates will grow at one percentage point per year from 1988 onward, and were one percentage point lower each year prior to 1988; (b) a 'medium HIV progression' model, which assumes HIV seroprevalence rates will increase at two percentage points per year from 1988 onward, and were two percentage points lower each year prior to 1988; and (c) a 'high progression' model, which assumes HIV seroprevalence rates will grow at three percentage points per year from 1988 onward, and were three percentage points lower each year prior to 1988. Reports from Uganda, Zaire, Malawi (Carswell, 1987; N'galy et al., 1988a; Ntaba et al., 1988) and other countries that have tracked HIV seroprevalence over time substantiate this range of between one and three percentage points increase per year.

A ceiling of 30% for seroprevalence rates was put into the model based on an assumption that HIV infection among adult women would eventually level off. While all urban and rural areas reach 30 per cent seroprevalence by the year 2000 in the 'high HIV progression' model, only one urban area and no rural areas reach that level in the 'low HIV progression' model.

Data/Assumptions Used to Estimate Under-five Mortality

Under-five mortality rates (U5MR) constructed before the AIDS epidemic for these ten countries were taken directly from the medium variant of the United Nations Population Division estimates (differential urban and rural rates are not available) (United Nations Department of International Economic and Social Affairs, 1989). United Nations urban and rural population estimates included the effect of anticipated urbanization, and were applied separately and weighted accordingly. The rapid urbanization expected in this region during the 1990s will exacerbate the AIDS epidemic because of significantly higher rates of HIV infection presently documented in urban areas. U5MR reduction targets were taken from the United Nations Third Development Decade goals (United Nations, 1980).

A vertical (perinatal) transmission rate of 30% was selected for this study. This rate is consistent with rates found in the United States (33%) (Willoughby et al., 1988), in Uganda (20–30%) (Mworozi et al., 1988) and in Zaire (30–40%) (Davachi and Kabena, 1988), but is lower than recent rates found in Zambia (45%) (Hira et al., 1988, 1989) and in the Congo (69%) (Lallement, 1989). Also, while not factored into this study, perinatal transmission rates in Africa could posibly rise over time as more HIV-positive mothers develop more advanced HIV infection, which may render them more infectious to their offspring (Ryder et al., 1989).

Progression of the disease in infants and children from HIV infection to HIV/

AIDS-related illness and death is rapid, owing to the vulnerability of infant immune systems, and to a lack of diagnostic capacity, clinical care, and pharmacological support. A 16% mortality rate per year for children born HIV-infected was selected, derived from WHO's estimate that 80% of all HIV infected newborns would die by age five (Chin *et al.*, 1989).

Data/Assumptions Used to Estimate Orphanhood

Annual population data for urban and rural woman aged 15–49 and children aged 0–15 were taken from the medium variant of the UN Population Division estimates (United Nations Department of International Economic and Social Affairs, 1989).

Assumptions of length of time between contracting HIV infection and developing AIDS were adapted from a San Francisco study in which it was found that 20% of HIV-infected women developed AIDS within five years and 50% within ten years after infection (Moss and Bacchetti, 1989). It was assumed for this paper that an average of 5% of each cohort of HIV-infected women will develop AIDS each year, and that after 20 years all the HIV-infected women in this region will develop AIDS.

Assumptions about the progression from AIDS to death were based on an adaptation of survival rates from black women in New York City (40.2% survival one year after diagnosis with AIDS, 20.9% after two years and 13.9% after three years) (Rothenberg *et al.*, 1987). For the present study it was assumed that, in any particular cohort of Central and East African women with AIDS, 65% will die after one year, 85% after two years and 100% after three years, a slightly higher rate of progression than that from the New York study.

To estimate the average number of children left behind by each woman who dies as a result of HIV/AIDS, data from the recent Uganda Demographic and Health Survey (Uganda Demographic and Health Survey, 1989) were used. After the effects of Ugandan under-five mortality are considered, this survey indicates that the average Ugandan woman aged 15–49 will have 2.83 surviving children. For the purposes of this paper, the figure of 2.83 was reduced by 30%, to 1.98, to reflect a 30% perinatal transmission rate (since 30% of children born to HIV-infected mothers will die). The present study does not attempt to estimate the proportion of children that will be born before as opposed to after the mother's infection; hence this model somewhat underestimates numbers of future AIDS orphans.

METHODOLOGY

Measuring Under-five Mortality

Approximately 80% of AIDS cases in children under age five in the United States occur through vertical transmission (from infected mother to fetus before or during birth) (Katz and Wilfert, 1989). Other modes of HIV transmission in the under-five age group (contaminated blood transfusions, other parenteral means, breastfeeding or sexual abuse) are considered to play comparatively minor roles. This study assumes a similar pattern in Africa and therefore only estimates under-five mortality resulting from vertical transmission of HIV.

Unlike in other developing country childhood disease patterns, more HIV-infected babies die from AIDS between the ages of two and five than during the first year of life. Consequently, HIV/AIDS has a higher impact on U5MRs than on infant (under age one) mortality rates; therefore, this study focuses on the impact of HIV/AIDS on under-five mortality.

Based on an adaptation of a WHO model (Chin *et al.*, 1989), the under-five mortality estimates given here, which include the impact of HIV/AIDS, were derived by considering, for urban and rural areas of each of the ten countries, the estimated level of HIV seroprevalence in women aged 15–49 and the estimated numbers of expected births to these women. The 30% rate of vertical transmission and the estimated mortality rate of 16% per year for vertically transmitted HIV-positive children aged 0–5 were applied to these data.

The resulting estimates of HIV/AIDS-related deaths in children were then reduced by deducting the number of children projected to die of HIV/AIDS who would have died anyway of competing causes according to the United Nations estimates of U5MRs (United Nations Department of International Economic and Social Affairs, 1989). Thus, the projections in this paper represent net additional child deaths as a result of HIV/AIDS. It was assumed that children born HIV-infected were neither more nor less likely to die of competing causes than those not HIV-infected.

United Nations estimates of numbers of births (United Nations Department of International Economic and Social Affairs, 1989) were multiplied by estimates of U5MRs (constructed before the AIDS epidemic) to obtain numbers of deaths anticipated without the effect of HIV/AIDS. These were added to estimates of HIV/AIDS-related under-five deaths to get total estimated child deaths. Finally, these estimates of total numbers of child deaths were divided by estimates of total births to arrive at estimates of U5MRs that take into account HIV/AIDS.

Measuring Orphanhood

For the purpose of this paper, AIDS orphans are defined as children under age 15 whose mothers have died of HIV/AIDS. Because of the likelihood of heterosexual transmission between mother and father, many fathers will also die of AIDS, if they have not already predeceased the mother. The mother is the primary provider for children in African culture, however, and even if the father survives the mother's HIV/AIDS death, experience with child care in Africa suggests that children do not usually receive sufficient care from their fathers alone (Nalwanga-Sebina and Sengendo, 1987; Bledsoe, 1989a).

Numbers of HIV-infected women were derived by applying estimated HIV seroprevalence rates for women aged 15–49 for urban and rural areas to the numbers of women in the cohort aged 15–49 in a given year. Five per cent of these

HIV-infected women are assumed to progress to AIDS each year. Assumptions of mortality from HIV/AIDS described above were then applied.

Each female death from HIV/AIDS was assumed to result in 1.98 surviving children. Numbers of surviving children were then reduced, based on the assumption that one-fifteenth (6.67%) of all orphans under age 15 would reach age 15 each year, and hence graduate from the orphan category.

This study, then, projects the cumulative number of children aged 0–15 who are orphans as a result of their mother's HIV/AIDS death in any given year during the 1990s.

RESULTS

Projections of Under-five Mortality

As Table 11.1 and Figure 11.2 illustrate, a dramatic increase in under-five deaths due to HIV/AIDS is projected during the 1990s, both in comparison with United Nations projections made before the AIDS pandemic and in comparison with United Nations targets for under-five mortality reduction.

Under the 'low HIV progression' model, this region will have 1.4 million additional under-five deaths due to HIV/AIDS during the decade of the 1990s, a 12% increase over the numbers of under-five deaths projected by the United Nations before the AIDS pandemic.

Under the 'medium HIV progression' model, this region will have 2.1 million additional under-five deaths due to HIV/AIDS during the decade of the 1990s, a 19% increase over the numbers of under-five deaths projected by the United Nations before the AIDS pandemic.

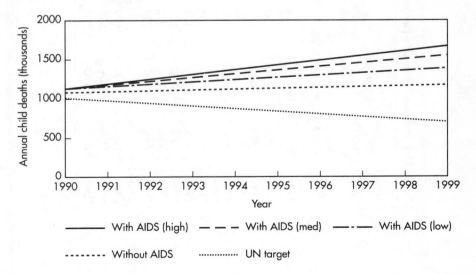

Figure 11.2 Projections of impact of AIDS on under-five deaths ('000s) in 10 African countries

Table 11.1 Projections of annual under-five deaths in ten African countries (1,000s)

Year	UN target for under-five deaths without AIDS (a)	UN projections of under-five deaths without AIDS (b)	Author's projections of under-five deaths due to AIDS (c)			Author's projections of total under-five deaths including AIDS (d)			Author's estimate of % increase in under-five deaths due to AIDS (e)=(c/b)		
			Low	Med	High	Low	Med	High	Low	Med	High
1990	1,008	1,070	44	52	60	1,114	1,122	1,130	4	5	6
1991	984	1,090	65	82	98	1,155	1,172	1,188	6	8	9
1992	956	1,100	90	119	147	1,190	1,219	1,247	8	11	13
1993	926	1,110	108	152	195	1,218	1,262	1,305	10	14	18
1994	892	1,120	127	187	246	1,247	1,307	1,366	11	17	22
1995	854	1,120	147	223	299	1,267	1,343	1,419	13	20	27
1996	815	1,130	168	262	353	1,298	1,392	1,483	15	23	31
1997	772	1,140	190	303	405	1,330	1,443	1,545	17	27	36
1998	726	1,140	213	346	452	1,353	1,486	1,592	19	30	40
1999	676	1,150	237	390	490	1,387	1,540	1,640	21	34	43
Subtotal urban	N/A	N/A	579	816	998	N/A	N/A	N/A	N/A	N/A	N/A
rural	N/A	N/A	810	1,300	1,747	N/A	N/A	N/A	N/A	N/A	N/A
Total	8,609	11,170	1,389	2,116	2,745	12,559	13,286	13,915	12	19	25

Under the 'high HIV progression' model, this region will have 2.7 million additional under-five deaths due to HIV/AIDS during the decade of the 1990s, a 25% increase over the numbers of under-five deaths projected by the United Nations before the AIDS pandemic.

Because this region is overwhelmingly rural, two-thirds of the additional deaths will be in the rural areas, despite the fact that the urban HIV infection rates are currently considerably higher than are the rural rates (Center for International Research, 1989) and despite rapid urbanization. Clearly, the future impact of HIV/AIDS in Africa cannot be seen as a primarily urban problem.

Table 11.2 Projections of impact of AIDS on annual under-five mortality rates (U5MR) in ten African countries (per 1,000 live births)

Year	UN U5MR target	UN project without AIDS	Author's est. including impact of AIDS		
			Low	Med	High
1990	149	158	165	166	167
1991	141	155	165	167	170
1992	133	153	165	169	173
1993	125	150	164	170	176
1994	117	147	163	171	179
1995	109	144	163	172	182
1996	101	141	161	174	185
1997	94	138	161	175	187
1998	86	135	160	176	189
1999	78	132	159	177	189

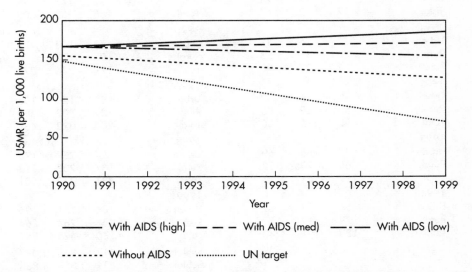

Figure 11.3 Projections of impact of AIDS on annual under-five mortality rates in 10 African countries

The United Nations has previously projected that the U5MR for this region will decline from 158 per 1,000 live births in 1990 to 132 by the year 1999 without the impact of HIV/AIDS (United Nations Department of International Economic and Social Affairs, 1989) and has set a target of a decrease to 149 in 1990 and 78 in 1999 (United Nations, 1980). As Table 11.2 and Figure 11.3 indicate, however, the U5MR is probably already between 165 and 167 per 1000 live birth in 1990 owing to the additional impact of HIV/AIDS (depending on which HIV progression model is used) and is predicted to fall only to 159 by 1999 under the 'low HIV progression' model and to rise to 177 and 189, respectively, under the 'medium' and 'high HIV progression' models.

Projected Numbers of Orphans

As Table 11.3 and Figure 11.4 indicate, the number of women aged 15–49 dying from AIDS in these ten countries will increase dramatically between 1990 and the end of 1999. By the end of the decade 1.5 million women will have died from HIV/AIDS under the 'low HIV progression' model, 2.2 million under the 'medium HIV progression' model and 2.9 million under the 'high HIV progression' model.

Table 11.3 Estimated AIDS mortality in women aged 15–49

	No. of annual deaths from AIDS in women aged 15–49 (1,000s)				No. of annual deaths from AIDS in women aged 15–49 (1,000s)		
	Low	Med	High		Low	Med	High
1990				**1995**			
Urban	27	25	24	Urban	63	86	110
Rural	30	27	25	Rural	92	146	199
Total	57	52	49	Total	155	232	309
1991				**1996**			
Urban	33	35	37	Urban	72	103	133
Rural	40	47	53	Rural	107	173	240
Total	73	82	90	Total	179	276	373
1992				**1997**			
Urban	39	46	52	Urban	82	120	156
Rural	53	69	86	Rural	122	202	282
Total	92	115	138	Total	204	322	438
1993				**1998**			
Urban	47	58	69	Urban	94	139	178
Rural	65	93	122	Rural	137	233	323
Total	112	151	191	Total	231	372	501
1994				**1999**			
Urban	54	72	89	Urban	106	161	195
Rural	79	119	159	Rural	154	264	364
Total	133	191	248	Total	260	425	559
				Subtotal urban	617	845	1,043
				Subtotal rural	879	1,373	1,853
				Total	1,496	2,218	2,896

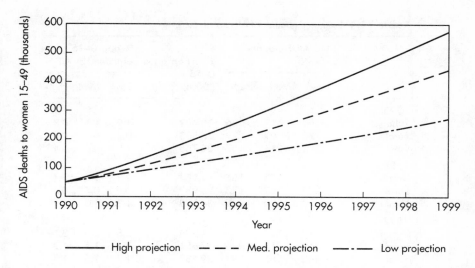

Figure 11.4 Projections of annual AIDS deaths in women aged 15–49 ('000s) in 10 African countries

As shown in Table 11.4 and Figure 11.5, under the low, medium and high HIV progression models, the number of AIDS orphans by the year 2000 will be 3.1 million, 4.3 million and 5.5 million, respectively. This will represent 6.1, 8.5 and 10.9% of the total population of children aged 0–15 in these countries, respectively.

In the 'high HIV progression' model, it was assumed that women became HIV-infected later in the epidemic, and infection was then spread more rapidly than under the 'low' and 'medium' models. Therefore, in the 'high HIV progression'

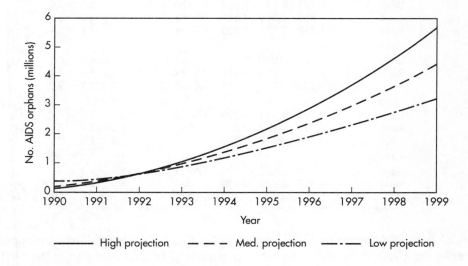

Figure 11.5 Projected number of AIDS orphans (millions) in 10 African countries

Table 11.4 Estimated number of AIDS orphans

	No. AIDS orphans ('000s)			Total pop. aged 0–15 ('000s)	% pop. 0–15 orphaned by AIDS		
	Low	Med	High		Low	Med	High
1990							
Urban	199	117	85	10,432	1.9	1.1	0.8
Rural	173	99	72	26,333	0.7	0.4	0.3
Total	372	216	157	36,765	1.0	0.6	0.4
1991							
Urban	261	183	156	11,184	2.3	1.6	1.4
Rural	249	187	173	26,989	0.9	0.7	0.6
Total	510	370	329	38,173	1.3	1.0	0.9
1992							
Urban	334	269	255	11,936	2.8	2.3	2.1
Rural	348	318	336	27,651	1.3	1.2	1.2
Total	682	587	591	39,587	1.7	1.5	1.5
1993							
Urban	421	378	386	12,689	3.3	3.0	3.0
Rural	470	494	566	28,315	1.7	1.7	2.0
Total	891	872	952	41,004	2.2	2.1	2.3
1994							
Urban	523	513	553	13,442	3.9	3.8	4.1
Rural	616	718	866	28,979	2.1	2.5	3.0
Total	1,139	1,231	1,419	42,421	2.7	2.9	3.3
1995							
Urban	640	675	758	14,194	4.5	4.8	5.3
Rural	789	990	1,240	29,643	2.7	3.3	4.2
Total	1,429	1,665	1,998	43,837	3.3	3.8	4.6
1996							
Urban	775	866	1,066	15,130	5.1	5.7	7.0
Rural	988	1,315	1,689	30,366	3.3	4.3	5.6
Total	1,763	2,181	2,755	45,496	3.9	4.8	6.1
1997							
Urban	929	1,090	1,297	16,067	5.8	6.8	8.1
Rural	1,215	1,693	2,218	31,089	3.9	5.4	7.1
Total	2,144	2,783	3,515	47,156	4.5	5.9	7.5
1998							
Urban	1,103	1,351	1,629	17,003	6.5	7.9	9.6
Rural	1,471	2,127	2,820	31,813	4.6	6.7	8.9
Total	2,574	3,478	4,449	48,816	5.3	7.1	9.1
1999							
Urban	1,300	1,652	1,993	17,939	7.2	9.2	11.1
Rural	1,757	2,620	3,499	32,536	5.4	8.1	10.8
Total	3,057	4,272	5,492	50,475	6.1	8.5	10.9

model, women progress to AIDS and death (and large numbers of orphans appear) later in the 1990s than under the other two models. In the latter part of the 1990s, however, numbers of female deaths and AIDS orphans under the 'high HIV progression' model far surpass those found in the other two models.

DISCUSSION

The projected HIV seroprevalence in women aged 15–49, combined with the large population base and high birth rates in this region, result in very large numbers of child deaths and in numbers of AIDS orphans that will swamp all existing forms of long-term child care. This is even true in countries like Zaire, where the rates of seroprevalence have apparently risen so slowly in the past two to three years that Zaire is held as a model of a country in which HIV seroprevalence rates may have nearly stabilized (N'galy *et al.*, 1988b).

While the impact will vary among countries, no rural or urban area of any country in the region will be untouched.

Under-five Mortality

Increased under-five mortality due to HIV/AIDS has come at a time when Central and East African countries were just beginning to see reductions in under-five mortality as a result, in part, of important child survival interventions such as control of diarrhoeal diseases, immunization against communicable diseases, nutrition interventions, family planning and so forth.

In terms of health service delivery, HIV/AIDS has also come at a time when many Central and East African countries are actually reducing expenditures in the social sectors, including health, owing to economic adjustment programmes. The enormous stress that HIV/AIDS-related child morbidity and mortality put on already overstretched health systems will make it increasingly difficult for health ministries to provide wide-reaching preventive and curative health care to children.

Maternal and child health services also risk threats to their credibility, as mothers associate important interventions such as breastfeeding and immunization with HIV transmission in children. Symptoms of AIDS resemble common child health problems, and children dying because of HIV/AIDS are not often diagnosed as such. Therefore, important interventions such as rehydration therapy and nutrition rehabilitation, which are so remarkably successful in saving children with life-threatening diarrhoea and malnutrition, will often not save children who actually have HIV/AIDS. If HIV infection is not identified and understood, mothers may lose confidence in other important efforts. African parents who perceive increasing child mortality may be less receptive to family planning, which is so critical to improving maternal and child health in Africa. Furthermore, interruption of lactational amenorrhoea in women whose children die because of AIDS before weaning could disturb an important natural birth spacing practice.

While industrialized countries are beginning to find clinical and pharmacological regimes such as azidothymidine (AZT), which prolong and improve the quality of life for a child with AIDS, lack of funding, weak distribution systems and inadequate clinical and laboratory services make these treatments largely inaccessible in Africa.

Prevention of HIV infection in women will be critical to reducing HIV/AIDS-related child mortality, as will breakthroughs in developing a vaccine against HIV and development of treatment modalities for HIV-infected children that are affordable and feasible in the African setting.

Orphanhood

Some orphans have always existed in Central and East Africa resulting from parents' deaths due to war, natural disasters, illness or abandonment for economic or other reasons. Historically, most widespread diseases and epidemics, unlike AIDS, have claimed the very young and elderly, rarely claiming both parents with young children. In wars and civil disturbance, fathers die in fighting but mothers are often spared. With famine or natural disasters, young children often die quickly, leaving few behind as orphans after their parents die. Despite high rates of maternal mortality in Africa, owing to the strong extended family system, orphans usually have been willingly and relatively easily adopted by other family members.

AIDS, however, presents a very different epidemiologic pattern. Major modes of HIV transmission in Africa are heterosexual and mother-to-child. HIV/AIDS claims the lives of infants and adults in their most productive years. Since transmission occurs within a couple, it will be rare to see one parent survive the epidemic when his or her partner or spouse has been HIV infected.

The implications for even the most basic long-term care of these orphans are enormous, both for the small minority of surviving children who are HIV positive and for the large majority who will be HIV negative but may be suspected of being infected. HIV-infected children and those ill with HIV/AIDS will have the greatest need for intensive care. To the extent that their infection or illness is recognized, they will find it most difficult to find homes, owing to fear and discrimination. This discrimination may be based on association of HIV/AIDS with promiscuity, prostitution or any behaviour deemed unacceptable by others (Bledsoe, 1990). The sheer numbers of AIDS orphans will inundate both institutional and non-institutional systems for care.

Four possible outcomes exist for AIDS orphans at present.

1 *Adoption by relatives or non-relatives.* In-country adoptions through the extended family system or by non-relatives are becoming more difficult with the economic and social problems created at the family level by HIV/AIDS and the general economic situation in Africa. Even when children are adopted or fostered, they often receive worse treatment than do natural-born children in the same family (Bledsoe, 1989a, b, 1990). Evidence from Uganda suggests that children who are adopted into an impoverished extended family often find that their education, nutrition and health status suffer acutely from lack of resources (Nalwanga-Sebina and Sengendo, 1987). Sending large numbers of African orphans to industrialized countries for adoption is unrealistic.

2 *Orphanages.* Owing to the extended family system, orphanages in Africa have been heretofore rare. Government orphanages are often poorly equipped and staffed and lack educational, nutritional and health services. Those run by private

organizations (religious or secular) have fared better, but they are expensive and rely upon continuous foreign funding.

While orphanages are often associated with Dickensian conditions, a study of war orphans in Uganda found that, on many criteria, children in orphanages lived in better circumstances than those in foster or adoptive families (Nalwanga-Sebina and Sengendo, 1987).

Orphanages may become increasingly reluctant to accept children whose parents have died of HIV/AIDS because: (a) they fear that HIV-positive children will contaminate the other children; (b) their donors feel HIV-positive children are not a 'good investment'; and (c) most institutions do not have the resources to cope with the special needs of chronically ill children.

3 *Abandonment.* Certainly a number of Central and East African AIDS orphans will join the ranks of the estimated 10 million 'street children' throughout the world (United Nations Children's Fund, 1989) who live in conditions of extreme hardship and, ironically, will become themselves highly vulnerable to HIV infection through the necessity to exchange sexual favours for food and money.

4 *Death.* There is evidence that the morbidity and mortality of young African orphans is higher than that of African infants and children who are in the care of their natural mother (Bledsoe *et al.*, 1988), especially if they are orphaned before they are weaned.

CONCLUSIONS AND RECOMMENDATIONS

In the ten Central and East African countries examined here, HIV/AIDS is projected to cause between one-quarter and half a million additional under-five deaths each year directly owing to HIV/AIDS by the year 2000 and between 1.4 and 2.7 million additional child deaths during the decade of the 1990s. With the additional burden of HIV/AIDS in these countries, under-five mortality rates are projected to be between 159 and 189 per 1,000 live births by the end of the decade – dramatically higher than the previous set UN target of 78 and the UN projection (without AIDS) of 132.

Child deaths from HIV/AIDS will be preceded by recurrent periods of severe morbidity, with HIV-infected infants presenting at health centres with symptoms which resemble common child health problems but which do not respond to standard treatment. The implications of HIV/AIDS-related child morbidity and mortality for the credibility, coverage, quality and impact of child survival programmes in the region are very large.

In terms of coping with this increased child morbidity and mortality, it is recommended that:

1 Increased educational and public health efforts to prevent HIV infection in women (which, in turn, leads to perinatal transmission) should be urgently undertaken.

2 All child health care workers should be trained in diagnosis and treatment of paediatric HIV/AIDS-related illness.

3 Primary health care services should be strengthened to enable them to preserve, if not expand, the coverage of critical child survival interventions such as immunization, control of diarrhoeal diseases, nutrition rehabilitation, family planning, etc., in the face of new demands for services created by HIV/AIDS. These interventions are critical for non-HIV-infected as well as HIV-infected children.

4 Within the existing framework of research, significant priority should be given to adapting HIV/AIDS-related technology initially developed for adults to paediatric AIDS cases, and to making therapeutic advances developed for industrialized countries available and affordable in Africa.

The cumulative number of children aged 0–15 whose mothers will die of AIDS in these ten countries, here defined as AIDS orphans, will increase to between 3.1 and 5.5 million by the year 2000, or between 6 and 11% of all children aged 0–15. These large numbers of orphans will overwhelm any and all historic institutional or informal systems of child care in this region.

Governments and non-governmental agencies must begin preparing now for the problem of AIDS orphans, although at present it has not yet become obvious or generally recognized. It is recommended that:

1 Governments should adopt an integrated policy and programme approach to AIDS orphans which involves all relevant ministries, including health, education, social welfare, rehabilitation, etc. No single sector can independently identify children in need or adequately address their multisectoral problems.

2 Governments and non-governmental organizations should focus on developing culturally acceptable solutions to the problems of AIDS orphans which are community based, as federal-level resources will be insufficient. This will require a more profound understanding of sociological and cultural patterns of family structure and child care in each country.

3 International donor agencies and governments should provide additional financial and technical support to Central and East African countries to enable them to begin to meet the basic needs of AIDS orphans.

4 Governmental and non-governmental inputs for AIDS orphans should be carefully coordinated to avoid duplication, delay and inappropriate or inefficient use of scarce resources.

REFERENCES

Bledsoe, C. (1989a) Differential care of children of previous unions within Mende households in Sierra Leone. Paper presented at the Rockefeller Foundation Exploratory Health Transition Programme, Workshop No. 1. Canberra.

Bledsoe, C. (1989b) Unravelling the trickle-down model within households: foster children and the phenomenon of scrounging. Paper presented at the Rockefeller Foundation Exploratory Health Transition Programme, Workshop No. 2, June 1989, London.

Bledsoe, C. (1990) The politics of AIDS and condoms for stable heterosexual relations in Africa: recent evidence from the local print media, in H. W. Penn (ed.) *Births and Power: The Politics of Reproduction* (Boulder, Colo., Westview Press).

Bledsoe, C. H., Ewbank, D. C. and Isiugo-Abanihe, U. C. (1988) The effect of child fostering on feeding practices and access to health services in rural Sierra Leone, *Social Science and Medicine*, 27, pp. 627–636.

Carswell, J. W. (1987) HIV infection in healthy persons in Uganda, *AIDS*, 1, pp. 223–227.

Center for International Research, US Bureau of the Census (1989) *HIV/AIDS Surveillance Data Base* (Washington, DC, US Bureau of the Census).

Chin, J., Sankaran, G. and Mann, J. M. (1989) Mother-to-infant transmission of HIV: an increasing global problem, in: E. Kessel and A. K. Awan (eds) *Maternal and Child Care in Developing Countries*, pp. 299–306 (Switzerland, Ott).

Davachi, R. and Kabena, M. (1988) Outcome of advanced maternal AIDS in offsprings. Abstract from the IVth International Conference on AIDS in Stockholm.

Hira, S., Bhat, G., Jamanga, J., Mwale, C., Luo, N. and Perine, P. *et al.* (1988) Perinatal transmission of HIV-1 in Lusaka, Zambia. Abstract from the IVth International Conference on AIDS in Stockholm.

Hira, S. K., Kamanga, J., Bhat, G. J., Mwale, C., Tembo, G., Guo, N. and Perine, P. L. (1989) Perinatal transmission of HIV-1 in Zambia, *British Medical Journal*, 299, pp. 1250–1252.

Katz, S.L. and Wilfert, C. M. (1989) Human immunodeficiency virus infection of newborns, *New England Journal of Medicine*, 320, pp. 1687–1689.

Lallement, M., Lallement-Le Coeur, S., Cheynier, D., Nzingoula, S., Jourdain, G., Dsinet, M., Dazza, M. C., Blanche, S., Griscelli, C. and Larouze, B. (1989) Mother–child transmission of HIV-1 and infant survival in Brazzaville, Congo, *AIDS*, 3, pp. 643–646.

Moss, A. R. and Bacchetti, P. (1989) Natural history of HIV infection, *AIDS*, 3, pp. 55-61.

Mworozi, E. A., Ndugwa, C. M., Kataaha, P. K. and Kiguli, S. (1988) Perinatal transmission of HIV infection in Uganda, 0–34 months follow-up. Abstract from the IVth International Conference on AIDS in Stockholm.

N'Galy, B., Ryder, R. W., Bila, K., Mwandagalirwa, K., Colebunders, R. L., Francis, H., Mann, J. M.
and Quinn, T.C. (1988a) Human immunodeficiency virus infection among employees in an African hospital, *New England Journal of Medicine*, 319, pp. 1123–1127.

N'Galy, B., Ryder, R., Francis, H., Hassig, S., Lubaki, M., Duma, M., Nguyen-Dinh, P. and Colebunders, R. (1988b) HIV prevalence in Zaire, 1984 to 1988. Abstract from the IVth International Conference on AIDS in Stockholm.

Nalwanga-Sebina and Sengendo, J. (1987) Orphaned and disabled children in Luwero and Kabale Districts and in Ugandan child care institutions. A comparative profile to the general child population (Kampala).

Norwood, C. (1989) AIDS orphans in New York City: projected numbers and policy demands. Abstract from the Vth International Conference on AIDS in Montreal.

Ntaba, H. M., Liomba, G. N., Schmidt, H. J., Scholhals, C., Gurtier, L. and Deinhardt, F. (1988) HIV-1 prevalence in hospital patients and pregnant women in Malawi. Abstract from the IVth International Conference on AIDS in Stockholm.

Rothenberg, R., Woelfel, M., Stoneburner, R., Milberg, J., Parker, R. and Truman, B. (1987) Survival with the acquired immunodeficiency syndrome – experience with 5,833 cases in New York City, *New England Journal of Medicine*, 317, pp. 1297–1302.

Ryder, R., Nsa, W. and Hassig, S. E. (1989) Perinatal transmission of the human immunodeficiency virus type 1 to infants of seropositive women in Zaire, *New England Journal of Medicine*, 320, pp. 1637–1642.

Uganda Demographic and Health Survey, 1988/89 (1989) *Preliminary Report*. Ministry of Health/Demographic and Health Surveys (DHS) (Columbia Institute for Resource Development).

United Nations (1980) Resolution 35/56, *International Development Strategy for the Third United Nations Development Decade* (New York, United Nations).

United Nations Children's Fund (1989) *Toward an Operational Strategy for Children in Especially Difficult Circumstances* (New York, UNICEF).

United Nations Department of International Economic and Social Affairs (1989) *World Population Prospects 1988*, Population Studies, 106, ST/ESA SER.A. 106 (New York).

Willoughby, A., Mendez, H., Goedert, J., Berthaud, M., Moroso, G., and Sunderland, A. *et al.* (1988) Natural history of infants born to HIV positive women. Abstract from the IVth International Conference on AIDS in Stockholm.

TWELVE

Psychosocial Needs Expressed by the Natural Care-Givers of HIV-Infected Children

Mary Reidy, Marie-Elizabeth Taggart and Line Asselin

INTRODUCTION

Vast, though perhaps inadequate, resources are being devoted to the prevention and cure of acquired immune deficiency syndrome (AIDS). However, little has been done to understand or develop one of our most essential resources: the natural care-givers of those who are infected by HIV. The infected person requires the help and support of someone close to him, if he is to avoid frequent lengthy hospitalizations and heavy dependence on costly health services, even early in the evolution of this disease. The child who is HIV positive, in his need for normal human nurturing and for the care necessitated by his illness, becomes doubly dependent and the natural care-giver who assumes his care becomes doubly burdened.

AIDS now affects an ever-increasing number of women and children all over the globe and it is estimated that during the 1990s this syndrome will be the cause of death of 3,000,000 women and children worldwide (Mann, 1989; Cabanes *et al.*, 1990). Chin (1990) has estimated, for women aged 15–49 years, a prevalence per 100,000 ranging from a low of 30 in Asia through 70 in Europe, 140 in North America and 200 in South America, to a high of 2,500 in Africa. In Europe, where more than 30,000 cases were declared in 1990, France had the greatest absolute number of women with AIDS, but Switzerland was equal in relative number (Cabanes *et al.*, 1990).

Maternal and infantile AIDS is also steadily increasing in both Canada and the United States (Ultmann *et al.*, 1987; Boland, 1987; Guyonet, 1991). In the latter, it is estimated that, by the end of the year 1991, 10,000–20,000 children will be infected by HIV and one paediatric bed in ten will be occupied by an infected child (Meyers and Weitzman, 1991; Oleske *et al.*, 1988). In Canada, the cumulative incidence of AIDS in women aged 18–44 reached a rate three to four times higher in the province of Quebec than in any other part of the country; and as might be expected it is in this province that one finds the greater proportion of infected children (Hankins and Lapointe, 1989; Centre Féderal sur le SIDA, 1990). The mode of transmission is in most cases (95%) perinatal, the infection is distributed more or less equally by sex, and fewer than one-third of these children will develop an immune deficit during the first year of their lives (Wishon and Gee, 1989; Blanche, 1990; Tricoire and Robert, 1990).

Whether in the adult or in the child, AIDS affects essentially the pulmonary, digestive, nervous and tegumentary systems and the reduction in immunity encourages the development of bacterial, viral, fungal and parasitical infections. The infected person suffers from such symptoms as weight loss, difficulty in swallowing, fatigue, recurrent diarrhoea and, in the later stages of the illness, possibly blindness and dementia (Ryan, 1984; Safai, 1985; Perry and Jacobsen, 1986). Further, the infected child is subject to retardation in growth and development, regression in behaviour, mental retardation, psychomotor and neurological disturbances and chronic encephalopathology (Crocker, 1989; Diamond, 1989; Harrison, 1989). While pain is often associated with such conditions as pneumonia, herpes, lymphadenopathy and attacks on the central nervous system (Durham and Cohen, 1987; Williams, 1989), current AIDS literature provides little information about its evolution. However, the paediatric literature concerning pain indicates that it is a complex phenomenon affecting both cognitive and psychomotor development (Dolgin and Phipps, 1989; Johnston, 1989; Varni *et al.*, 1989), which can be evaluated in infants and young children through the systematic observation of its clinical manifestation (Gauvain-Piquard, 1990).

AIDS is, on the one hand, a terminal disease with severe signs and symptoms which requires frequent and intensive medical intervention; and on the other hand, it is a progressive chronic disease which necessitates long-term family commitment and involvement. Meyers and Weitzman (1991) suggest that the health system should begin thinking of and responding to AIDS as a major chronic childhood illness. However, the very nature of the disease, its cause and transmission, and the particular relationship between sick child and his natural care-giver, necessarily makes the problems of AIDS different from that of other chronic childhood diseases. The presence of an infected child in a family (with perhaps the exception of the small number of haemophiliacs and transfusion-infected children) means almost necessarily the presence of one or more infected adults, one of whom is almost always the mother. The problem, in such a situation, is not primarily that of a child and his illness but rather that of an entire family (Weil-Halprin, 1989). Authors, discussing this phenomenon, describe the difficulties of a parent's caring for a child when she herself is frightened of being sick or is already sick and facing frequent hospitalizations. These difficulties are often increased by a conspiracy of silence in the face of a positive diagnosis of either parent or child and the social isolation attendant on maintaining such a silence (Kübler-Ross, 1988; Cooper *et al.*, 1988; Lewis and Thomson, 1989). As the burden of care becomes heavier, as anxiety for the future increases and as intrafamilial conflicts are heightened, the family closes in on itself, deprived of most sources of information and of external aid and support (Tiblier, 1987; Kübler-Ross, 1989; Mansour, 1990). While family organization tends to become nuclear, with a poor support system, those close to them are called upon to contribute to the care of infected family members and to form a new family structure (Iazetti, 1986; St-Jacques, 1988; Lloyd, 1988; Flaskereud, 1989).

NEEDS OF THE NATURAL CARE-GIVER OF THE CHILD WITH HIV INFECTION

The emotional reactions and the needs of these care-givers is believed to be similar to those of parents of children suffering from other fatal diseases such as cancer (Boland and Gaskill, 1984; Klug, 1986). However, the added burden of the mother's actual or anticipated illness and the possibility of either socio-cultural divergence from the cultural mainstream or of a high-risk lifestyle make it difficult to either identify or to meet the needs of the natural care-givers of the child faced with AIDS (Coates *et al.*, 1984). These needs have, to some extent, been described in the American literature on paediatric AIDS (Boland and Gaskill, 1984; Klug, 1986; Bennett, 1987; Belfer *et al.*, 1988). However, these reports tend to be fragmented in scope and limited in content and are often based on clinical observations of a small number of clients rather than on systematic investigation (Christ and Weiner, 1985; Cohen and Weisman, 1986; Salisbury, 1986).

The needs model, developed by Henderson (1966) to guide nursing practice, provides a conceptual framework which permits a heuristic classification of this diverse literature. This framework, based on Thorndike's needs theory (1940), views human functioning in terms of 14 basic needs, each of which possesses, to a greater or lesser extent, a psychosocial component. It provides the nurse with a structure for classification and evaluation of the fundamental needs of the client in sickness and in health. The role of the nurse, apart from the co-identification of needs with the client, is that of helping the client to meet current needs while developing strategies for meeting these or other emerging needs in the future.

The stress and distress felt by the natural care-giver faced with the evolution of a chronic and fatal illness in a dependent family member constitutes one of the most acute problems in the domain of paediatric AIDS (Lapointe, 1988; Kübler-Ross, 1989; Flaskereud, 1989; Schwartz, 1989). In keeping with the conclusions of these authors and with the literature concerning parents of children with other life-threatening disorders, we focused our inquiry on the five primarily psychosocial, fundamental needs (Henderson, 1966; as adapted by Adam, 1983) which are amenable to intervention by the health professional. Consequently, we have classified and presented the following literature according to the needs of the natural care-giver, to feel useful, to learn to communicate, to know how to maintain physical integrity and to act according to personal beliefs and values.

The need 'to maintain physical integrity' is broad in scope and encompasses many physiological aspects (Adam, 1983). Here, because of our focus on the psychosocial, we have retained only its cognitive component. It might be restated more specifically as the need to possess that knowledge which is fundamental to the maintenance of bodily integrity in this particular situation. The natural care-giver needs to understand the threat posed by AIDS as well as the susceptibility of family members to this disease, and to know the daily precautions necessary to prevent the spread of the infection to others in the household or in the child's social environment, and the hygienic measures needed to reduce the secondary infections associated with this virus (Nelson and Album, 1987; St Jacques, 1988).

The fulfilment of the need 'to learn' implies continued acquisition of knowledge and information, whether necessary to satisfy curiosity or to understand, evaluate and deal with life events (Adams, 1983). A seropositive diagnosis, with or without symptoms, provokes a multitude of questions as the natural care-giver struggles to cope, and to help the family and the child live with this devastating event. Many are troubled by unanswered questions about the clinical manifestations and the evolution of the infection, the care required by the child and the way in which death would come (Bennett, 1987; Tiblier, 1987; Mansour, 1990). Granting the variation introduced by intellectual development, interest, openness and education, a failure to meet this need serves to increase tension and to reduce the ability to cope with a threatening situation (Waters *et al.*, 1988).

The strength of the need 'to act according to a set of beliefs and values' is associated with the degree of internalization of a more or less explicit ideology or philosophy. This need is related to the moral or spiritual life, whether or not of a religious nature, which guides life decisions and supports the individual in times of trouble (Adams, 1983). The acceptance of the responsibility to care for a child with AIDS, or likely to develop AIDS, is in itself a statement of values and attitudes. However, this task easily leads to feelings of helplessness and often to a questioning of previous beliefs or sources of inner strength. In other cases this feeling of helplesness and the approach of death for themselves or a loved one led to a renewal of religious practices or to a re-examination of beliefs and values (St Jacques, 1988; Weil-Halpern, 1988). These sentiments are accentuated by a very real fear of death and the unknown (Iazetti, 1986; St Jacques, 1988).

The need 'to communicate' is concerned with interpersonal relationships and encompasses all verbal and non-verbal conveyance of ideas, opinions, feelings, attitudes and demands for and offers of help (Adams, 1983). However, the reaction engendered by the presence of this infection in a family member makes it difficult on the part of a natural care-giver to have this need fulfilled. Not only are feelings of shame and guilt provoked by the social stigma associated with this illness, but also certain care-givers, because of their high-risk lifestyles, feel directly responsible for the transmission of this childhood infection (Klug, 1986). These feelings on the part of the child's immediate family group are well justified by the ostracism often imposed by the extended family, friends, health professionals and the general public. Such reactions contribute to social isolation and reduce both the availability of social support and their ability to ask for help (Iazetti, 1986; Lloyd, 1988; Mansour, 1990).

The need 'to feel worth while and useful' encompasses the process of self-realization and the feeling of accomplishment of an individual in the role of a family member, at work or during social activities (Adam, 1983). However, the energies and resources of a family are quickly strained when the AIDS virus infects a child; the natural care-giver is easily overwhelmed and paralysed by the demands put on her, and soon tends to feel useless (Bennett, 1987). Difficult conjugal situations (such as single parenthood, abandonment or the death of an AIDS-infected spouse), frequently coupled with the incertitude of a high-risk lifestyle, entailing feelings of uselessness and a loss of control in child raising, accentuate a lack of confidence in parental abilities. Such parents or care-givers suffer from a lack of confidence in their abilities, feelings of powerlessness and loss of control in the care and raising of both their infected and non-infected children (Klug, 1986; Waters *et al.*, 1988; Lewis and Thomson, 1989).

Paediatric AIDS, with the likely infection of both mother and child, evinces further loss of autonomy and an increase in financial dependence. If the mother is the primary wage earner, she faces loss of income for time taken from work for treatment or diagnosis; if in addition she herself is infected, she faces eventual loss of employment and the need for financial assistance in the form of welfare. Further, with time, the demands of the child's, and of her own, condition will increase as her human and financial resources decrease. Her feelings of worth are further threatened as she, if she is not to abandon the child, relinquishes to another family member, fully or in part, the role of natural care-giver (Boland 1987; Tiblier, 1987). If this role is assumed by a grandmother or aunt, the stresses and conflicts in the family are in turn reintensified as she assumes, more or less willingly, the double burden of care. Her needs are similar and no more likely to be met than those of the natural mother (Flaskereud, 1989).

THE PRESENT STUDY

Despite this mosaic of information from a variety of sources, there appeared to be little systematic research reported on the needs of the care-givers as they themselves perceive such needs, and none available particular to the needs of a francophone, in part Haitian, population of natural care-givers of children infected by the retrovirus. We felt that a more global approach would provide the type of knowledge basic to the development of intervention strategies tailored to the needs of such families. We therefore carried out a comprehensive analysis of psychosocial needs of the natural care-givers of children infected or in danger of being infected perinatally by HIV, as reported by these natural care-givers themselves.

METHODS

The aim of our study was to describe, according to their perceptions, the psychosocial needs of these care-givers. By the term natural care-giver, we mean any person, whether biological parent or other adult in a non-professional relationship (aunt, grandmother, friend, etc.), who cares for or who participates in the care of the child on a regular basis, at home.

While the sample of children were of three sub-types, unknown serology, seropositive non-symptomatic and seropositive symptomatic, the source of infection or possible infection was in all cases perinatal. The availability sample of 30 natural care-givers consisted of mothers ($n = 13$), other significant persons ($n = 12$) and fathers ($n = 5$). They were recruited from 21 families followed by the multidisciplinary team of a paediatric AIDS research unit at a large urban hospital in the province of Quebec.

Because of the nature and subject of this research and the current availability of pertinent scientific writings, we were unable to find an already validated instrument for data collection. We, therefore, developed and validated a questionnaire proper to this study. The preliminary part of the instrument was designed to amass the usual socio-demographic information, the main body to collect data concerning the target variables of the study. The concepts (or specific needs) included were first identified through an intensive review of the paediatric AIDS literature. Next, these concepts were reclassified according to the five general fundamental needs, which include a strong psychosocial component (Henderson, 1966). The final instrument consisted of 35 items, each representing a specific need, each completed by a four-level Likert scale of 'importance' and of 'satisfaction'. Finally a series of open-ended questions were integrated into the questionnaire. This was done in order to allow the subjects to elaborate further, when desired, on the pre-coded responses and to discuss such needs as had not been included in the itemized list of specific needs.

Content validity was assured by submitting the instrument to two separate groups of judges. The first was composed of five health professionals working in the domain of AIDS; the second included 18 master's level nursing students. Each group looked at the universality of the set of items and the exclusivity and clarity of individual items. The former group also paid particular attention to the appropriateness of language, with consideration of the socio-economic characteristics of the target population. Minor modifications were carried out according to their recommendations. Taking into account the limited number of target families at the time the study was begun (1989), the final version of the instrument was pre-tested with only two natural care-givers. Each came from a family of a different ethnic origin: one French-Canadian, the other Haitian.

Data collection, using this questionnaire in the form of a semi-structured interview, was carried out in the respondents' homes or at the hospital clinic which followed the sick children (according to the preference of the respondents). Their verbal answers to the open-ended questions were recorded by the interviewer. She also read to them the scaled items and then recorded their responses. This approach was adopted in order to humanize the exploration of the needs of a fragile population as well as to take into account the presence of illiteracy in about one-third of our sample.

The importance and the satisfaction of specific needs were calculated in terms of each of the five general fundamental needs mentioned above. Analyses of variance for repeated measures (ANOVA) permitted us to determine if there were significant differences in the importance and in the level of satisfaction of these specific needs. These analyses were carried out by means of the Reliability Procedure of SPSS, and are justified by the fact that they are applicable to a test of comparison of means of items. They are more powerful than non-parametric methods, and with a sample of 30 subjects they are robust with regard to the postulate relative to the form of the distribution, even according to the principle of the theorem of central limits. Finally, pairwise comparisons (TUKEY-HSD) permitted us to identify which of the specific needs were seen as the most important and as the most satisfied by the natural care-givers. Tables 12.1 to 12.6 illustrate the most important results concerning the specific needs, grouped according to the five general fundamental needs retained in this study. It should be noted in the interpretation of mean scores of both importance and satisfaction that the range of possible scores for each item is 1 to 4.

RESULTS

Profile of the Care-givers

The natural care-givers who participated in this study care for children who are HIV-positive or who are at risk of becoming positive. They live in greater Montreal and they are either the mothers of the infected children (43%), other significant persons such as a grandmother or feminine member of a foster family (40%) or fathers (17%). The families are equally distributed between two ethnic groups: Haitians and French-Canadians. Fifty per cent are single-parent families headed by mothers, most of whom were abandoned by their partner within the 18 months following the diagnosis of AIDS within the family. Incomes ($5,000–10,000/year) are below the mean of $19,177 reported for Canadian single-parent families (Statistics Canada, 1986). The source of this income is, for the most part, either revenue from the work of one family member (48%) or welfare (33%). Most of the children from these families (76%) are aged between one month and two years. Where the family has only one child, 62% of these children are still in the indeterminate stage of seroposivity because of their age.

General and Specific Fundamental Needs

THE NEED 'TO MAINTAIN PHYSICAL INTEGRITY'
In this study, the natural care-givers identified three specific cognitive needs associated with the general fundamental need 'to maintain physical integrity' (Table 12.1). They state that they need to know the modes of transmission of HIV infection, how to prevent the spread of the infection and how to protect the infected person from other types of infection. There is little difference in the importance

accorded to each of these needs. However, the need to know how to protect the child from other possible infections is the least studied of these three specific needs, whatever its importance.

Table 12.1 Perception of the importance and of the level of satisfaction of the need 'to maintain physical integrity'

Specific need (n = 30)	Importance of the need		Satisfaction of the need	
	Mean	s.d.	Mean	s.d.
Need to:				
Understand the means of transmission of HIV	3.43	4.92	3.53	0.78
Know how to prevent the transmission of HIV	3.10	1.18	3.10	1.18
Know how to protect the person infected by HIV from other types of infection	3.30	1.08	2.73	1.26
Results of ANOVA	$F(2.58) = 2.5$ not significant		$F(2.58) = 5.2$ $P < 0.05$	
Results of pairwise comparisons (TUKEY, HSD)	–		need 1 > 3	

THE NEED 'TO LEARN'

As concerns the general need 'to learn' the natural care-givers of this study (Table 12.2) accord great importance to the specific needs: to obtain honest answers to their questions; to be informed and kept up to date on the evolution and treatment of AIDS; to know the different roles of the health professional with whom they come into contact; to have written information made available to them; and to learn how to deal with stress. According to the pairwise comparisons the first three of these needs are better met by the multidisciplinary team than the other four needs. The last two needs, according to the spontaneous comments made during the

Table 12.2 Perception of the importance and of the level of satisfaction of the need 'to learn'

Specific need (n = 30)	Importance of the need		Satisfaction of the need	
	Mean	s.d.	Mean	s.d.
Need to:				
Obtain honest answers	3.73	0.69	3.27	0.98
Be informed of the evolution, the prognosis and the treatments for AIDS	3.63	0.76	2.83	1.15
Have written information about AIDS	3.10	1.29	1.77	1.30
Known how to cope with the stress associated with the condition	2.50	1.48	1.43	0.82
Learn the role(s) of the various health professionals at the hospital	3.13	1.19	2.43	1.33
Be informed about the availability of support groups	2.20	1.40	1.93	1.26
Be consulted about who will be included in the discussion of their family problem with HIV	1.80	1.16	1.20	0.66
Results of ANOVA	$F(7.202) = 11.2$ $P < 0.05$		$F(7.203) = 12.0$ $P < 0.05$	
Results of pairwise comparisons (TUKEY, HSD)	needs 1, 2 > 4, needs 3, 5 > 6, 7 6, 7		needs 1, 2 > 3, need 5 > 4, 7 4, 6, 7	

interviews, tended to be met in those cases where a special endeavour was made on the part of the care-givers to seek help.

A comparison of the importance of the specific need 'to deal with stress' in terms of the sex of the care-giver reveals that it is more often the women of the study who consider it to be very important ($P = 0.034$). Nevertheless, it was the mothers of single parent families who expressed the lowest level of satisfaction of this particular need ($P = 0.077$). It is plausible to accept that this reflects the reality of their lives, where the multiple stresses of a financial, psychological, pathological and social nature emerge.

THE NEED 'TO ACT ACCORDING TO A SET OF BELIEFS AND VALUES'

The need to be respected by the hospital personnel, for doing what they believe is 'right', is both the most important of the specific needs identified by the care-givers and the best met within this category of general fundamental needs (Table 12.3). The discussion of death is seen, on the other hand, as both the least important and the least well met. The spontaneous comments of several natural care-givers during the interview would lead one to believe that the relative importance of these two needs reflects the worth accorded to living with the stricken member of the family as compared with that of coming to terms with the approaching death of that member.

Table 12.3 Perception of the importance of the level of satisfaction of the need 'to act according to a set of beliefs and values'

Specific need (n = 30)	Importance of the need		Satisfaction of the need	
	Mean	s.d.	Mean	s.d.
Need to:				
Discuss beliefs and values	2.77	1.38	2.40	1.35
Be respected by the hospital personnel	3.37	1.07	3.40	1.00
To discuss death with health professionals	1.73	1.26	1.57	1.07
Results of ANOVA	$F(2.58) = 14.4$		$F(2.58) = 18.2$	
	$P < 0.05$		$P < 0.05$	
Results of pairwise comparisons (TUKEY, HSD)	needs 1, 2 > 3		need 1 > 3	
			need 2 > 1, 3	

THE NEED 'TO COMMUNICATE'

In this needs analysis, communication with both the formal (Table 12.4) and the informal (Table 12.5) networks of resource persons was considered. The results presented in Table 12.4 indicate that the care-givers perceive that being kept up to date on the condition of the child and being able to speak of their feelings and reactions are the most important and best satisfied of the specific needs associated with the formal network of resource persons. It is interesting to note that, according to their comments, none of the natural care-givers belong to a parental self-help group and that being part of such a group is not seen as important.

Table 12.4 Perception of the importance and of the level of satisfaction of the need 'to communicate' with a formal network of resource persons

Specific need (n = 30)	Importance of the need		Satisfaction of the need	
	Mean	s.d.	Mean	s.d.
Need to:				
Be kept up to date on the child's condition	3.70	0.70	3.27	1.06
Discuss feelings and reactions	3.13	1.14	2.48	1.15
Be helped to face the reactions of those close to them	1.97	1.35	1.31	0.81
Be helped with their financial problems	2.03	1.30	1.62	1.01
Be part of a group of parents	1.83	1.20	1.00*	0.00
Results of ANOVA	$F(4.116) = 18.0$ $P < 0.05$		$F(3.84) = 23.4$ $P < 0.05$	
Results of pairwise comparisons (TUKEY, HSD)	needs 1, 2 > 3, 4, 5		needs 1, 2 > 3, 4	

* Item not integrated into the analysis because the variance is null.

Within the informal social network, the care-givers see it as most important to be able to count on those closest to them, and on their families. Being integrated into their religious community comes next, and their perception of the importance of the support of a spouse is found to be fourth in importance. The level of satisfaction of these needs seems congruent with the reported levels of importance, except for that of being able to count on those near to them. It is interesting to note that none of the care-givers feel that this need has been satisfied.

Table 12.5 Perception of the importance and of the level of satisfaction of the need 'to communicate' with an informal network of resource persons

Specific need (n = 30)	Importance of the need		Satisfaction of the need	
	Mean	s.d.	Mean	s.d.
Need to:				
Be close to a 'mate'	2.20	1.45	2.04	1.30
Be close to their family of origin	2.53	1.31	2.13	1.22
Be close to a friend	1.93	1.36	1.61	1.12
Be close to a neighbour	1.20	0.66	1.08	0.29
Be close to a religious group	2.47	1.50	1.52	1.50
Be able to count on those close to them	3.27	1.00	–	–
Results of ANOVA	$F(5.145) = 11.38$ $P < 0.05$		$F(4.85) = 6.8$ $P < 0.05$	
Results of pairwise comparisons (TUKEY, HSD)	needs 1, 2, 5 > 4 need 6 > 1, 3, 4		needs 1, 2, 5 > 4 need 5 > 3	

THE NEED 'TO FEEL WORTH WHILE AND USEFUL'

In order to feel useful and of some worth, the natural care-givers of this study accord the greatest importance to the need to be supported by the personnel of the hospital who follow the infected children, as they continue to give the care these children need (Table 12.6). They also rate the need for a low-cost day nursery as being very important. In comments made to the interviewers, this was seen as a way to give them some time to be free to 'feel like a person again', 'to get away for bit', 'to be able to go on coping' or to have a chance 'to work a little'. Both of these needs seem to be satisfied in direct proportion to their importance. However, the need to continue social activities is considered to be neither very important nor to be well satisfied. Comments made by certain of the care-givers indicate that in the family crisis situation provoked by the AIDS infection, it seems more important 'to ration energies' or 'to stick with the family' than to socialize.

Table 12.6 Perception of the importance and of the level of satisfaction of the need 'to feel worth while and useful'

Specific need (n = 30)	Importance of the need		Satisfaction of the need	
	Mean	s.d.	Mean	s.d.
Need to:				
Be supported by the health professionals maintaining their ordinary life and care of the infected child	3.27	0.94	3.33	1.03
Have day care services made available	3.00	1.26	2.63	1.27
Maintain their social activities	1.70	1.06	1.43	0.82
Results of ANOVA	$F(2.58) = 22.9$		$F(2.58) = 2.33$	
	$P < 0.05$		$P < 0.05$	
Results of pairwise comparisons (TUKEY, HSD)	needs 1, 2 > 3		need 1 > 2, 3 need 2 > 3	

Other Needs Expressed by the Natural Care-givers

The care-givers, in responding to a series of open-ended questions, identified 24 different needs. While most of these were already included in the scaled items of the questionnaire, certain do not even seem to have been discussed, as yet, in the paediatric AIDS literature. These needs can be grouped into three main categories: needs for formal support, needs of an emotional nature and needs of an instrumental or functional nature. The first of these categories incorporates the need for continuity of care. They feel that they need to see and develop a relationship with the professionals who follow their family; they need to see the same individual, not just the same type of professional. They also indicate that they require the help of a professional such as a psychologist to help them deal with their feelings and fears.

Needs of an emotional nature include the need to be helped to react appropriately to the changes in the child's behaviour following numerous hospitalizations, to be supported and guided in explaining the repercussions of the disease to the child when he reached an appropriate age and, for the mothers who were sick, to know who would look after their children after their death. Seropositive fathers whose partners had already died feel the need for a new partner to share their lives and to regain an active sex life.

Instrumental needs expressed by the care-givers consist of the need for: aid with household tasks (particularly by the mothers who were seropositive and who wished to remain at home as long as possible in a calm environment); transport for their children for their consultations at the hospital; help in writing letters and paying bills; and monetary aid in order to reduce the chronic penury in which they live.

DISCUSSION

The results of our study underline the fact that the natural care-givers of children infected or at risk of being infected by AIDS are cognitively, socially and financially circumscribed by the impact of AIDS. As seen in the literature, hard pressed as these care-givers are, they try to ignore all but the most basic or immediate of their personal needs, and tend to organize family life around the most urgent needs of the infected child (St Jacques, 1988). These observations parallel those of American authors, who conclude that such care-givers are in danger of becoming burned out, physically and emotionally, by the stress brought on by this infection (Krener, 1987; Kübler-Ross, 1988; Waters *et al.*, 1988). This process is intensified by isolation and by the tendency to communicate only with those closest to them. This conspiracy of silence is noted by other authors in the domain of AIDS generally, as well as that of paediatric AIDS (Iazetti, 1986; Klug, 1986; Nelson and Album, 1987).

It is important to note that many of the subjects of this study try simultaneously to come to terms with the sick role as well as that of care-giver and parent of a sick child. This double burden, personal and familial, increases the magnitude of their reaction to the illness. In sum, they must cope with the diagnosis of an HIV infection not just in themselves but also in another member of their family.

In brief, the distress engendered by the presence of this chronic and fatal viral illness provokes a reaction, on the part of the natural care-giver of the HIV-positive child, which is concretized in the form of a series of specific needs. According to Henderson (1966), the role of the nurse is to help maintain or restore the client's independence in the meeting of his needs. The results of this study allow a better understanding of the psychosocial aspects of the fundamental needs of a specific target population. It would seem appropriate, given these results, to begin to develop strategies of intervention, proper to the nurse of the interdisciplinary health team, and to study the impact of such strategies in the form of a quasi-experimental evaluative research. Any such intervention must take into account the needs for knowledge, support and communication, which are intensified by the circumstances of the life of the natural care-giver and of the illness of the infected family members.

Further, the family situation of the care-giver of the HIV-infected child, as discussed in this study, leads us to the recommendation that it is important and timely to consider at least three longitudinal studies. The first should study the evolution of the health (physical, psychological and social) of the natural care-giver, whether as parent or as an individual who assumes the role; the second should describe the mourning process of the mother who is losing both herself and her child to AIDS; and the third should investigate the parenting and nurturing patterns within the HIV-infected family, considering the needs imposed by the illness and by the growth and development of the HIV-positive child. Other interesting directions for research would be the comparison of the needs of care-givers who are themselves positive with those who are not infected, of the needs of care-givers of single-child families with those of families with more than one child or of the needs of foster care-givers with those of the biological parent care-giver.

In conclusion, this research is a study of the psychosocial needs of a particular sub-population of natural care-givers of chronically ill children. It was intended to be systematic, comprehensive and global in light of the fragmentary nature of much of the current literature. However, we have found that the identified needs tend to be both congruent with much of this literature and fundamental to the general population of care-givers rather than being specific to our group of care-givers of AIDS-infected children. Further, the great range and variety of needs described by different researchers and clinicians documented are substantiated by the perceptions of the care-givers themselves.

REFERENCES

Adam, E. (1983) *Etre infirmière* (Montréal, HRW Ltée).

Belfer, L. M., Krener, K. P. and Miller, B. F. (1988) AIDS in children and adolescents, *Journal of American Academy of Child and Adolescents Psychiatry*, 27 (2), pp. 147–151.

Bennett, K. (1987) A generation of children at risk, *Journal of Psychosocial Nursing*, 25 (12), pp. 32–34.

Blanche, S. (1990) Profil évolutif de l'infection à VLH de l'enfant, *La revue du practicien*, 40 (2), pp. 124–126.

Boland, G. M. (1987) The child with AIDS: Special concerns, in: D. J. Durham and L. F. Cohen (eds) *The Person with AIDS, Nursing Perspective*, pp. 192–210 (New York, Springer).

Boland, G. M. and Gaskill, T. (1984) Managing AIDS in children, *Men: The American Journal of Maternal Child Nursing*, 9 (6), pp. 384–389.

Cabanes, P. A. and Chevalier, E. (1990) Epidémiologie de l'infection à VIH et du SIDA chez la femme et l'enfant, in: Centre international de l'enfance (eds) *SIDA enfant famille: les implications pour l'enfant et la famille*, pp. 17–35 (Paris).

Centre Fédéral sur le SIDA (1990) *Mise à jour de surveillance: le SIDA au Canada* (Ottawa).

Chin, J. (1990) Current and future dimensions of the HIV/AIDS pandemic in women and children, *Lancet*, 336, pp. 221–224.

Christ, G. H. and Weiner, L. S. (1985) Psychosocial issues in AIDS, in: J. R. Vincent, S. Devita and A. S. Rosenberg (eds) *AIDS: Etiology, Diagnosis, Treatment and Prevention*, pp. 275–297 (Philadelphia, J. B. Lippincott).

Coates, J. T., Temoshok, L. and Mandel, J. (1984) Psychosocial research is essential to understanding and treating AIDS, *American Psychologist*, 39 (11), pp. 1309–1314.

Cohen, M. A. and Weisman, W. H. (1986) A biopsychosocial approach to AIDS, *Psychosomatics*, 27 (4), pp. 245–249.

Cooper, E. R., Pelton, S. L. and Lemay, M. (1988) Acquired immunodeficiency syndrome: a new population of children at risk, *The Pediatric Clinics of North America*, 35 (6), pp. 1365–1387.

Crocker, A. E. (1989) Developmental services children with HIV infection, *Mental Retardation*, 27, pp. 223–225.

Diamond, G. W. (1989) Developmental problems in children with HIV infection, *Mental Retardation*, 27, pp. 213–217.

Dolgin, M. J. and Phipps, S. (1989) Pediatric pain: the parent's role, *Pediatrician*, 16, pp. 103–109.

Durham, J. and Cohen, F. L. (1987) *The Person with AIDS: Nursing Perspectives* (New York, Springer).

Flaskereud, J. H. (1989) Psychosocial and neuropsychiatric aspects in: J. H. Flaskereud (ed.) *AIDS/ HIV Infection: A Reference Guide for Nursing Professionals*, pp. 145–168 (Philadelphia, W. B. Saunders).

Gauvain-Piquard, A. (1990) Le nourrisson qui a mal, *L'enfant*, 2, pp. 101–111.

Guyonnet, M. (1991) L'enfant atteint du SIDA, *L'infirmière canadienne*, 1, pp. 38–42.

Hankins, C. and Lapointe, N. (1989) Epidémiologie de l'infection VIH, *Revue canadienne de santé publique*, 80, S24–S26.

Harrison, T. (1989) Children with AIDS, *Nursing Times*, 85 (43), pp. 64–65.

Henderson, V. (1966) *The Nature of Nursing* (New York, Macmillan).

Iazetti, L. (1986) Nursing management of the pediatrics AIDS patient, *Issues in Comprehensive Pediatric Nursing*, 9 (2), pp. 119–129.

Johnston, C. C. (1989) Pain assessment and management in infants, *Pediatrician*, 16, pp. 16–23.

Klug, R. (1986) Children with AIDS, *American Journal of Nursing*, 86, pp. 1126–1132.

Krener, G. P. (1987) Impact of the diagnosis of AIDS on hospital care of an infant, *Clinical Pediatrics*, 26 (1), pp. 30–34.

Kübler-Ross, E. (1989) *SIDA, un ultime défi à la société* (Canada, Editions Alain Stanké).

Lapointe, B. (1988) L'approche psychosociale du patient séro-positif au VIH, *L'actualité médicale*, March, pp. 25–30.

Lewis, K. B. and Thomson, H. B. (1989) Infants, children, adolescents, in: J. H. Flaskereud (ed.) *AIDS/HIV Infection: A Reference Guide for Nursing Professionals*, pp. 111–127 (Philadelphia, W. B. Saunders).

Lloyd, G. A. (1988) HIV infection, AIDS and family disruption, in: A. F. Fleming *et al.* (eds) *The Global Impact of AIDS*, pp. 183–190 (New York, Alan R. Liss).

Mann, J. (1989) La mère, l'enfant et la stratégie mondiale de lutte contre le SIDA. *Actes de la Conférence internationale sur les implications du SIDA pour la mère et l'enfant*, Paris.

Mansour, S. (1990) Les retentissements psychologiques de l'infection à VIH sur l'enfant et sa famille in: *Synthèses bibliographiques: SIDA, enfant, famille*. Centre international de l'enfance, pp. 75–83.

Meyers, A. and Weitzman, M. (1991) Pediatric HIV disease: the newest chronic illness of childhood, *Pediatric Clinics of North America*, 38 (1), pp. 169–172.

Nelson, P. L. and Album, M. M. (1987) Children with HIV infection and their families, *Journal of Dentistry for Children*, 54 (5), pp. 353–358.

Oleske, J. J., Connor, M. and Boland, M. (1988) A perspective on pediatric AIDS, *Pediatric Annals*, 17, 319–321.

OMS/GPA (1989) La santé des mères et des enfants dans le contexte de l'infection à VIH/SIDA. Genève.

Perry, S. and Jacobsen, P. (1986) Neuropsychiatric manifestations of AIDS, Spectrum disorders, *Hospital and Community Psychiatry*, 37, pp. 135–142.

Ryan, L. J. (1984) AIDS: a threat to physical and psychological integrity, *Topics in Clinical Nursing*, 7, pp. 19–25.

Safai, B. (1985) The natural history of Kaposi's sarcoma in acquired immunodeficiency syndrome, *Annals of Internal Medicine*, 103 (5), pp. 744–750.

St-Jacques, A. (1988) Families sans espoir, *Nursing Québec*, 8 (3), pp. 50–53.

Salisbury, M. D. (1986) AIDS: psychosocial implications, *Journal of Psychosocial Nursing*, 24 (12), pp. 13–16.

Schwartz, T. (1989) Caring for the HIV child: the identification of family stressors to target and improve nursing interventions, *Résumé de la 5ième Conférence nationale sur le SIDA pédiatrique*, Los Angeles (6–8 Sept.), p. 82.

Statistics Canada (1986) *Santé et bien-être social Canada* (Ottawa).

Tiblier, K. (1987) Intervening with families of young adults with AIDS, in: M. Leahy and M. L. Wright (eds) *Families and Life Threatening Illness*, pp. 250–270 (Springhouse, Pa., Springhouse Corporation).

Tricoire, J. and Robert, A. (1990) La sémiologie de l'infection par le VIH chez l'enfant, *La revue du praticien*, 40 (2), pp. 120–123.

Ultmann, M. H., Diamond, G. A., Ruff, H. A., Belhaw, A. L. *et al.* (1987) Developmental abnormalities in children with acquired immunodeficiency syndrome (AIDS): a follow-up study: *International Journal of Neuroscience*, 32, pp. 661–667.

Varni, J. W., Walco, G. A. and Katz, E. R. (1989) Assessment and management of chronic and recurrent pain in children with chronic diseases, *Pediatrician*, 16, pp. 56–63.

Waters, B. G. H., Ziegler, J. B., Hampson, R. and McPherson, A. H. (1988) The psychosocial consequences of childhood infection with human immunodeficiency virus, *Medical Journal of Australia*, 149 (4), pp. 198–202.

Weil-Halpern, W. H. (1988) Nourrissons hospitalisés victimes d'infection à virus VIH ou SIDA: prise en charge psychosociale, *Soins: gynécologie, obstétrique, puériculture, pédiatrie* (87–88), pp. 17–20.

Weil-Halpern, F. (1989) Problèmes psychosociaux posés par les families ayant un nourrisson victime de l'infection au virus VIH ou du SIDA, *Annales pédiatriques*, 36, pp. 409–412.

Williams, A. D. (1989) Nursing management of the child with AIDS, *Pediatric Nursing*, 15, pp. 259–261.

Wishon, S. L. and Gee, G. (1989) Children and HIV infection, in: G. Gee and A. Moran (eds) *AIDS: Concept in Nursing Practice*, pp. 41–61 (Baltimore, Williams & Wilkins).

CHOICE
OF PARTNERS

THIRTEEN

The Impact of HIV Antibody Status on Gay Men's Partner Preferences: A Community Perspective

Colleen C. Hoff, Leon McKusick, Bobby Hilliard and Thomas J. Coates

The decision as to whether or not one should be tested for HIV antibodies is complex. Prior to the availability of medical drug therapies for HIV-infected individuals, health professionals were divided in their recommendations about whether or not gay men should be tested (Weiss and Hardy, 1990; Perry and Markowitz, 1988; Centers for Disease Control, 1988; Coates et al., 1988). High rates of sexual behaviour change among gay men have been documented in many studies (Stall et al., 1988; Becker and Joseph, 1988). Many, but not all, studies showed that men who knew they were HIV-positive were more likely to practise safer sex than those who did not know their antibody status or who had not been tested, thus supporting the use of testing in primary prevention safer sex campaigns (McKusker et al., 1988; Coates, et al., 1987; Fox et al., 1987; Coates et al., 1988; McKusick et al., 1990).

With the advent of early medical intervention for HIV (i.e. AZT, DDI and other approved and experimental drug therapies), there has been an increase in the number of professionals advocating testing – and of gay and bisexual men who have been tested – for antibodies to HIV. People infected with HIV are living longer as a result of drug interventions and other, less conventional interventions (Lemp et al., 1990; San Francisco City Cohort Study, 1990; Volberding et al., 1990).

It may be said generally that relationships are difficult, but gay relationships can be especially difficult and gay relationships in which one or both partners is infected with HIV much more so. An increase in HIV testing in the gay community has resulted in the disclosure of HIV antibody status becoming a relevant issue in relationship and friendship formation. Levinger (1974) suggested that exchange of intimate disclosures is necessary for the development of close relationships. Some feel it is a requirement for a strong attraction to emerge (Derlega et al., 1976). The fundamental premise of social exchange theory is that relationships that provide more rewards and fewer costs will be more satisfying and will endure longer (Brehm and Kassin, 1990). Once a couple moves beyond the honeymoon phase of the relationship, where costs may be relatively unimportant (Hays, 1985), the fact that one or both partners is HIV positive could be considered quite costly. Costs may appear even more amplified if one of the partners has lost a previous partner or friend(s) to AIDS (McKusick and Hilliard, 1991).

Has antibody testing had an impact on partner selection and relationship development? In a recent survey of male homosexual and heterosexual bar patrons in San Francisco, McKusick and Hoff (1989) found that gay men were more likely than heterosexual men and women to rely on knowledge of antibody status as a prevention strategy. In a nationwide survey of its readers, *Partners Newsletter for Gay and Lesbian Couples* (Bryant and Damian, 1990) reported that 8% of gay male respondents indicated that AIDS had a major role and 21% indicated that AIDS had a minor role in their decisions *to form relationships*. In addition, 14% reported that AIDS had a major role and 34% reported that AIDS had a minor role in *continuing a relationship*. Couples who gave their relationship the highest quality rating were those least likely to consider AIDS a factor in forming or continuing their relationship (Bryant and Damian, 1990). Clearly, the threat of AIDS is a factor in gay relationships.

The objective of this study was to determine the degree to which antibody status was a consideration in selection preferences for friends or romantic partners in a sample of gay men in San Francisco. We hypothesized that seropositive individuals would prefer seropositive partners and seronegative individuals would prefer seronegative partners or romantic relationships. Further, we hypothesized that HIV status would not influence friendships.

METHODS

The AIDS Behavioral Research Project (ABRP) is a longitudinal cohort of gay men originally recruited in 1983 and 1984 at bath houses and bars and by advertising for individuals who were in committed relationships or who did not use bars or baths. A total of 754 men, or 51% of those approached, were enrolled in the sample in 1984 (Coates *et al.*, 1987; 1988; Ekstrand and Coates, 1990; Hays *et al.*, 1990; McKusick *et al.*, 1985a, b, 1990; Pollack *et al.*, 1990; Stall *et al.*, 1986, 1990). Subjects were mailed a self-administered questionnaire each November and asked to return it by mail to the investigators. As of Wave 5 of data collection (November 1988), 71% ($n = 540$) of the original cohort had responded to the survey. Another 8% ($n = 61$) were known to have died (either through report or their friends or through matching in the California Death Registry).

Included in the survey were measures of *sexual behaviour* (subjects were asked how often they had engaged in each of 22 sexual behaviours in the previous 30 days), *antibody testing status* (subjects were asked if they had been HIV tested and to report their test results, if known), *prodromal symptoms* (respondents were asked to indicate which, if any, of the 11 symptoms listed they had experienced in the last year), *AIDS loss* (respondents were asked to report how many of their friends or acquaintances had been diagnosed with AIDS or had died of it) and *relationship status* (all respondents were asked if they were in a primary relationship, defined as a relationship with a man to whom they felt committed more than anyone else and with whom they had had sex: McKusick *et al.*, 1990).

Specifically we were interested in HIV antibody status preferences in potential romantic relationships and friendships. We asked respondents to indicate whether they preferred romantic partners to be HIV seropositive or HIV seronegative or to indicate that HIV status did not matter. The question was repeated to indicate preferences for friendships and again for sexual partners. Subjects were also asked to make open-ended comments regarding their responses. All subjects were asked to complete the item, regardless of relationship status. The items were placed several pages before questions asking the participants about their own HIV antibody status and more general questions about antibody testing to reduce possible feelings of fear or anxiety concerning personal health status.

STATISTICAL ANALYSIS

Participants were categorized by their reported HIV antibody status (HIV negative, HIV positive, untested). Responses to partner preferences based on serostatus were dichotomized and analysed using χ^2 analysis. Tabled data show percentages of those in the sample preferring HIV-seropositive partners, HIV-seronegative partners, or those who reported HIV status having no influence on their preferences for romantic partners or friendships. *Post hoc* contingency analyses were performed on paired group comparisons to examine further statistically significant differences between groups.

RESULTS

Participants

Respondents were largely white (93%) and college-educated (69%). The mean age of respondents was 35 years (s.d. = 8.37) and 57% reported an annual income of over $30,000 (McKusick *et al.*, 1985a, b, 1990). The sample is representative of the San Francisco gay community, with data from this project being consistent with two random samples surveying similar variables and populations (Bye, 1984; Winkelstein *et al.*, 1987; Ekstrand and Coates, 1990).

Twenty-nine per cent of respondents reported having tested HIV antibody seropositive ($n = 157$), 38% reported being seronegative ($n = 205$) and 29% had not been tested ($n = 158$). Fifty-four per cent ($n = 230$) of the sample reported being currently in a primary relationship.

There were no differences in subject responses to the items regarding romantic partner preferences and sex partner preferences. Thus, sex and romance categories were collapsed and will be referred to as romance. As Table 13.1 shows, seronegative and untested men preferred HIV-negative partners for romantic relationships (83% and 74% respectively), whereas HIV-positive men were more likely to report that antibody status did not matter (68%). Of the seropositive men who expressed a preference, 24% preferred an HIV-positive partner (χ^2 = 194.855, P = 0.0001). Responses of seronegative and untested men did not differ significantly from each other. Seropositive men were more likely to respond, 'it doesn't matter' (68%) than seronegative (16%) and untested (24%) individuals (χ^2 = 192.125, P = 0.0001), further substantiating similarities of HIV-negative and untested men. Seropositive men were less likely to prefer seronegative romantic partners (8%) than seronegative and untested men (χ^2 = 181.234, P = 0.0000). Finally, seropositive men were more likely to prefer seropositive romantic partners (24%) than seronegative and untested men, 0.6 and 2% respectively (χ^2 = 59.871, P = 0.0000).

Table 13.1 Preferences for romantic relationships

	Prefer HIV-negative		Doesn't matter		Prefer HIV-positive	
	%	n	%	n	%	n
Seropositive men	8%	(10)	68%	(84)	24%	(29)
Seronegative men	83%	(144)	16%	(27)	0.6%	(1)
Untested men	74%	(82)	24%	(27)	2%	(2)

Seropositive men were less likely to report antibody status preferences for friendships. 89% of those who tested seropositive, 76% of those who tested seronegative, and 79% of those untested individuals did not have preferences for friendships based on antibody status (χ^2 = 10.8118, P = 0.0288) (see Table 13.2). Again, there were no significant differences between seronegative and untested individuals' responses; seronegative and untested men were more likely to prefer seronegative friendships (15% and 12%, respectively) than were seropositives.

Table 13.2 Preferences for friendships

	Prefer HIV-negative		Doesn't matter		Prefer HIV-positive	
	%	n	%	n	%	n
Seropositive men	5%	(7)	89%	(125)	6%	(8)
Seronegative men	15%	(30)	76%	(149)	8%	(16)
Untested men	12%	(17)	79%	(111)	9%	(13)

Further χ^2 analyses were performed to examine the influence of *relationship status* on partner preference. We found no significant difference in preference for romantic relationships based on the respondent's current relationship status. The majority of participants, regardless of relationship status, reported they did not have preferences for friendship. However, single men (24%) were more likely than men in relationships (15%) to have a preference for friendship based on antibody status ($\chi^2 = 8.288$, $P = 0.0159$). Thirteen per cent of singles preferred HIV antibody seronegative friends and 11% preferred seropositive friends.

DISCUSSION

Seronegative and untested men were more likely to prefer seronegative men for romantic relationships. Seropositive men were more likely to report that serostatus did not matter or to prefer other seropositive men for romance. The vast majority of men reported that serostatus was not an issue in friendship selection. However, single men were more likely to have preferences than those in relationships, and seronegative and untested men were more likely to prefer seronegative men than seropositive men for friendship. Two common reasons given by HIV-seropositive men who prefer HIV-seropositive partners were that they desire a 'common bond' or they are afraid of infecting a partner. One participant wrote, 'I generally feel a kinship with people who are HIV positive. Many HIV negatives don't understand what we are dealing with as positives. Intellectually they may understand but they don't grasp the impact on one's life.' Another said, 'I don't have sex with him [a seronegative lover] since I found out I was positive. I know what safe sex is but I couldn't live with myself if I infected him.' Fear and stigmatization are common feelings among HIV-seropositive men, a finding that anecdotally supports our hypothesis that HIV-seropositive men would tend to prefer HIV-seropositive partners. Yet the data suggest that most seropositive men did not have a preference. One person wrote, 'As I refuse to do anything unsafe, HIV status doesn't matter.' Another wrote, 'I assume everyone is positive, therefore HIV has no effect.' This unwillingness to discriminate could also be an unwillingness to perpetuate the all-too-familiar feelings of internalized fear and stigmatization. Perhaps confronting one's own mortality allows a person the freedom to reflect on life itself and, through this, the freedom to appreciate the importance of human relationships regardless of HIV antibody status.

Seronegative men preferring seronegative partners are typically burdened by fear of infection and fear of loss. One man indicated, 'After having more than 20 friends and close acquaintances die of AIDS, I avoid new relationships with people I know to have AIDS or are HIV positive.' Another expressed wariness: 'Just about anybody could lie about their antibody status. I am a little suspicious of anyone not in a primary relationship who tells me they are seronegative.' Some feel more conflicted, for example the person who said, 'I was seriously interested in someone until he tested and the result was positive. I cooled the relationship to a friendship but don't feel altogether good for having done so.'

A division of romantic partner and friendship selection is a concern in a community where, regardless of antibody status, gay men seek support from friends more than any other source of social support (Hays et al., 1990). Even those who claim to be unbiased show subtle signs of community divergence. A participant wrote, 'HIV does not affect my value of people or friends but sometimes the tragedy of it all makes it hard to deal with *them*, but I try not to let it influence my behaviour towards them.'

These data also show that men not yet tested are likely to prefer seronegative men for romance and friendship. From a public health standpoint, HIV-seronegative individuals seeking partners with similar HIV antibody status may reduce transmission, assuming that the relationship eventually becomes monogamous. However, untested individuals who prefer seronegative romantic partners could be making incorrect assumptions, since they themselves might be seropositive. Since 42% of this sample had unsafe anal intercourse between 1988 and 1989 (Pollack *et al.*, 1990), it is very likely that HIV transmission is still occurring – despite one's estimation of one's own and one's potential partner's antibody status. This raises concern as to why this group is not tested; why are they behaving as though they are seronegative? Although there are a multitude of reasons why men are not being tested, could one be that these men fear being rejected and stigmatized by their community, particularly if they have participated in the overt or covert rejection of another owing to his HIV status? Denial of one's own mortality and one's ability to transmit the virus is likely to be a factor with this group. Historical patterns of self-hatred, in this case manifested by not being tested and not seeking medical treatment, could also be a factor for some. Although we have learned a tremendous amount about motivations in being tested for HIV in recent years, there is still resistance by many who are at risk for HIV, thus supporting the need for continued outreach programmes targeted on 'hard to reach' individuals.

There are several limitations to the findings here. Members of the San Francisco gay community are very 'out' about homosexuality and about HIV status. The level of openness in this community has allowed health professionals to obtain information and to address problems as they develop. This close monitoring has been beneficial to community organizations in their prevention efforts. There are also support groups and mental health professionals available to attend to many issued raised by the AIDS epidemic. In gay communities and other high-risk communities that are less cohesive and more restricted, open disclosure of serostatus is not as forthcoming. Is San Francisco's openness a developmental stage of a community ravaged by disease? Will other high-risk communities reach this developmental stage? If so, is there a measurable impact on AIDS prevention? As more interventions are developed and targeted on specific communities, it is safe to assume that HIV status divisions will be present but, more than likely, hidden. In order to detect these divisions, intervention teams must be sensitive to community and cultural norms, customs, religions and taboos.

Although determination of antibody status has become a desirable secondary prevention tool, we cannot overlook the inevitable social and psychological consequences of advocating the test, as in this instance, for partner selection. Further investigation is needed to determine whether pairing people by antibody status has any relevance to primary prevention and to examine any ill-effects such pairing may have on relationships and community bonds. Meanwhile, we need to work to prevent undue stigmatization of those infected with HIV, continuing to provide support and friendship despite our losses and our fears. The amount of loss and grief inflicted on the gay community in San Francisco is massive. In the next few years, *everyone* in the gay community will know someone with AIDS – be it a neighbour, an employer or a clerk at the corner store. Current efforts must focus on coping with our losses so we can keep the gay community as a community.

REFERENCES

Becker, M. H. and Joseph, J. G. (1988) AIDS and behavioral change to reduce risk: a review, *American Journal of Public Health*, 78 (4), pp. 394–410.

Brehm, S. S. (1985) *Intimate Relationships* (New York, Random House).

Brehm, S. S. and Kassin, S. M. (1990) *Social Psychology* (Boston, Houghton Mifflin).

Bryant, S. and Damian (1990) *Partners Newsletter for Gay and Lesbian Couples* (Seattle, Sweet Corn Productions).

Bye, L. (1984) A report on designing an effective AIDS prevention campaign strategy for San Francisco. Report for the San Francisco AIDS Foundation by Research and Design Corporation, San Francisco.

Centers for Disease Control (1988) Update: serologic testing for antibody to human immunodeficiency virus, *Morbidity and Mortality Weekly Report*, 36 (52), pp. 833–844.

Coates, T. J., Morin, S. F. and McKusick, L. (1987) Behavioral consequences of AIDS antibody testing among gay men, *Journal of the American Medical Association*, 258 (14), p. 1989.

Coates, T. J., Stall, R. D., Kegeles, S. M., Lo, B., Morin, S. F. and McKusick, L. (1988) AIDS antibody testing: will it stop the AIDS epidemic? Will it help people infected with HIV? *American Psychologist*, 43 (11), pp. 859–864.

Derlega, V. J., Wilson, M. and Chakin, A. L. (1976) Friendship and disclosure reciprocity, *Journal of Personality and Social Psychology*, 34, pp. 578–582.

Ekstrand, M. I. and Coates, T. J. (1990). Maintenance of safer sexual behaviors and predictors of risky sex: the San Francisco men's health study, *American Journal of Public Health*, 80 (8), pp. 973–977.

Fox, R., Ostrow, D., Valdiserri, R., VanRaden, B. and Polk, B. (1987) Changes in sexual activities among participants in the Multicenter AIDS cohort study. Presented at the IIIrd International Conference on AIDS in Washington, DC.

Hays, R. B. (1985) A longitudinal study of friendship development, *Journal of Personality and Social Psychology*, 48, pp. 909–924.

Hays, R., Catania, J., McKusick, L. and Coates, T. J. (1990). Help-seeking for AIDS-related concerns: a comparison of gay men with various HIV diagnoses, *American Journal of Community Psychology*, 18, pp. 743–755.

Hendrick, C. and Hendrick, S. (1983) *Liking, Loving and Relationships* (Monterey, Calif., Brooks/Cole).

Lemp, G. G., Payne, S. F., Neal, D., Temelso, T. and Rutherford, G. W. (1990) Survival trends for patients with AIDS, *Journal of the American Medical Association*, 263, pp. 402–406.

Levinger, G. (1974) A three-level approach to attraction: toward an understanding of pair relatedness, in: T. L. Huston (ed.), *Foundations of Interpersonal Attraction* (New York: Academic Press).

McKusick, L., Coates, T. J., Morin, S. F., Pollack, L. and Hoff, C. (1990) Longitudinal predictors of reductions in high risk sexual behaviors among gay men in San Francisco: the AIDS Behavioral Research Project, *American Journal of Public Health*, 80 (8), pp. 1–6.

McKusick, L. and Hilliard, R. (1991) Multiple loss accounts for worsening distress in a community heavily hit by AIDS. Presented at the VIIth International Conference on AIDS, Florence, Italy.

McKusick, L. and Hoff, C. C. (1989) Relationship between HIV awareness, partner selection criteria, and early relationship formation in two groups of San Francisco bar patrons. Presented at the Vth International Conference on AIDS in Montreal.

McKusick, L., Horstman, W. and Coates, T. J. (1985a) AIDS and sexual behaviour reported by gay men in San Francisco, *American Journal of Public Health*, 75 (5), pp. 493–496.

McKusick, L., Wiley, J. A., Coates, T. J., Stall, R., Saika, G., Morin, S., Charles, K., Horstman, W. and Conant, M. (1985b) Reported changes in the sexual behaviour of men at risk for AIDS, San Francisco, 1982–84. The AIDS Behavioral Research Project, *Public Health Reports*, 100 (6), pp. 622–628.

McKusker, J., Stoddard, A., Mayer, K., Zapka, J., Morussen, C. and Saltzman, M. (1988) Effects of HIV antibody test knowledge on subsequent sexual behaviors in a cohort of homosexual men, *American Journal of Public Health*, 78, pp. 462–467.

Perry, S. W. and Markowitz, J. C. (1988) Counselling for HIV testing, *Hospital and Community Psychiatry*, 39 (7), pp. 731–739.

Pollack, L., Ekstrand, M. L., Stall, R. and Coates, T. J. (1990) Current reasons for having unsafe sex among gay men in San Francisco: the AIDS Behavioral Research Project. Presented at the VIth International Conference on AIDS in San Francisco.

San Francisco City Cohort Study (1990) The San Francisco city cohort study: progression to HIV disease and the need for intervention, *San Francisco Epidemiologic Bulletin*, 6 (9).

Stall, R., Coates, T. J. and Hoff, C. (1988) AIDS risk reduction for HIV infection among gay and bisexual men, *American Psychologist*, 43 (11), pp. 878–885.

Stall, R., Ekstrand, M. and McKusick, L. (1990). Relapse from safer sex: the next challenge for AIDS prevention efforts, *Journal of Acquired Immune Deficiency Syndrome*, 3, pp. 1181–1187.

Stall, R., McKusick, L., Wiley, J., Coates, T. and Ostrow, D. G. (1986) Alcohol and drug use during sexual activity and compliance with safe sex guidelines for AIDS, *Health Education Quarterly*, 13, p. 4.

Volberding, P. A., Lagakos, S. W., Koch, M. A., Pettinelli, C., Myers, M. W., Booth, D. K., Balfour, H. H., Reichman, R. C., Bartlett, J. A., Hirsch, M. S., Murphy, R. L., Soeiro, R., Fischl, M. A., Bartlett, J. G., Merigan, T. C., Hyslop, N. E., Richman, D. D., Valentine, F. T. and Corey, L. (1990) Zidovudine in asymptomatic human immunodeficiency virus infection, *New England Journal of Medicine*, 322 (14), pp. 941–949.

Weiss, R. and Hardy, L. M. (1990) HIV infection and health policy, *Journal of Consulting and Clinical Psychology*, 58 (1), pp. 70–76.

Winkelstein, W., Lyman, D. M., Padian, N., Grant, R., Samuel, M., Wiley, J. A., Anderson, R. E., Lang, W. and Riggs, J. A. (1987) Sexual practices and risk of infection by the Human Immunodeficiency Virus: the San Francisco men's health study, *Journal of the American Medical Education*, 257, pp. 321–325.

FOURTEEN

Maintenance of Open Gay Relationships: Some Strategies for Protection against HIV

Ford C. I. Hickson, Peter M. Davies, Andrew J. Hunt, Peter Weatherburn, Thomas J. McManus and Anthony P. M. Coxon

INTRODUCTION

In the early years of AIDS, there was much speculation that the pandemic would force gay men to abandon their 'promiscuous' lifestyles and embrace sexual monogamy as a risk-reduction strategy. In 1983 Blumstein and Schwartz wrote:

> some of this pattern of casual sex may be changing because of a terrible disease which non-monogamous gay men run a particular risk of contracting, it is called AIDS. (p. 174)

Some writers actually thought that they had detected such a trend. In 1984, McWhirter and Mattison claimed:

> we believe there is a trend towards more sexual exclusivity in the future amongst gay men. Currently it is being propelled by fear of AIDS and more and more individuals are expressing the desire for sexual exclusivity with one other man. (p. 291)

The claim, it seems, was mistaken, or perhaps the trend has petered out. As this paper will show, in the 1990s, many gay male couples in England and Wales – as elsewhere – do not choose monogamy.

From work done in the 1970s and 1980s, it is clear that sexual exclusivity was neither a reality nor an ideal for most coupled gay men before AIDS (Blumstein and Schwartz, 1983; Harry and De Vall, 1978; Saghir and Robins, 1973). The most common reasons given for non-monogamy were sexual variety and the sense of personal independence attained by not confining sexual activity to one person (Blasband and Peplau, 1985). That open relationships are a positive choice on the part of gay men seemed, however, to be too simple an explanation for some researchers, who saw openness as evidence of a failed closed relationship. Blumstein and Schwartz (1983), for example, talk of the 'threat' of openness to relationships and Bell and Weinberg (1978, p. 138) suggest that 'a monogamous quasi-marriage between homosexual men is probably difficult to achieve'.

With the advent of AIDS, this implicit moral agenda becomes explicit with calls for a return to monogamy as an effective HIV prevention strategy (Watney, 1987). This 'advice' ignored the epidemiological evidence – which was available at the time (Coxon, 1988; van Griensven *et al.*, 1987) – that the number of sexual partners is not, in itself, an accurate determinant of HIV risk, but only when the type of sex is taken into account (see, more recently, Hunt *et al.*, 1991; Jenkins *et al.*, 1991).

The identification of anal intercourse as the most efficient sexual transmission route of HIV between men (Darrow *et al.*, 1983; van Griensven *et al.*, 1987) and the often replicated finding that anal intercourse was more common in regular relationships than with casual partners (Connell *et al.*, 1989; Davies *et al.*, 1990; Fitzpatrick *et al.*, 1989) have led at least one study (McKirnan *et al.*, 1991) to identify the move to regular relationships as a 'part of a syndrome of denial'. This bizarre idea leaves gay men in an insoluble dilemma: choose to enter a regular relationship and stand accused of denying the risk of HIV; remain uncommitted and perpetuate the notion of promiscuity.

That non-exclusive relationships are, for many men, simply more fulfilling than monogamous ones leads us to ask about the ways in which non-exclusivity can be combined with a strategic regard for safer sex.

Among couples who chose an open relationship, past researchers have found a number of regulatory mechanisms. These mechanisms take the form of rules and guidelines, either explicitly negotiated between the partners or implicitly understood by them, and have been found between heterosexual couples (e.g. Buunk, 1980) as well as homosexual couples (e.g. Blumstein and Schwartz, 1983; McWhirter and Mattison, 1984). These rules have both manifest and functional components. A manifest component is about, for example, whom sex is allowed with; where it may take place; what kinds of sex are permitted; where the other partner is at the time; what is said between the partners about the sex; the number of times sex is allowed with the same third party, etc.

A functional component can be thought of as the effects of rules facilitate; for example, there are those rules that are concerned with maintaining the primacy of the relationship, which assert it as separate and different from other sexual encounters. Another example is rules which function on a day-to-day basis to avoid confrontations and irritation (akin to agreeing to put the toothpaste top back on, or taking turns to wash the dishes).

There need be no direct correspondence between the manifest content of rules and their functions. Indeed two contradictory rules – for example, (a) to tell the partner when extra-relational sex has taken place and (b) not to talk about sex with third parties – may be used for the same purpose: to minimize jealousy. Furthermore, a manifest rule may function, possibly unintentionally, in more than one way. For example, a rule about engaging in anal intercourse only with the primary partner is a rule that makes sex safer in terms of infections, for both partners, but it may also function in keeping the relationship special, given the emotional significance attached to anal intercourse (Prieur, 1990).

A literature review on sexual non-exclusivity and rule making, along with a discussion of definitional problems associated with open and closed relationships, can be found in Hickson (1991). The current paper reports on some of the rules used by gay men in open relationships, with particular reference to those rules concerned with safer sex.

METHODS

Data presented here arise from Project SIGMA's third wave of interviews conducted in 1990, with 387 men who have sex with men and who currently take part in a five-wave, six-year socio-sexual study.

The majority of these men are single (88.4%); currently have sex only with men (90.1%); rate their feelings as mainly or exclusively homosexual (93.2%); and most of their family, friends and work colleagues know of their homosexuality. The median age of the sample is 32 years, range 18–33 years. (For a more detailed description of this group of men, see Weatherburn et al., 1991.)

For the purposes of standardization, after respondents were given the opportunity to describe in their own words the state of their current gay sexual relationships (i.e. whether they were in an open, closed or no relationship), they were given definitions of regular and casual sexual partners, and asked if they were currently in a regular relationship. A regular partner is defined by the Project as 'someone you have had sex with more than once where the second and subsequent meetings were not accidental, and with whom you regularly have sex or currently intend to have sex in the near future'. For each regular partner the respondent had, they were asked the partner's sex, age, residence and occupation, whether the partner was, to their knowledge, sexually exclusive to them, the length of their relationship, and who else the respondent had had sex with over that period.

The classificatory system for open and closed relationships initially used the respondents' own assessment of the relationships. If the respondent said that he and his partner had sex with other people as well as each other, the relationship was considered open. For the relationship to be classified as closed, the sexual activity of those respondents who said they were in sexually exclusive relationship was examined. A relationship was considered closed if the respondent had not had sex with a third party in the preceding month. If he had, it was classified as open, irrespective of the respondent's assessment. Having no independent verifier for the partner's exclusivity, it was assumed that the respondents' assessment of their partners' sexual activity was correct. In fact, those respondents who claimed to be in a closed relationship, but who had had sex with someone other than their partner in the preceding month, comprised only 3% of those with regular partners. This is in accord with Blasband and Peplau's (1985) observation of the congruence of gay men's self-reports and actual behaviour.

RESULTS

Proportion of Men in Open and Closed Relationships

Of the 387 men interviewed, 252 (65.1%) had one or more regular sexual partner at the time of interview. One hundred and ten men (43.7% of those in relationships) were in relationships designated at the time to be closed (monogamous). More (142; 56.3%) were in open relationships; that is, either the respondent or his partner or both were having sex with other people. This finding is consistent with previous studies (Bell and Weinberg, 1978; Blasband and Peplau, 1985; Blumstein and Schwartz, 1983; Harry and De Vall, 1978; Mendola, 1980; Peplau, 1981; Peplau and Cochran, 1981; Saghir and Robins, 1973) in that open relationships are more common than closed ones. Further, at least one regular sexual partner plus other partners is the most common sexual relationships configuration for all the men (36.7% of all respondents were in open relationships, 28.4% in closed relationships and 34.9% had no regular partner).

Numbers of Regular Partners

Between them, the 252 men had 382 regular partners (see Table 14.1). The modal number of regular partners (192 respondents) was one. The distribution is highly skewed. The largest number of regular relationships (using the Project's wide definition), sustained by any one individual was ten.

Table 14.1 Distribution of numbers of regular partners

	Number of respondents with that number of regular partners ($n = 252$)	% of respondents
1	192	76.2
2	24	9.5
3	19	7.5
4	5	2.0
5	4	1.6
6	2	0.8
7 or more	4	1.6

Details of the length of the relationship, the ages of the two partners, the type of sex that had occurred within the relationship and any rules or guidelines for sex outside the relationship were available for 255 of the 382 partners (88 closed and 154 open relationships), to which the rest of this paper refers.

Length of Relationships

The median length of relationship was 21 months (mean, almost four years), the maximum being 38 years.

McWhirter and Mattison's (1984) analysis of the relationships of 156 couples leads them to state that none of the relationships over five years in length were monogamous, and similar time-scales have been put forward for a change to open marriages in heterosexual couples (Ramey, 1975). In this study relationships over five years in length are more likely to be open than those less than five years ($\chi^2 = 4.782$, $P<0.05$). Of the relationships of five years or longer 72.6% were open, compared to only 57.0% of those under five years. An analysis of variance of the lengths of the relationships by the type of relationship also proved significant ($F = 7.938$, $P<0.05$), confirming a trend towards sexual non-exclusivity over time.

Age Differences between Partners

The majority of work on age differences within gay relationships has concentrated on partner selection and the role of age differences in decision making. Lee's (1988) analysis of *Advocate* personal advertisements points towards men preferring, on the whole, partners about the same age as themselves, while Harry and De Vall (1978) found that the age range 25–35 years was most desirable to all age groups. Men in their early twenties prefer older partners, those aged 25–35 prefer partners about the same age, and over 35s younger or age-egalitarian relationships.

The median age difference between partners in the current group of men was six years (mean, nine years), the maximum difference being 53 years. Just over 43% of the couple's ages were within five years of each other (compare Bell and Weinberg's (1978, p. 319) figure of 48%).

In terms of type of relationship, the present data suggest an association between age difference and open and closed relationships. Of those couples who were contemporaries within one year, 48% were maintaining open relationships, this figure rises to 55% for those within ten years of each other, and 72% for those with an age difference of over ten years ($\chi^2 = 8.230$, $P<0.02$).

Sex Rules

Those respondents with at least one regular sexual partner were asked:

> Do you currently have any rules, guidelines or understandings about sex outside your relationship?

Considering first the 88 relationships that were closed, although the majority of respondents said that there were no rules or guidelines as they did not have sex with other people, some talked about discussions that anticipate the rules of the open couples:

> We have an understood rule not to have other partners. My partner was away for four months and it was understood that he might, and I might, have other partners then, but neither of us did.

> We had threesomes before 1986, but not since then. If either of us had sex with someone else in the future it would have to be a threesome. We understood that from the beginning.

These rules are anticipatory. Neither partner expects to have sex with other people in the future, but they acknowledge the possibility. What these men highlight is that their monogamy is not a restrictive rule but an active choice.

Some undertandings are explicit that HIV is an issue to be considered if outside sex does take place:

> We agreed that if we strayed there would be no fucking or cumming in anyone, or vice versa.

> If he does it must be safe . . .

The most common agreement within a closed relationship was that if extra-relational sex did occur, that the partner would be told about it;

> If he does . . . he must tell me.

> If we had another partner we'd tell each other afterwards.

These men view their sexual exclusivity as contingent, not necessary: open to the possibility of sex with someone else. In principle, this minimizes the emotional disturbance should one of them have sex with another, while also developing strategies that minimize the risk of HIV infection.

Of the 154 *relationships* that were open, 72.7% ($n = 112$) had some agreement between the partners as to the nature of sex with third parties. One feature of these rules and guidelines is their diversity. Some of the rules reverse rules within other relationships. Consider the following pairs:

> (a) My partner can bonk women but not men.
> (b) Generally, not to have sex with women as it's found more threatening.

> (a) If we pick someone up it must always be in our flat and never theirs . . .
> (b) Never at our home . . .

> (a) We should tell each other.
> (b) Not to talk about it.

The following analysis of the rules concentrates on their manifest rather than functional content. As mentioned previously, the same rule may function in two opposing ways. Conversely, two rules that appear contradictory, for example the pairs above, may facilitate the same outcome.

RULES ABOUT INFORMATION AND HONESTY

The first type of rule is about information and honesty. Twenty-eight open relationships involved such an understanding. Anticipated by the pre-emptive rule within the closed relationship mentioned earlier, these agreements often take the form of telling the partner when sex has occurred:

> ... being totally honest.

> I do not like to be deceived and we don't pretend that nothing has happened.

> ... we're supposed to tell the truth.

In this last quote, we see a recognition of the fragility of the rules.

Some rules demand that the partner knows before the sex occurs:

> The partner must know and give permission ...

> We have to tell each other first or immediately afterwards.

Some rules concerning information are more pragmatic and aim at reducing worry:

> We must tell each other what's happening, e.g. if we stay out all night.

> If I go out I must tell him where I am so he doesn't worry.

Yet others suggest a sharing of the sexual experience by recounting the session in some detail:

> Each tells the other exactly what happened.

> ... if I take someone back for sex I must give my partner an account in the morning.

RULES ABOUT REGULARITY AND EMOTIONAL DISTANCE

While rules about information and honesty can serve different functions, the following set concentrates on maintaining the primacy of the partnership. They were present in 20 relationships. These rules emphasize that other sexual relationships are different; that they are 'only sex'. Often they prohibit seeing another partner more than a set number of times, or curtail the regularity of seeing them:

> Casuals are OK, one-offs. We must not go back to someone twice; that would be a relationship.

> We're not allowed to have partners we see more than once.

> We can go with others as long as it's not more than two or three times.

> I imposed a rule on myself never to date anyone else on a regular basis.

Another rule found that kept extra-relational sex 'just sex' was:

> No sleeping with anyone else.

Other respondents couched this rule in more explicit terms, concentrating on the partner's feelings for, and emotional attachment to, the other partners:

> That outside relationships are not threatening.
>
> We think it's important for us to have sex with other people, that way our needs are met. Our relationship is central though, our prime loyalty. If someone gets too close it will be discussed. It doesn't happen for me so it's no problem, but for him it does because he forms deeper relationships.
>
> The unwritten rule is no emotional involvement.

RULES ABOUT DISCRETION AND POLITENESS

Rules about regularity and emotional distance are aimed at sustaining the relationship as primary to both members. They concern themselves with making sure no major friction occurs that could damage the stability of the relationship. A third group of rules aims at avoiding irritation and hurt feelings out of thoughtlessness:

> We mustn't offend each other's sensibilities in the execution of infidelities.
>
> Don't bring people back to the house when the other is there. It's an implicit rule out of politeness.

These rules can come into conflict with the sharing of information and being honest with each other, in which case one principle must yield to the other:

> We don't discuss other partners with each other, and we don't introduce them.

In some cases a mode of operation has developed that bridges both the underlying principle of prohibitions on regularity, that of keeping the relationship primary, and also facilitating discretion:

> We wouldn't walk off with someone in front of each other.
>
> If we go out together we go home together.

The problem of not been seen to choose someone else over the partner can also be achieved more simply:

> We don't go cruising together.

Or it can be achieved by restricting extra-relational sex to times when sex between the partners is not possible, for example:

> We wouldn't have sex with people in Britain, but we're allowed casuals in Amsterdam or Thailand.
>
> . . . only away from our own town.

These last two examples, while involved with issues of discretion, also safeguard the primacy of the partnership. Eighteen relationships had negotiated rules about discretion and politeness.

RULES ABOUT THREESOMES

Seven couples had found that they could both have sex with other people, without having to think about their partner having sex with someone else instead of them, by doing it at the same time:

> We only sleep with other people if it's a threesome. This was a joint discussion when we discussed the possibilities of dos and don'ts.
>
> No outside partners unless it's in a threesome. We decided that this was OK and not threatening.

This rule can be part of a larger objective that satisfies both partners:

> The rules are: (1) we work as a team; (2) we have to both pick someone up or go as a threesome; (3) no fucking with others without a condom . . .

RULES ABOUT SAFER SEX

By far the most common type of rule among these couples concerned safer sex. Many (43%) open relationships had some kind of agreement as to what kind of sex partners could have outside that relationship, usually based on perceived safer sex guidelines.

These rules take a variety of forms and illustrate the different ways people construe 'safer sex'. They included acts prohibited:

> He doesn't like me to fuck or have someone come in my mouth.
>
> Always safe sex, no fucking even with condoms.
>
> Sexually, no fucking at all.

And they included acts prescribed;

> It has to be incredibly safe, mutual wanking only, as we don't have safe sex ourselves.

Where there was no restriction on anal intercourse with others *per se*, many men mentioned an agreement about condom use with outside partners:

> It must always be safe sex, I'm allowed to fuck and be fucked with condoms.

> No fucking with others without a condom and obey all safer sex rules.

> It must all be safe; always with a condom and no taking of semen.

Some of these rules were occasionally elaborated on, the respondent going on to say that he did not have safer sex with his partner.

> We screw each other but have safer sex with other people. This has been the case since we met. We both knew the realities of the risks.

Rules about anal intercourse did not always develop because of safer sex. The symbolic importance of this act in a regular relationship, as an act of love and/or trust, can result in partners not wishing to perform this sexual act with others:

> We've both talked about sex with other people. My partner wouldn't fuck because of his love for me; having a wank is OK.

Owing to the diversity of these rules about safer sex, there is also a diversity of their epidemiological relevance. This point will be returned to in the discussion.

OTHER RULES

The preceding rules cover the majority of responses. There were, however, a few rules, each mentioned by only one respondent, that illustrate their diversity:

> He doesn't mind me having sex with other people, but I've told him he can't have sex with anyone else.

This rule indicates an imbalance in ascriptions of trust to the two partners. Other rules included: not to go cottaging; to have sex only with prostitutes; and to have sex with other people only when accepting money from them.

DISCUSSION

In terms of the socio-sexual organization of gay men, these data suggest a structure predominantly comprising of regular couples who are also having casual sexual partners. This is in distinction to a network of men regularly having sex with each other. As the type of relationship between two people is the strongest predictor of the type of sex they may engage in (Connell *et al.*, 1989; Davies *et al.*, 1990; Fitzpatrick *et al.*, 1989), understanding this point is essential to an accurate sexual epidemiology of HIV among gay men.

Although in many cases sex with others only occurred after discussion, and taking only the form agreed upon, some statements made by respondents give an indication of the dynamics of rule making and breaking. After initial discussions about ground rules and the form the guidelines will take, implementation and experimentation takes place:

> We arrived at these rules by trial and error, by going too far sometimes.

Here the rules are developed in tandem with sex outside the relationship, rules being formed or amended dependent on the reaction of the participants. This may be motivated by both partners, or one may take the lead:

> There was a rule with my second partner about one-off sex, but I always break the rule. I'm talking established rules – I broke them and we established new ones.

Also, some of the possible barriers to rule making were indicated:

> No, we don't have rules, he drinks too much and wouldn't abide by them.

> No, because he doesn't know I have other contacts. If he did he would be very upset, he gets very jealous. It's something I have to learn to live with.

An intentional agreement mentioned by Blumstein and Schwartz (1983), but neither McWhirter and Mattison (1984) nor Buunk (1980), was 'not to bring home sexually transmitted diseases', but they do not make clear the manifest content of this rule. Possible forms of this may be: taking into consideration the appearance of prospective partner; asking questions about their sexual history; avoiding, or using condoms for, penetrative sex. These manifest contents obviously have different utilities in fulfilling their common function. Similarly, different rules about safer sex with others have different epidemiological relevance. The implications for sex within a regular relationship when partners are not having penetrative sex with others and when they are having protected penetrative sex are different. If a couple are having unprotected penetrative sex with each other, a broken condom when either is having penetrative sex with someone else may elicit a drastic reassessment of their sexual life. Highlighting the possible consequences of different types of sex rules among couples is an area for health education to cover.

Many gay men choose to continue to fuck. Given the physical pleasure of the act, its cultural symbolism and emotional significance, this is not surprising. That most fucking takes place within regular relationships (Connell *et al.*, 1989; Davies *et al.*, 1990; Fitzpatrick *et al.*, 1989) is testimony to this. The endorsement of sexual exclusivity within these relationships is neither realistic nor necessary, and any calls for it must be seen as morally guided. That sexual exclusivity among these gay men is not a norm indicates that these points are being recognized by them. It would appear that alternative strategies, rule making that takes account of HIV, are developing. That more and continued health education with particular reference to relationships is needed is beyond doubt. It may be said that health education tools that have so far proved useful in information dissemination, e.g. poster and leaflet campaigns, are inadequate for the complexity of safer sex strategies where couples are concerned. If this is the case, we should be looking more towards workshop and discussion groups. We must question campaigns aimed at gay men in relationships that carry mixed messages, continue using the term 'safer sex' as a homogeneous behavioural category, and implicitly validate sexual exclusivity (as, for example, in the Health Education Authority's recent 'If your sex life is unprotected, so is your relationship' campaign).

Endorsement of sexual exclusivity over other lifestyle choices has little, if any, part to play in empowering and effective health education. We need to highlight the potential risks of new and continuing sexual partners within an atmosphere of sexual openness in which people can make decisions for themselves. A prescriptive model, morally and puritanically motivated, which tells people what, and what not, to do is patronizing, unrealistic and ultimately ineffective. We must acknowledge, validate and encourage rule making as a strategic response of couples to HIV, and encourage discussion of their epidemiological relevance, so that informed and effective choices can be made. Maintaining condom use while fucking within regular relationships must also be addressed, and epidemiologically safe strategies for their disuse made common knowledge.

REFERENCES

Bell, A. P. and Weinberg, M. S. (1978) *Homosexualities: A Study of Diversity among Men and Women* (London, Mitchell Beazley).

Blasband, D. and Peplau, L. A. (1985) Sexual exclusivity versus openness in gay male couples, *Archives of Sexual Behaviour*, 14, pp. 395–412.

Blumstein, P. and Schwartz, P. (1983) *American Couples* (New York, William Morrow).

Buunk, B. P. (1980) Sexually open marriages: ground rules for countering potential threats to marriage, *Alternative Lifestyles*, 3, 312–328.

Connell, R. W., Crawford, J., Kippax, S., Dowsett, G. W., Baxter, D., Watson, L. and Berg, R. (1989) Facing the epidemic: changes in the sexual lives of gay and bisexual men in Australia and their implications for AIDS prevention strategies, *Social Problems*, 36, pp. 384–402.

Coxon, A. P. M. (1988) The numbers game: gay lifestyles, epidemiology of AIDS and social science, in: P. Aggleton and H. Homans (eds) *Social Aspects of AIDS* (Lewes, Falmer Press).

Darrow, E., Jaffe, H. and Curran, J. (1983) Passive anal intercourse as a risk factor for AIDS in homosexual men, *Lancet*, 2, p. 160.

Davies, P., Hunt, A., Macourt, M. and Weatherburn, P. (1990) Longitudinal study of the sexual behaviour of homosexual males under the impact of AIDS. A final report to the Department of Health.

Fitzpatrick, R., Boulton, M., Hart, G., Dawson, J. and McLean, J. (1989) Variations in sexual behaviour in gay men, in: P. Aggleton, P. M. Davies and G. Hart (eds) *AIDS: Individual, Cultural and Policy Dimensions* (Lewes, Falmer Press).

Harry, J. and De Vall, W. B. (1978) *The Social Organization of Gay Males* (New York, Praeger).

Hickson, F. C. I. (1991) Sexual exclusivity, non-exclusivity and HIV. Project SIGMA Working Paper No. 31.

Hunt, A. J., Davies, P. M., Weatherburn, P., Coxon, A. P. M. and McManus, T. J. (1991) Changes in sexual behaviour in a large cohort of homosexual men in England and Wales, 1988–9, *British Medical Journal*, 302, pp. 505–506.

Jenkins, P., Hill, A. M., Gompels, M. S., Anderson, R. M. and Pinching, A. J. (1991) Synergistic effects of behaviour change among gay men on the risk of HIV-1 transmission. Poster presented at the VIIth International Conference on AIDS, Florence.

Lee, J. A. (1988) Forbidden colours of love: patterns of gay love and gay liberation, in: J. P. DeCecco (ed.) *Gay Relationships* (London, Harrington Park Press).

McKirnan, D., Doll, L., Harrison, J., Delgado, W., Doetsch, J., Mendoza, G. and Burzette, R. (1991) Primary relationships confer risk of HIV exposure among gay men. Paper presented at the VIIth International Conference on AIDS, Florence.

McWhirter, D. P. and Mattison, A. M. (1984) *The Male Couple: How Relationships Develop* (Englewood Cliffs, NJ, Prentice-Hall).

Mendola, M. (1980) *The Mendola Report: A New Look at Gay Couples in America* (New York, Crown).

Peplau, L. A. (1981) What homosexuals want in relationships, *Psychology Today*, 15, pp. 28–38.

Peplau, L. A. and Cochran, S. (1981) Value orientation in the intimate relationships of gay men, *Journal of Homosexuality*, 6, pp. 1–19.

Prieur, A. (1990) Gay men: reasons for continued practice of unsafe sex, *AIDS Education and Prevention*, 2, pp. 110–117.

Ramey, J. W. (1975) Intimate groups and networks: frequent consequences of sexually open marriages, *Family Coordinator*, 24, pp. 515–530.

Saghir, M. T. and Robins, E. (1973) *Male and Female Homosexuality: A Comprehensive Investigation* (Baltimore, Williams & Wilkins).

van Griensven, G. J., Tielman, R. A. P. and Goudsmit, J. (1987) Prevalence of LAV/HTLV III antibodies in relation to lifestyle characteristics in homosexual men in the Netherlands, *American Journal of Epidemiology*, 125, pp. 1048–1057.

Watney, S. (1987) *Policing Desire* (Comedia, London).

Weatherburn, P., Hunt, A. J., Davies, P. M., Coxon, A. P. M., and McManus, T. J. (1991) Condom use in a large cohort of homosexually active men in England and Wales, *AIDS Care*, 3, pp. 31–41.

FIFTEEN

Anthropology and AIDS: The Cultural Context of Sexual Risk Behaviour among Urban Baganda Women in Kampala, Uganda

Janet W. McGrath, Charles B. Rwabukwali, Debra A. Schumann,
Jonnie Pearson-Marks, Sylvia Nakayiwa, Barbara Namande,
Lucy Nakyobe and Rebecca Mukasa

INTRODUCTION

Because of the importance of human behaviour in HIV transmission, the AIDS epidemic has posed multiple research questions about the social and cultural context of sexual behaviour that constitutes a risk of HIV infection (e.g. Hrdy, 1987; Brokensha, 1988; Caldwell et al., 1989; Larson, 1989). Since the epidemic of AIDS was recognized in Africa in the early 1980s anthropologists have been active in African AIDS research (e.g. Feldman et al., 1987; Hrdy, 1987; Brokensha, 1988; Conant, 1988a, b; de Zalduondo et al., 1988; Obbo, 1988; Schoepf et al., 1988a, b; Caldwell et al., 1989; Larson, 1989; Feldman, 1990; Hunter, 1990; McGrath, 1990; Valleroy et al., 1990). One contribution of anthropologists to research on AIDS in Africa has been to stress the importance of the cultural and biological diversity of the populations of the continent (de Zalduondo et al., 1988). We have been caught short as a discipline, however, by the relative dearth of ethnographic research that can help to describe the current cultural context of sexual risk behaviour in Africa. While there are many ethnographies of Africa, there are fewer recent ones, especially in areas at the heart of the epidemic in East and Central Africa. The reasons for this are manifold and include war, decreased access to research sites and changing funding opportunities for ethnographic fieldwork. Nevertheless, with few exceptions (Obbo, 1980; Kilbride and Kilbride, 1990) there is sparse recent ethnographic information that can contribute to our understanding of the culturally relevant variables influencing behaviours that are associated with HIV infection. This paper reports on a study of the cultural determinants of sexual behaviour and risk of HIV infection in urban Baganda women in Kampala, Uganda, and uses the AIDS Risk Reduction Model (ARRM) (Coates et al., 1988; Catania et al., 1990) as a framework to examine sexual behaviour change for risk reduction.

Epidemiology of AIDS in Africa

Numerous summaries of the epidemiology of AIDS in Africa have been published (McGrath, 1990; Mann *et al.*, 1986, 1988; Quinn *et al.*, 1986; Torrey *et al.*, 1987; Piot and Carael, 1988; Piot *et al.*, 1988). As of 1 March 1991 there have been 83,749 cases of AIDS reported to the World Health Organization for the continent of Africa, with estimates for the number of individuals in Africa who may already be infected running as high as 5–6½ million (WHO, 1990, 1991; Palca, 1991).

HIV infection in Africa is focused in Central and East Africa. It is spread primarily through heterosexual contact, with perinatal and blood transmission constituting secondary routes of infection (pattern II; Piot *et al.*, 1988). Seroprevalence surveys indicate that up to 17–20% or more of the populations of some African urban areas may already be infected, but there are difficulties in interpreting seroprevalence surveys (Torrey *et al.*, 1987). Data from rural areas reports considerably lower infection rates, although this is not universally true (Torrey *et al.*, 1987; Nzilambi *et al.*, 1988; WHO, 1990, 1991; Palca, 1991). While it is true that high seroprevalence rates may primarily reflect the adequacy of reporting (Lamptey and Piot, 1990), it is clear that HIV infection rates are high in some areas and that AIDS is a common reason for hospital admissions (Sewankambo *et al.*, 1990; Goodgame, 1990; Muller *et al.*, 1990).

AIDS in Uganda

The first case of 'slim' disease or AIDS was identified in Uganda in 1981 (Serwadda *et al.*, 1985). On the basis of current reporting programmes, Uganda is second only to the United States in number of AIDS cases in the world. By 31 December 1990, 21,179 cases of AIDS had been reported to the AIDS Control Programme in Uganda (AIDS Control Programme, 1990). It has been estimated that a million or more people in Uganda may be infected with HIV (Asedri, 1989), including more than 20% of the population of the city of Kampala (Goodgame, 1990).

The highest rates of infection and disease in Uganda occur in women aged 20–30 (Asedri, 1989; Berkley *et al.*, 1989; AIDS Control Programme, 1990), many of whom are likely to have been infected in their early teens. In addition, HIV-infected women who bear children have as much as a 40% likelihood of infecting their child (Guay *et al.*, 1991), producing a high prevalence of paediatric AIDS.

In Africa the first identified groups at high risk of HIV infection were commercial sex workers, truck drivers and other mobile male workers known to have a large number of sexual partners. In Uganda up to 67% of the barmaids and 32% of the truck drivers were reported infected in 1987 (Carswell, 1987). Today, however, 28% of the mothers attending a prenatal clinic at Mulago Hospital in Kampala are reported to be HIV-infected (Hom *et al.*, 1991) and 16.6% of blood donors in Kampala were HIV-infected during the period 1986–9 (AIDS Control Programme, 1990). These data support the position that focusing on 'risk groups' is no longer appropriate. As Goodgame (1990) notes, and these figures confirm, once the prevalence in a community exceeds 10% 'knowing a patient's social history rarely helps in making a diagnosis of HIV infection' (see also Berkley, 1990). With high baseline seroprevalence rates essentially every sexually active person is at risk of becoming HIV-infected.

In response to the epidemic the Ugandan government has responded through, first, an active National AIDS Control Programme (Okware, 1987, 1988) and, more recently, established the AIDS Commission, which utilizes a 'multisectorial' approach that encompasses programmes in communication, rehabilitation, education, community services, defence and economic planning (Museveni, 1991). These programmes have resulted in a high level of awareness about AIDS which appears to have resulted in a decline in other sexually transmitted diseases (Museveni, 1991). But the epidemic is far from over. Therefore, continued focus on behaviour, specifically behaviours that pose a risk of HIV infection, is essential to understand the future course of the epidemic in this setting.

Behavioural Determinants of HIV Risk

Extensive research has been conducted on the determinants of preventive health measures and behavioural risk reduction in populations at risk for HIV infection in the United States (e.g. McKusick and Coates, 1985; Emmons *et al.*, 1986; Joseph *et al.*, 1987; Becker and Joseph, 1988; Coates *et al.*, 1988; Stall *et al.*, 1988). General models of health behaviour have been used for some time (e.g. the Health Belief Model: Rosenstock, 1974). The only model of the determinant of behavioural risk reduction that has been published to date specifically for HIV/ AIDS is the AIDS Risk Reduction Model (ARRM) (Coates *et al.*, 1988; Catania *et al.*, 1990). This model has been applied to several different populations in the USA. In addition, Lindan *et al.* (1991) used the ARRM to identify variables predicting behaviour change in women in Kigali, Rwanda.

Models of health behaviour have had some success in predicting the initial decision to change behaviour, but have not been predictive of maintenance of these changes (Becker and Joseph, 1988). In a study of Joseph *et al.* (1987), for example, the only variable consistently related to risk reduction behaviours six months after the first interview was the presence of social norms supporting such behaviour change. What these results suggest is that the cultural and social context within which the person operates is critical to understanding the likelihood of sustained behaviour change, since the social norms occur within a cultural system. Therefore, individual actions with respect to behaviour change must be examined within the cultural setting within which they occur.

In a context in which HIV infection is transmitted primarily through heterosexual contact a specific risk reduction strategy or strategies is also affected by gender relations. Socio-cultural norms and values regarding sexuality often differ for males and females (Larson, 1989; Kilbride and Kilbride, 1990) and therefore the specific costs and constraints of a specific risk reduction strategy may be gender-specific. In addition, specific status and power in sexual and social relationships may condition the ability of individuals to alter traditional patterns of sexual communication and ability to introduce innovative behaviours into sexual relationships (Obbo, 1980; Frankenberg, 1988), skills that may be necessary to reduce the risk of becoming infected with HIV. Patterns of sexual and marital relationships are strongly influenced by culture. As such, gender relations are conditioned by factors such as the relative economic independence of women, rights to land and inheritance, patterns of bridewealth, etc. (Obbo, 1980; Larson, 1989).

This study examines the cultural factors that influence sexual risk behaviour of Baganda women in Kampala, Uganda. The focus of this paper is the examination of the cultural rules and values governing sexual relations and their implications for risk reduction in this population.

Cultural Background of the Baganda

The Baganda are the predominant ethnic group in Kampala, which lies in the heart of what was once the Kingdom of Buganda, one of the most powerful of the Bantu kingdom states. The ethnography of the Baganda has been recorded by many anthropologists (e.g. Roscoe, 1911; Mair, 1934; Southall and Gutkind, 1957; Fallers, 1960, 1964; Southwold, 1965, 1972, 1973; Richards, 1966; Perlman, 1970; Kisekka, 1972a, b, 1973; Obbo, 1980; Kilbride and Kilbride, 1990).

The Baganda method of recognizing descent is patrilineal and individuals are traditionally associated with the clan of their father, although this association need not include residence in the clan village (Richards, 1966; Perlman, 1970; Southwold, 1965; Kilbride and Kilbride, 1990). Subsequent to marriage a couple is expected to establish a household separate from their parents. Even early accounts of foreign researchers indicate that multigenerational extended family households were rare (Fallers, 1964; Southwold, 1973).

Buganda was ruled by the Kabaka or king. The organization of the kingdom is thought to have been, in part, responsible for the high degree of physical and social mobility in the Baganda (Fallers, 1964; Southwold, 1965, 1972, 1973; Richards, 1966; Kilbride and Kilbride, 1990). This mobility in Baganda social organization applies to sexuality and marriage as well. Movement between sexual partners was and is reportedly frequent for both males and females (see Roscoe, 1911; Mair, 1934; Parkin, 1966; Mandeville, 1975, 1979). Anthropologists have commented on what they perceive to be the impermanence of Baganda marriages (e.g. Roscoe, 1911; Mair, 1934; Fallers, 1960; Southwold, 1965, 1972, 1973; Perlman, 1970; Kisekka, 1972a, b, 1973; Mandeville, 1975), linking this to, among other things, bridewealth rules that discourage stable partnerships (Fallers, 1964). Traditionally, bridewealth was returned to the husband if the marriage ended, through the initiation of either party, so that marital dissolution was a simple transaction between the two families (Mair, 1940; Fallers, 1960; Kisekka, 1972b). These authors argue that there appear to be no significant institutional constraints on marital separation among the Baganda, so that high rates of marital dissolution are not unexpected.

Objectives

In 1987 Case Western Reserve University in Cleveland, Ohio, and Makerere University in Kampala, Uganda, began a multi-year research collaboration in cooperation with the Ugandan Ministry of Health. One component of that project was the examination of the cultural context of sexual risk behaviour of those in the population who appear, in epidemiological terms, to be at high risk – women aged 17–30. The objective of the study was to ascertain the cultural context of sexual behaviours that place Baganda women living in Kampala, the primary urban area in Uganda, at risk of HIV infection.

Models of health and risk behaviours have often failed to examine the cultural context of health behaviours (e.g. Rosenstock, 1974). Many of the important barriers to behaviour change can only be understood in the context of norms and values influencing behaviour within a particular social group. Although the cross-cultural applicability of the ARRM has not been firmly established, Lindan *et al.*'s (1991) work in Rwanda suggests that the ARRM is a useful framework in which to explore the variables associated with behaviour change in different populations. Use of the ARRM as a framework for examining sexual risk behaviour in Baganda women doesn't constitute a formal test of the ARRM, but may offer further insight into the cross-cultural validity of the variables employed in the ARRM.

MATERIALS AND METHODS

Subjects for this study were recruited from the Case Western Reserve University–Makerere University collaborative paediatric follow-up study at Mulago Hospital in Kampala (K. Olness and C. Ndugwa, Project Directors). As participants in the paediatric study, each woman was given an HIV antibody test at an antenatal visit to Mulago Hospital (the exact stage in pregnancy of this visit varied), at the time of delivery at Mulago Hospital, and a proportion of the women were tested again at 10–12 weeks post-partum. Classification of HIV antibody status is based on consistent results on at least two blood draws. There is the possibility of seroconversion between that time and enrolment in the behavioural risk study. Most of the women chose not to be informed of their serostatus, despite being fully informed concerning the procedure (L. Guay, personal communication).[1]

Subsequent to HIV testing and enrolment in the paediatric project, women were recruited into the behavioural risk study at the clinic through the cooperation of the clinic staff. Women were eligible for inclusion in the behavioural study if they were Baganda, aged 15–30, and at least three months post-partum. Clinic staff prepared a list of potential subjects that was presented to the interviewers. Interviewers did not review clinical records and were not informed of the serostatus of the individual women. The women were approached by one of four Luganda-speaking female interviewers (SN, BN, LN, RM) who explained the objectives of the study. Each woman was asked if she was willing to participate through extensive interviews in her home. It was emphasized that participation was voluntary, all responses would remain confidential, and that refusal would not jeopardize access to clinic or home medical care. If the women consented, the interviewer collected specific information on the location of the respondent's home and made an appointment to visit her at home. The record of each interview includes a study identification number but no name. Subjects' names and identification numbers were only linked on a master list retained by the senior Ugandan investigator (CBR).

Demographic information was collected either at the clinic or during the first home visit. Information included age, marital status, income, education and religion. Subsequently, each woman was interviewed in her home over a period of several days. Interview topics included: cultural rules regarding sex, marriage and fidelity; individual sexual attitudes and behaviours; contraceptive knowledge and use; self-reported history of sexually transmitted diseases (STDs); AIDS knowledge and practices; and preferences and patterns of health treatment (Appendix). Questions about specific sexual practices and risk factors for HIV infection were constructed based on other studies of AIDS in Africa and Uganda (Quinn *et al.*, 1986; Berkley *et al.*, 1989; Simonsen *et al.*, 1990). Interviews were conducted in Luganda and translated into English by the interviewers. Complete sets of interviews are on file at Makerere University and the Johns Hopkins University Case Western Reserve University.

Analysis of the interviews focused on themes identified in the Appendix. Descripive statistics from the demographic questionnaire were coded and then analysed using Epi-Info and SPSS/PC+. Relationships were tested using χ^2 statistics, t test statistics, and Pearson's correlation coefficients generated by SPSS/PC+. Other quantitative findings are forthcoming (Schumann *et al.*, in press).

RESULTS

Table 15.1 presents the socio-demographic characteristics of the sample.[2] The mean age of the sample was 21 years (range 15–30). Forty-two cases (65%) and 41 controls (64%) have completed primary school or less, compared to 55.4% of the general population of women in Kampala (Kaijuka *et al.*, 1989). Thirty-seven (57%) of cases of 41 (64%) of controls reported earning less than 3,000 Ugandan shillings a month (approx $4.30 at a rate of 700 shillings to the dollar). Twelve (19%) cases and 17 (26%) controls are Muslims, 21 (32%) cases and 30 (47%) controls are Catholic and 27 (42%) cases and 15 (23%) controls are Protestant ($P = 0.07$) (Schumann *et al.*, in press).

Ninety-four (73%) of the women reported that they are currently living with a sexual partner. These sexual unions take several forms, including civil or church marriages, consensual unions and visiting unions. Twelve (18%) cases and seven (11%) controls have been married previously. Polygyny is common among the

Table 15.1 Socio-demographic data

Socio-demographic factors	Cases (n = 65)		Controls (n = 64)	
	n	%	n	%
Education				
None	4	6.2	0	0.0
Some primary	27	41.5	23	35.9
Primary completed	11	16.9	18	28.1
S3 completed	21	32.3	22	34.3
S4-S6	1	1.5	1	1.6
Teacher's training/technical school	1	1.5	0	0.0
Income (Ugandan Shillings per month)*				
None	32	49.2	36	56.3
1–3,000	5	7.7	5	7.8
3,001–5,000	9	13.8	2	3.1
5,001–7,000	10	15.4	4	6.3
7,001–10,000	2	3.1	12	18.8
>10,001	5	7.7	2	3.1
Unknown	2	3.1	3	4.7
Religion				
Muslim	12	18.5	17	26.6
Catholic	21	32.3	30	46.9
Protestant	27	41.5	15	23.4
Other	5	7.7	2	3.1
Marital status†				
Legal marriage	21	32.3	24	37.5
Consensual union	26	40.0	24	37.5
Visiting union	14	21.5	10	15.6
Formerly married	2	3.1	4	6.3
Single	2	3.1	2	3.1

*$P = 0.008$.

†Legal marriage is defined as one involving a religious or civil ceremony. Consensual unions exist when the couple live together with no such ceremonies. Visiting unions exist when one partner comes and goes from the household. The remaining categories are self-explanatory.

Baganda: 31% of urban Ugandan women reported that they are currently in a polygynous union (Kaijuka *et al.*, 1989), while 25 cases (39%) and 24 controls (38%) in this study reported that their husband has more than one wife. In addition, 44 (68%) cases and 35 (56%) controls reported that their husband has children with other women. It was not ascertained whether these children were born prior to their current marriage. Therefore, this measure cannot serve as a measure of previous or 'extramarital' sexual activity.

Both cases and controls reported an average of only one sexual partner in the last year. Over the past five years cases reported an average of 2.5 partners and controls reported an average of two partners ($P = 0.001$) (Schumann *et al.*, in the press). Cases and controls had the same mean age at first intercourse (15 years; range for cases 12–19 years, range for controls 10–20 years) and years of sexual activity (5.7 years). We recognize that the number of sexual partners over the past five years is a measure that may be confounded by years of sexual activity. Because the average age of the women is 21 years, this sample represents primarily women who are at the beginning of their sexual lives. The older women in the sample (who have been sexually active longer) may have had more lifetime partners than the other women. Therefore, for some younger women this measure represents lifetime partners, while for the older women it represents only the sexual partners over the past five years.

Cultural Rules and Values Regarding Sexual Behaviour

Insight into the sexual values of this sample is gained from examining responses to three specific questions. First, subjects were asked to name occasions when a woman should not have sex with any man, even her husband. Occasions named include during menstruation, after delivering a baby, when a child is sick, particularly with measles, and during mourning, especially for a close family member. Second, women stated that it is wrong to have sex with men other than one's husband during pregnancy, immediately after delivery and while breast feeding. Violation of these prohibitions is believed to lead to the death of the child, unless appropriate preventive actions, such as herbal baths from a traditional healer, are taken. Finally, 24 (37%) cases and 13 (20%) controls (P <0.05) identified occasions when a women is traditionally expected to have sex with men other than her husband. These occasions include: rituals around the birth of twins; funerals, especially the funeral of her husband, when a woman might be expected to have sex with the husband's brother; and weddings, when the parents of the bride (whether currently married or not) might have sex, or the bride's paternal aunt might have sex with the groom before the bride does. This sample of urban women widely regard these as traditional practices that are generally ignored today. The importance of these findings, however, is that they identify a set of cultural rules about sex, including when it is or is not acceptable, expected or appropriate to have more than one sexual partner.

Women reported that a woman's infidelity is a common reason for a man to leave his wife, while it is less often the case that a wife leaves her husband because of his extramarital sexual partners. This difference in the impact of infidelity for males and females stems from the fact that it is acceptable, even expected, for Baganda males to have more than one sexual partner (e.g. Southall and Gutkind, 1957; Mandeville, 1979; Obbo, 1988), while women are expected to remain faithful to their husbands.

The sanctions against a woman's infidelity include beatings, divorce or being chased from the home, or withdrawal of monetary support. Nevertheless, subjects gave several reasons why women have partners outside of their primary union, despite these cultural prohibitions (Table 15.2). Men are expected to provide material assistance to their girlfriends. Women often stated that if a husband fails to provide properly for his wife she is justified in having sex with a man who will provide either money or items such as clothing. Eighty-two (63%) of the women state that women have other partners for economic reasons, with cases significantly more likely to state this reason ($P < 0.05$). Subjects also reported that women have additional sexual partners in order to obtain greater sexual satisfaction (36 (28%) total, 25 (39%) cases and 11 (17%) controls, $P < 0.01$); to revenge on a philandering husband (18; 14%); and because some women are just born 'sex maniacs' ('abakasagazi' – literally 'itchy like elephant grass' (41; 32%)).

Table 15.2 Reasons why women have partners outside their primary union

	Cases (n = 65)		Controls (n = 65)		Total (n = 130)	
	n	%	n	%	n	%
Economic reasons	47	72	35*	54	82	63
Lack of sexual satisfaction	25	39	11**	17	36	28
Some women are naturally promiscuous ('sex maniacs')	23	35	18	28	41	32
Revenge on a promiscuous husband	8	12	10	15	18	14

*Significant at the 0.05 level.
**Significant at the 0.01 level.

Response to AIDS

All of the 130 women have heard of AIDS. Subjects were asked to name any routes of HIV transmission of which they were aware (Table 15.3). There were no significant differences between cases and controls in the modes of transmission named. Sixty-three (97%) cases and 65 (100%) controls mentioned sexual activity as a means of transmission of AIDS. Other methods of transmission mentioned include: blood transfusions (14 (22%) cases, 12 (18%) controls, $P > 0.5$), unsterile needle use (13 (20%) cases, 9 (14%) controls, $P > 0.3$), mother to child (6 (9%) cases, 3 (5%) controls, $P > 0.2$), breast feeding (4 (6%) cases, 1 (2%) controls, $P > 0.1$), witchcraft (2 (3%) cases, 0 controls, $P > 0.1$), and houseflies (1 (2%) cases, 0 controls, $P > 0.3$).

Sixty-three (97%) cases and 62 (95%) controls have heard of ways to protect themselves from getting AIDS (Table 15.3). There are no significant differences between cases and controls in the means of protection they named. Of these, 47 (75%) cases and 42 (68%) controls mentioned 'zerograzing' or 'stick to one partner' ($P > 0.3$).[3] Fourteen (22%) cases and 12 (19%) controls mentioned reducing the number of partners ($P > 0.5$) and 22 (35%) cases and 14 (23%) controls mentioned abstinence ($P > 0.1$). Nineteen (30%) cases and 25 (40%) controls specifically mentioned using condoms as a means of protection against infection ($P > 0.2$) (Rwabukwali *et al.*, 1993).

Fear of AIDS is high in this population. Fifty-six (86%) cases and 50 (77%) controls feared getting AIDS through sexual activity. Of those stating this fear, 32 (57%) cases and 31 (62%) controls gave a reason related to their male partner's

Table 15.3 Knowledge of HIV transmission and prevention

	Cases (n = 65)		Controls (n = 65)	
	n	%	n	%
HIV transmission				
Through sexual activity	63	97	65	100
Blood transfusion	14	22	12	18
Unsterile needles	13	20	9	14
From mother to child	6	9	3	5
Breast-feeding	4	6	1	2
Witchcraft	2	3	0	0
Houseflies	1	2	0	0
Knowledge of HIV prevention				
'Stick to one partner'	47	75	42	68
Abstinence	22	35	14	23
Condoms	19	30	25	40
Decrease number of partners	14	22	12	19

sexual behaviour, such as his having more than one partner ($P > 0.8$). This finding parallels that of Lindan *et al.* (1991) in Rwanda, who report that 62% of the women in their sample who perceive themselves at risk of HIV infection report that their risk is due to their partner's behaviour. In the current study, when women were asked how many partners they think that their sexual partner has had in the past year the cases reported an average of 1.8 and the controls 1.9. They reported that they think that their partners have had 3.6 partners (cases) and 3.4 partners (controls) in the past five years. These figures represent only the woman's opinion about her partner's number of partners, but nevertheless they indicate at least part of the basis for the women's perception that they are at risk of infection because of their male partner's behaviour.

What are these Baganda women doing to protect themselves against AIDS? Forty-one (63%) cases and 23 (35%) controls ($P > 0.01$) explicitly stated that they have changed their behaviour in order to reduce their risk of getting AIDS. Of these women (i.e. those who stated that they have changed their behaviour), 29 (71%) cases and 18 (78%) controls state that they are now 'sticking to one partner' and five (12%) cases and two (9%) controls now abstain from sexual activity altogether. Seven (17%) cases and three (13%) controls named other ways in which they had changed their behaviour (such as avoiding injections) to reduce their risk of infection. Of those women who reported that they have not changed their behaviour because of AIDS (15 (23%) cases and 24 (37%) controls), all cases and 19 (79%) controls reported that they have not changed their behaviour because they *already* had only one partner. Only three (5%) cases and two (3%) controls reported ever having used a condom and no women reported that they were currently using them (Rwabukwali *et al.*, 1993).

DISCUSSION

There are no significant differences between cases and controls with respect to AIDS knowledge and prevention strategies in this sample of Baganda women. The women in this study reported an average of only one sexual partner in the last year, a fact that may be related to two things. First, the women described a strong cultural belief that having sexual intercourse with a man other than the baby's father during pregnancy and lactation leads to the baby's death ('makiro' (Obbo, 1988); 'amakiro' (Roscoe, 1911; Orley, 1970)), unless appropriate actions (such as ritual baths in traditional herbs) are undertaken as protection. Therefore, it is not unexpected that this sample of women reported that they did not have additional partners in the 12 months preceding this study, a time which coincided with pregnancy and nursing. A second important reason for this finding is that some of the women reported that they have changed their behaviour out of fear of AIDS, and therefore have remained faithful to one partner.

This group of Baganda women have a high level of knowledge about AIDS, regardless of their serostatus. Their primary response to the threat of AIDS is to limit the number of partners by remaining faithful to their current partner. Despite these attempts by some of the women to reduce the risk of infection, subjects expressed fear that their partner is not practising similar risk reduction strategies. This fear stems from the cultural value described above, which deems that men can (and should) have multiple sexual partners. This, in combination with the women's own fears and concerns about using condoms (Rwabukwali *et al.*, 1993), limits the extent to which women can control their own risk of infection. The women, therefore, perceive themselves to be at risk of infection *despite* their own behaviour change.

These results indicate the difficulty of only examining what women know about HIV/AIDS, for it is not knowledge of the disease alone that reduces the risk of infection, but rather a combination of knowledge and culturally permissible behaviour change. In addition, in order for behaviour change successfully to reduce risk of infection it is necessary for both partners to change. In other words, even if the women change their behaviour there is a need for partners to change their behaviour as well.

Interestingly, McCombie (1990) found that males and females in a sample of Ugandans are equally likely to report that they feared AIDS because they did not trust their partners. Although we only have data on women it is clear that the issue of a *partner's risk-reducing behaviours* is an important one in this population. These findings, therefore, support earlier work (e.g. Lindan *et al.*, 1991) that suggests that a focus on individual sexual behaviour alone is insufficient – as both partners must respond to risk reduction messages for the risk reduction to be effective.

AIDS prevention advice usually involves two messages: be faithful to one partner and use condoms. The results of this study suggest two dilemmas for Baganda women in responding to this advice. First, although subjects report limiting their number of partners at the present time, they emphasize that there are situations, such as economic need, when a woman is justified in having another partner or partners. For women who employ multiple partner strategies out of economic need, advising them to reduce their sexual contacts, without recognizing the potential economic harm to them, is unlikely to result in behaviour change. Second, in a context in which males frequently have multiple partners, women can only control their exposure to infection to a limited extent. The reasons for this include the expectation that Baganda males will have more than one sexual partner, while women will not. The result of this cultural pattern is that women feel that they can only reduce their risk of infection to a certain extent, because of their inability to alter male behaviour.

The AIDS Risk Reduction Model

It is useful to explore these data in the context of the AIDS Risk Reduction Model proposed by Catania *et al.* (1990). The model proposes three stages of risk reduction: (1) The presence of variables supporting change, (2) a decision to change, and (3) taking action.

Variables identified in the ARRM as relevant to supporting change include: perception of the morbid event as problematic; perception of associated behaviours as problematic; knowledge of behaviours involved in disease transmission; perceived susceptibility; perceived norms; and aversive emotional states associated with problem behaviour. Our study population has a high perception of the morbid event (AIDS) as problematic, as well as a high perception of associated behaviours as problematic and a depth of knowledge about behaviours that transmit the disease. In addition, these women express a high degree of perceived susceptibility to infection. Perceived norms place women at risk of HIV infection, however, by sanctioning non-monogamous male sexual practices, thus limiting female control over sexual behaviour. Yet despite the cultural values that limit their options in terms of *specific behavioural changes*, these data suggest that the women in our sample may be in a strong position to *decide in favour of behaviour change* owing to their high perception of susceptibility to risk of infection. That is, according to the ARRM framework these urban Baganda women are in a situation that is supportive of behaviour change, based on their education about HIV and AIDS.

The decision to change one's behaviour according to the ARRM involves perceived costs of low versus high risk behaviours; perceived benefits of low versus high risk behaviours; skills and self-efficacy; and perceived norms. The women in our study perceive multiple sexual partnerships to be a 'high cost behaviour' and perceive a reduction in partners as a benefit in terms of risk for contracting AIDS. While they state that they have chosen to reduce their number of partners, they do not express the skills necessary to achieve any further reduction in risk of infection through negotiations with their sexual partner. This is linked to the women's limited ability to control their sexuality. These data suggest *that while women may make the decision to change their own behaviour this results in only a partial removal of the risk of infection.*

Taking action to change behaviour involves help-seeking behaviour; skills in healthful sexual behaviour; sexual communication skills; and perceived norms. Despite a high perception of risk of infection and personal decisions to reduce such risk, these women report little ability to take action beyond the step of reducing their number of partners, because this is the only action that is within their control. However, despite the fact that traditional values favour a woman's fidelity to her primary union, women report that the realities of economic needs may cause some women to seek outside partners. The value of single partnerships as 'safer sex' has not yet been fully operationalized in this population.

What does examination of the AIDS Risk Reduction Model tell us about risk behaviour in this population? By consideration of these data, in association with the elements of ARRM, it is clear that cultural values regarding sexuality serve as significant barriers to further risk reduction in this population of women. Risk of infection is, therefore, not reduced despite high levels of perception of risk of infection, susceptibility and benefits of behaviour change. This suggests that the ARRM may need to be modified for use in this context because it overemphasizes individual behaviour and choices without fully recognizing the influence of social-cultural factors on behaviour choices. Furthermore, our data demonstrate clearly that while education may have laid the foundation for a 'decision to change', other factors are now critical in achieving behaviour change.

CULTURE, SEX AND AIDS: POLICY IMPLICATIONS

The policy implications of these findings are clear although not startling: education about risk of infection is not sufficient. Cultural determinants of health behaviours serve as important barriers to health behaviour change. The ramifications of this as regards AIDS in Uganda have yet to be fully explored.

The women we studied have heard of AIDS and know the messages for reducing risk of infection. These messages include practising partner reduction in the form of 'zerograzing' and 'loving carefully'. Despite somewhat different interpretations of these messages, these women believe that they are acting upon them. It is clear, however, that *the women do not believe that their male partners have received or acted upon the same messages* (McGrath *et al.*, 1991, 1992). Without data on males we cannot directly address the degree to which this perception is accurate. However, the women we interviewed clearly state that they are afraid of getting AIDS because of their partner's behaviour. No comparable study on Baganda males has been published to date, but the data presented in this paper stress the urgency of understanding male sexual behaviour that poses a risk of infection in this context. Our data clearly indicate that focusing only on women is not sufficient.

The importance of knowledge alone in reducing risk of HIV infection seems to decrease over time (Becker and Joseph, 1988). Therefore, while it may be true that knowledge about AIDS has been important in reducing risk of infection in this population of Baganda women, it is now clear that knowledge alone cannot overcome barriers to further behaviour change. The implication of this for planning education and intervention programmes is that emphasis should now be on programmes that will teach about *how* to accomplish risk reduction and programmes that make such changes possible. These programmes will have the maximum value in this group.

Because Baganda women have limited ability to reduce their risk of HIV infection owing to prevailing cultural values with respect to sexual behaviour, policy makers are faced with the dilemma of how to alter the sexual norms and values of a cultural group. To reduce risk for HIV infection it would appear to be necessary to promote better sexual communication, faithful sexual unions and increased sexual decision-making powers for women.

At the present time behaviour change for risk reduction is the only available response in the fight against AIDS. This study illustrates the complexities of sexual behaviour, which is linked to economics, gender relations and a host of other socio-cultural factors. To say simply that we must increase women's sexual decision-making powers glosses over these complexities. But AIDS educators must now realize that AIDS control programmes must move beyond teaching facts of AIDS if AIDS prevention is to be achieved.

APPENDIX: INTERVIEW TOPICS

1 Cultural rules regarding sex, marriage and fidelity.
   - Sex inside marriage.
   - Sex outside marriage.
   - Attitudes toward fidelity and infidelity.
   - Sexual behaviour in general.
2 Individual behaviour.
   - Sex inside marriage.
   - Sex outside marriage.
   - Attitudes to fidelity and infidelity.
   - Sexual behaviour (including age at first intercourse, sexual practices, frequency of intercourse, etc.)
3 Contraceptive knowledge and use.
4 Sexually transmitted diseases.
   - Women's history.
   - Women's report of her husband's history.
5 AIDS knowledge and practices.
   - Knowledge about AIDS.
   - Knowledge of methods of prevention.
   - Knowledge about causation.
   - Attitudes and practices regarding condoms.
   - Personal risk reduction behaviours.
6 Preferences and patterns for health treatment.

NOTES

1 All study procedures involving testing and information of patients were approved by human subjects review committees in the United States and Uganda and were undertaken in accordance with the PHS policy for informing those tested for HIV status (National Institutes of Health, Policy on informing those tested about HIV serostatus. PRR Report 10 June 1988)

All the women participating in the paediatric follow-up study were informed that they would receive an HIV test. This information was transmitted to them in their native language at the time of enrolment. Participation in that study included a blood test at the times described in the text plus continued medical follow-up for the infant. Owing to the inability to diagnose HIV infection in infants prior to 18 months infants were not given HIV tests until their 12 and 18 month clinic visit. Prior to this time they were given continuous clinical follow-up and may have shown symptoms of clinical AIDS, in the absence of serodiagnosis. At the time that this behavioural study was completed only a proportion of the infants had reached 12 and 18 months.

It is important to note that at the time that the Case Western Research University – Makerere University collaborative study began the Ugandan policy in general and at Mulago Hospital in particular was not to inform patients of their HIV status, unless they had advanced clinical AIDS. This policy was based on a complex set of parameters, including lack of adequate counselling facilities and lack of adequate facilities for confirmatory tests. Policies worldwide require that positive serotests be confirmed using a Western Blot serotest, and technical difficulties in Uganda delayed attainment of confirmatory results. In the absence of proper confirmatory tests and adequate counselling, Case Western Reserve–Makerere University researchers were not permitted to inform patients of their serostatus unless they specifically asked for the results. All the women attending the clinic received AIDS education in Luganda, following the UNICEF model for AIDS education. As the study progressed, more and more of the women requested their test results, usually because they or their child has fallen sick. Today in Uganda, counselling services are more widely available and informing patients of their serostatus is acceptable. In addition, it is the policy of Mulago Hospital, in accordance with the World Health Organization, not to recommend that HIV-infected women in developing countries discontinue breastfeeding. The data on transmission of HIV by breast milk, while inconclusive, suggests that the risk of HIV transmission is small, while the risk of infant mortality from cessation of breastfeeding remains high. As a result, the policy has been not to discourage women from breastfeeding at this time (see, for example, S. J. Heymann, Modeling the impact of breastfeeding by HIV-infected women on child survival, *American Journal of Public Health*, 80, pp. 1305–1309, 1990).

2 One control subject was removed from quantitative analysis because she was identified as an extreme outlier. Quantitative analysis was therefore performed on 64 controls and 65 cases. This subject was retained for quantitative analysis of cultural themes and rules as she did not constitute an outlier with respect to this analysis.

3 'Stick to one partner' or 'zerograzing' are messages from the Ugandan government AIDS Control Programme. 'Stick to one partner' promotes monogamy and is interpreted as such by the respondents. 'Zerograzing' is a term taken from herd management theory. The idea is to 'graze' only within your own compound. The interpretation of this slogan varies from 'have only one partner' to 'have fewer partners, whom you know well'. A less frequent interpretation is 'abstinence'.

REFERENCES

AIDS Control Programme (1990) *AIDS Surveillance Report, Fourth Quarter* (Entebbe, Ministry of Health).

Asedri, V. (1989) 790,522 Ugandans are HIV positive, *The New Vision*, 4, p. 271.

Becker, M. H. and Joseph, J. G. (1988) AIDS and behavioral change to reduce risk: a review, *American Journal of Public Health*, 70, pp. 394–410.

Berkley, S. F. (1990) AIDS in Africa: a personal perspective, *Rhode Island Medical Journal*, 73, pp. 309–315.

Berkley, S. F., Widy-Wirski, R., Okware, S. I., Downing, R., Linnan, M. J., White, K. E. and Sempala, S. (1989) Risk factors associated with HIV infection in Uganda, *Journal of Infectious Diseases*, 160, pp. 22–30.

Brokensha, D. (1988) Overview: social factors in the transmission and control of AIDS, in N. Miller and R. C. Rockwell (eds) *AIDS in Africa: The Social and Policy Impact*. Studies in African Health and Medicine, 10, pp. 167–173 (Lewiston, Edwin Mellen Press).

Caldwell, J. C., Caldwell, P. and Quiggin, P. (1989) The social context of AIDS in sub-Saharan Africa, *Population and Development Review*, 15, pp. 185–234.

Carswell, J. W. (1987) HIV infection in healthy persons in Uganda, *AIDS*, 1, pp. 223–227.

Catania, J. A., Kegeles, S. M. and Coates, T. J. (1990) Towards an understanding of risk behaviour: an AIDS risk reduction model (ARRM), *Health Education Quarterly*, 17, pp. 53–72.

Coates, T. J., Stall, R. D., Catania, J. A. and Kegeles, S. M. (1988) Behavioural factors in the spread of HIV infection, *AIDS*, 2, Suppl., S239–246.

Conant, F. P. (1988a) Social consequences of AIDS: implications for East Africa and the eastern United States, in: R. Kulstad (ed.) *AIDS 1988*, AAAS Symposium Papers, pp. 147–156 (Washington, DC, American Association for the Advancement of Science).

Conant, F. P. (1988b) Using and rating cultural data on HIV transmission in Africa, in: R. Kulstad (ed.) *AIDS 1988*, AAAS Symposium Papers, pp. 199–204 (Washington, DC, American Association for the Advancement of Science).

De Zalduondo, B., Msamanga, G. I. and Chen, L. C. (1988) AIDS in Africa: diversity in the global pandemic, *Daedalus*, pp. 165–204.

Emmons, C. A., Joseph, J., Kessler, R., Wortman, C. B., Montgomery, S. B. and Ostrow, D. G,. (1986) Psychosocial predictors of reported behaviour change in homosexual men at risk for AIDS, *Health Education Quarterly*, 13, pp. 331–345.

Fallers, L. A. (1964) *The King's Men: Leadership and Status in Buganda on the Eve of Independence* (East African Institute of Social Research, Oxford University Press).

Fallers, M. C. (1960) *The Eastern Lacustrine Bantu* (London, International African Institute).

Feldman, D. A. (1990) Assesing viral, parasitic, and socio-cultural co-factors affecting HIV-1 transmission in Rwanda, in: D. A. Feldman (ed.) *Culture and AIDS*, pp. 45–54 (New York, Praeger).

Feldman, D. A., Friedman, S. R. and Des Jarlais, D. C. (1987) Public awareness of AIDS in Rwanda, *Social Science and Medicine*, 24, pp. 97–100.

Frankenberg, R. (1988) Social and cultural aspects of the prevention of the three epidemics (HIV infection, AIDS, and counterproductive societal reaction to them), in: A. F. Fleming, M. Carballo, D. W. FitzSimons, M. R. Bailey and J. Mann (eds) *The Global Impact of AIDS*, pp. 191–199 (New York, Alan R. Liss).

Goodgame, R. (1990) AIDS in Uganda – clinical and social features, *New England Journal of Medicine*, 323, pp. 383–389.

Guay, L. A., Ball, P., Ndugwa, C., Kenya-Mughisa, N., Hom, D., Kataaha, P., Olness, K. and Goldfarb, J. (1991) Vertical transmission of HIV infection in Ugandan infants. Paper presented at the 31st meeting of ICAAC, Chicago, Illinois.

Hom, D., Guay, L., Mmiro, F., Ndugwa, C., Goldfarb, J. and Olness, K. (1991) HIV-1 seroprevalence rates in women attending a prenatal clinic in Kampala, Uganda. Presented at the VIIth International Conference on AIDS, Florence.

Hrdy, D. B. (1987) Cultural practices contributing to the transmission of human immunodeficiency virus in Africa, *Review of Infectious Diseases*, 9, pp. 1109–1119.

Hunter, S. (1990) Orphans as a window on the AIDS epidemic in sub-Saharan Africa: Initial results and implications of a study in Uganda, *Social Science and Medicine*, 31, pp. 681–690.

Joseph, J., Montgomery, S., Emmons, C. A., Kessler, R., Ostrow, D., Wortman, C., O'Brien, M. and Eshleman, S. (1987) Magnitude and determinants of behaviour risk reduction: longitudinal analysis of a cohort at risk for AIDS, *Psychological Health*, 1, pp. 73–96.

Kaijuka, E. M., Kaija, E. Z. A., Cross, A. R. and Loaiza, E. (1989) *Uganda Demographic and Health Survey, 1988/1989* (Entebbe, Uganda, Ministry of Health).

Kilbride, P. L. and Kilbride, J. C. (1990) *Changing Family Life in East Africa: Women and Children at Risk* (University Park, University of Pennsylvania Press).

Kisekka, M. (1972a) Attitudes and values related to love, sex and marriage, in: A. Molnos (ed.) *Cultural Source Materials of Population Planning in East Africa*, I, pp. 162–166 (Review of Sociocultural Research 1952–1972) (Institute of African Studies, University of Nairobi).

Kisekka, M. (1972b) The Baganda of central Uganda, in: A. Molnos (ed.) *Cultural Source Materials of Population Planning in East Africa*, II, pp. 171–180 (Innovation and Communication) (Institute of African Studies, Univerity of Nairobi).

Kisekka, M. (1973) The Baganda of central Uganda, in: A. Molnos (ed.) *Cultural Source Materials of Population Planning in East Africa*, III, pp. 148–162 (Beliefs and Practices) (Institute of African Studies, University of Nairobi).

Lamptey, P. and Piot, P. (1990) *The Handbook of AIDS Prevention in Africa* (Durham, NC, Family Health International).

Larson, A. (1989) Social context of human immunodeficiency virus transmission in Africa: historical and cultural bases of East and Central African sexual relations, *Review of Infectious Diseases*, 11, pp. 716–731.

Lindan, C., Allen, S., Carael, M., Nsengumuremyi, F., Van de Perre, P., Serufiliria, A., Tice, J., Black, D., Coates, T. and Hulley, S. (1991) Knowledge, attitudes, and perceived risk of AIDS among urban Rwandan women: relationship to HIV infection and behaviour change, *AIDS*, 5, pp. 993–1002.

McCombie, S. (1990) Beliefs about AIDS prevention in Uganda. Paper presented at the American Anthropological Association meetings, November 1990.

McGrath, J. W. (1990) AIDS in Africa: a bioanthropological perspective, *American Journal of Human Biology*, 2, pp. 381–396.

McGrath, J. W., Schumann, D. A., Rwabukwali, C. B., Carroll-Pankhurst, C. and Marks, J. (1991) 'Zerograzing' and 'loving carefully': Baganda women's response to AIDS. Presented at the Society for Applied Anthropology meetings, March 1991.

McGrath, J. W., Schumann, D. A., Rwabukwali, C. B., Pearson-Marks, J., Mukasa, R., Namande, B., Nakayiwa, S. and Nakyobe, L. (1992) Cultural determinants of sexual risk behaviour among Baganda women, *Medical Anthropology Quarterly*, 6, pp. 153–161.

McKusick, J. W. and Coates, T. (1985) Reported changes in the sexual behaviour of men at risk for AIDS, San Francisco, 1982–1984. The AIDS Behavioral Research Project, *Public Health Reports*, 100, pp. 622–629.

Mair, L. (1934) *An African People in the Twentieth Century* (New York, Russell & Russell).

Mair, L. (1940) *Native Marriage in Buganda*, International Institute of African Language and Cultures, XIX, pp. 1–33 (London, Oxford University Press).

Mandeville, E. (1975) The formality of marriage: a Kampala case study, *Journal of Anthropological Research*, 31, pp. 183–195.

Mandeville, E. (1979) Poverty, work, and the financing of single women in Kampala, *Africa*, 49, pp. 42–52.

Mann, J. M., Chin, J., Piot, P. and Quinn, T. (1988) The international epidemiology of AIDS, in: *The Science of AIDS*, pp. 50–61 (New York, W. H. Freeman).

Mann, J. M., Francis, H., Quinn, T., Asila, P. K., Bosenge, N., Nzilambi, N., Bila, K., Tamfum, M., Ruti, K., Piot, P., McCormick, J. and Curran, J. W. (1986) Surveillance of AIDS in a Central African city, *Journal of American Medical Association*, 255, pp. 3255–3259.

Muller, O., Musoke, P., Okong, P., Duggan, M. and Moser, R. (1990) The presentation of adult HIV-1 disease in Kampala hospitals, *AIDS*, 4, pp. 601–602.

Museveni, Y.K. (1991) AIDS and its impact on the health, social and economic infrastructure in developing countries, in: G. B. Rossi, E. Beth-Giraldo, L. Chieco-Bianchi, F. Dianzani, G. Giraldo and P. Verani (eds) *Science Challenging AIDS*, pp. x–xvi (Basel, Karger).

Nzilambi, N., Decock, K. M., Forthal, D. N., Francis, H., Ryder, R. W., Malebe, I., Getchell, J., Laga, M., Piot P. and McCormick, J. B. (1988) The prevalence of infection with human immunodeficiency virus over a 10-year period in rural Zaire, *New England Journal of Medicine*, 318, pp. 276–279.

Obbo, C. (1980) *African Women: Their Struggle for Economic Independence* (London, Zed Press).

Obbo, C. (1988) Is AIDS just another disease? in: R. Kulstad (ed.) *AIDS 1988*, AAAS Symposium Papers, pp. 191–197 (Washington, DC, American Association for the Advancement of Science).

Okware, S. I. (1987) Towards a national AIDS-control programme in Uganda, *Western Journal of Medicine*, 147, pp. 726–729.

Okware, S. I. (1988) Planning AIDS education for the public in Uganda, in: *AIDS: Prevention and Control*, pp. 32–36 (Geneva, World Health Organization).

Orley, J. H. (1970) *Culture and Mental Illness. A Study from Uganda* (Nairobi, East African Publishing House).

Palca, J. (1991) The sobering geography of AIDS, *Science*, 252, pp. 372–373.

Parkin, D. J. (1966) Types of African marriage in Kampala, *Africa*, 36, pp. 269–285.

Perlman, M. L. (1970) The traditional systems of stratification among the Ganda and the Nyoro of Uganda, in A. Tuden and L. Plotnikov (eds) *Social Stratification in Africa*, pp. 125–161 (New York, Macmillan).

Piot, P. and Carael, M. (1988) Epidemiological and sociological aspects of HIV-infection in developing countries, *British Medical Bulletin*, 44, pp. 68–88.

Piot, P., Plummer, F. A., Mhalu, F. S., Lamboray, J. L., Chin, J. and Mann, J. M. (1988) AIDS: an international perspective, *Science*, 239, pp. 573–579.

Quinn, T. C., Mann, J. M., Curran, J. W. and Piot, P. (1986) AIDS in Africa: an epidemiologic paradigm, *Science*, 234, pp. 955–963.

Richards, A. I. (1966) *The Changing Structure of a Ganda Village* (Nairobi, East Africa Institute Press).

Roscoe, J. (1911) *The Baganda: Their Customs and Beliefs* (New York, Barnes & Noble).

Rosenstock, I. (1974) Historical origins of the health belief model, *Health Education Monographs*, 2, pp. 328–335.

Rwabukwali, C. B., Schumann, D. A., McGrath, J. W., Carroll-Pankhurst, C., Mukasa, R., Nakayiwa, S., Nakyobe, L. and Namande, B. (1993) Culture, sexual behaviour and attitudes towards condom use among Baganda women, in: D. A. Feldman (ed.) *Global AIDS Policy* (New York, Bergin & Garvey).

Schoepf, B. G., Wa Nkara, R., Ntsomo, P., Engendu, W. and Schoepf, C. (1988a) AIDS, women, and society in Central Africa, in: R. Kulstad (ed.) *AIDS 1988*, AAAS Symposium Papers, pp. 175–181 (Washington, DC, American Association for the Advancement of Science).

Schoepf, B. G., Wa Nkara, R., Schoepf, C., Engendu, W. and Ntsomo, P. (1988b) AIDS and society in Central Africa. A view from Zaire, in: N. Miller and R. C. Rockwell (eds) *AIDS in Africa: The Social and Policy Impact*, Studies in African Health and Medicine, 10, pp. 211–235 (Lewiston, Edwin Mellen Press).

Schumann, D. A., McGrath, J. W., Rwabukwali, C. B., Carroll-Pankhurst, C., Mukasa, R., Namande, B., Nakyobe, L. and Nakayiwa, S. Poverty and the risk of HIV infection in Kampala, Uganda (manuscript).

Serwadda, D., Mugerwa, R. D., Sewankambo, N. K., Lwegaba, A., Carswell, J. W., Kirya, G. B., Bayley, A. C., Downing, R. G., Tedder, R. S., Clayden, S. A., Weiss, R. A. and Dalgleish, A. G. (1985) Slim disease: a new disease in Uganda and its association with HTLV-III infection, *Lancet*, ii, pp. 585–852.

Sewankambo, N. K., Carswell, J. W., Mugerwa, R. D., Lloyd, G., Kataaha, P., Downing, R. G. and Lucas, S. (1987) HIV infection through normal heterosexual contact in Uganda, *AIDS*, 1, pp. 113–116.

Simonsen, J. N., Plummer, F. A., Ngugi, E. N., Black, C., Kreiss, J. K., Gakinya, M. N., Waiyaki, P., D'Costa, L. J., Ndinya-Achola, J. O., Piot, P. and Ronald, A. (1990) HIV infection among lower socioeconomic strata prostitutes in Nairobi, *AIDS*, 4, pp. 139–144.

Southall, A. W. and Gutkind, P. C. W. (1957) Townsmen in the making: Kampala and its suburbs (Kampala, East African Institute of Social Research).

Southwold, M. (1972) The Baganda of Central Uganda, in: A. Molnos (ed.) *Cultural Source Materials of Population Planning in East Africa*, Innovation and Communication, II, pp. 171–180 (Institute of African Studies, University of Nairobi).

Southwold, M. (1973) The Baganda of Central Uganda, in: A. Molnos (ed.) *Cultural Source Materials of Population Planning in East Africa*, Beliefs and Practices, III, pp. 163–173 (Institute of African Studies, University of Nairobi).

Southwold, M. (1965) The Ganda of Uganda, in J. L. Gibbs (ed.) *Peoples of Africa*, pp. 41–78 (New York, Holt, Rinehart, & Winston).

Stall, R. D., Coates, T. J. and Hoff, C. (1988) Behavioral risk reduction for HIV infection among gay and bisexual men: a review of results from the United States, *American Psychologist*, 43, pp. 878–885.

Torrey, B. B., Way, P. O. and Rowe, B. M. (1987) Epidemiology of HIV and AIDS in Africa: emerging issues and social implications, in: N. Miller and R. C. Rockwell (eds) *AIDS in Africa: The Social and Policy Impact*, Studies in African Health and Medicine, 10, pp. 31–54 (Lewiston, Edwin Mellen Press).

Valleroy, L. A., Harris, J. R. and Way, P. O. (1990) The impact of HIV-1 infection on child survival in the developing world, *AIDS*, 4, pp. 667–672.

World Health Organization (1990) The global AIDS situation: September 1990, *World Health Forum*, 11, pp. 341–342.

World Health Organization (1991) *Weekly Epidemiological Record*, 66, p. 73.

COUNSELLING

SIXTEEN

Application of a Family Systems Approach to Working with People Affected by HIV Disease

Riva Miller, Eleanor Goldman and Robert Bor

INTRODUCTION

HIV disease, like many other medical conditions, has a profound impact not only on the individual but also on significant others, affecting their relationships with each other, particularly within the family. Psychotherapeutic[1] support for those affected by illness traditionally focuses on the individual and his or her psychological symptoms. Psychosocial research, in the first decade since HIV became a major health and social problem in 1981, has focused mainly on the individual (Bor *et al.*, 1989a). Since 1990 there has been an emerging interest in the impact of HIV on the family (Bor *et al.*, 1993) and in translating this knowledge into therapeutic practice (Bor *et al.*, 1992; Walker, 1991). This paper describes the application of a family systems approach to psychotherapy for people affected by HIV. Two case studies illustrate some of the main themes and problems that may emerge in the course of therapy.

Who Constitutes 'the Family'?

The advent of HIV has prompted a redefinition of the family, taking into account the diverse social networks affected by the disease. Both biological (blood) relations and social (chosen) relationships are viewed within this context of *the family*, whether or not they are legally defined as a family. Same-sex relationships are therefore included under this definition.

Why a Family Systems Approach?

A family systems approach has particular relevance in the field of HIV disease. Individuals are part of social systems that may overlap, including their family of origin, family of choice, networks of friends, school, work and other organizations.

The interaction of these systems with health care systems, as well as the changing position of the individual in those systems of which he or she is part, need to be taken into account in planning and in conducting therapy (Miller and Bor, 1988).

Any physical illness may have implications for relationships whether they are within the family or in other support systems. Illness may bring about changes in relationships for the individual and those connected with him or her (McDaniel *et al.*, 1992). The traditional life stages in individual and family development (Carter and McGoldrick, 1980) may be disrupted by a diagnosis of HIV disease. Death may come sooner to young people who, hitherto, may not have seriously contemplated their mortality. Traditional patterns of caring may be reversed in families as children come home to their parents to convalesce or die. The hopes that people have for themselves and others close to them may be replaced with feelings of uncertainty, hopelessness about the future and remorse about the past.

There is a good 'fit' between a family systems approach and the nature of HIV infection, which involves multisystems: both may be characterized by interrelated systems (Engel, 1992). HIV can affect any organ or system in the body. Many different medical teams may be involved in the care of a patient at one time and through different stages of illness. At all stages of HIV disease, from infection, through the symptomatic and asymptomatic phases, to terminal illness and death, different issues may have to be considered in relation to clinical monitoring and treatment, sexual relationships, roles within the family and the patient's ability to function in work and social settings (Miller and Bor, 1988).

While there is as yet no cure or effective treatment for the virus there is also uncertainty as to whether all those infected with HIV will develop AIDS and die. Some techniques inherent in the systems approach, such as hypothesizing and the use of circular, hypothetical and future-oriented questions, may help to address the fine balance between such certainties and uncertainties.

How Did a Family Systems Approach Arise in Our Own Setting?

The approach to treatment and care discussed in this paper was first introduced in the Haemophilia Centre of the Royal Free Hospital, London. It was then applied to the development of the HIV/AIDS Unit in the same teaching hospital and medical school. A family systems approach was incorporated into the counselling in the HIV Testing Clinic and the AIDS Counselling and Social Care Unit. The evolution and development of a Milan-systemic approach to care in the HIV counselling service was itself an important intervention in the wider system and is discussed in greater detail in two previous publications (Bor *et al.*, 1988; Bor and Miller, 1990).

Some Aims of a Family Systems Approach in HIV Care

As is common with psychological problems, particularly in medical settings, patients with HIV disease are usually referred on their own for therapy. Connections between their apparent problem and family and social relationships are initially rarely made. A family systems approach may prompt individuals to view some problems and their solutions in a wider context of family and other relationships. While psychological adjustment to HIV can be the presenting problem, it often reveals previously repressed problems pertaining to relationships, particularly secrets within the family. HIV can also bring forth new problems stemming from a role reversal in an established pattern of relationships. The individual with HIV can be helped to consider how others might react and adjust to the diagnosis, and how they can be supported by them. Such connections help patients to identify and mobilize their own resources, thereby reducing some of the effects of social isolation experienced by those infected with HIV (Bor *et al.*, 1992). By engagement of the patient's wider network, demands on professionals to provide social support can be reduced.

A family systems approach may help to address the effects of secrecy about HIV in families, and between the family and others, such as health carers and schools. Patients can be helped to prepare for the future if they consider the implications of maintaining secrets in the family or disclosing sensitive information (Karpel, 1980). Collaborative teamwork between professionals comprising the health system can enhance comprehensive care and reduce the detrimental effects of secrets, such as tension between patients and staff who do and do not know the diagnosis.

The approach described focuses on *ideas* and *beliefs* relating to health care, and how people respond to illness in the family. The therapist may be interested in the patient's view of him or herself in relation to having a potentially fatal medical condition (Rolland, 1984). A family systems approach to medical problems emphasizes a time perspective to perceptions of relationships. This in turn may have implications for current relationships. Some examples of past actions that may emerge through the diagnosis of HIV infection include themes and ideas pertaining to 'infidelity', 'promiscuity', 'unacceptable lifestyle', 'misfortune' (transfusion-associated infection) and risk-taking activities, including sharing intravenous needles, having unprotected sexual intercourse or accidents in the occupational setting. These revelations mean that patients and their families may have to discuss and confront both HIV disease *and* the circumstances that have led to infection.

Patients who were infected with HIV as a consequence of infidelity in marriage or drug use might experience guilt and remorse. On the other hand, patients who have become infected through contaminated blood or blood products (prior to HIV screening for blood in 1985 in the UK) might be resentful of the doctors who inadvertently caused their disease, but at the same time have to reconcile this with their dependence on the medical system for their clinical care. This can add complexity to the patient's relationship with his or her doctor and the health care team (Kernoff and Miller, 1986).

In addition to issues in therapy stemming from the meaning of this illness, there are the ideas created in the mind of the patient at the time of diagnosis, and in the course of his or her clinical care. The language used in conveying diagnoses, prognoses and clinical information to patients may either create unrealistic feelings of hope or destroy any hope in the minds of patients and others. Prefaces of 'I'm afraid to tell you . . .' or 'It's nothing that should worry you now,' create meanings about illness at the time 'bad news' is given to patients. Perhaps one of the most difficult tasks in the psychological care of people affected by HIV disease is to address the delicate balance between the reality of the disease and its implications, and helping the patient and other to maintain hope (Bor *et al.*, 1992).

The authors have found a family systems approach to be adaptable to different cultures. HIV infection disregards ethnicity, social class and gender. For example, fears of disclosing HIV in cultures where arranged marriages are the norm poses particular challenges to both patients and health care workers. Health carers have a responsibility both to the index patient and for the health and welfare of others. Failure to ensure that patients understand the risks that they might take in transmitting the virus to others would mean neglecting a public health responsibility.

HIV infection can precipitate a crisis in all systems. The task is to help the patient manage the perturbations and the inconsistencies that emanate from the crisis in such a way that the individual continues to find ways of coping even when facing death.

The approach to therapy was adapted from the techniques of the Milan Associates. This enabled the therapists to develop a map of therapeutic practice and to conceptualize problems in a systemic framework (Miller and Bor, 1988). The salient features of the approach are:

1 There is a structure to the therapy session to ensure that important issues are addressed in the context of busy medical outpatient settings.
2 Before the start of each session a hypothesis is made about the impact of HIV problems and other related issues on relationships.
3 A focus is given to the session by setting small, achievable goals.
4 Patients' main concerns are elicited early in sessions and ranked in order of importance or severity to enable the most pressing issues to be addressed in the time available.
5 Questions are asked of the patient to test the hypothesis and to elicit and impart information.
6 Hypothetical, future-oriented questions are especially used to address concerns and people's perceptions of each other as well as their beliefs about HIV and medical care.
7 Problems may be reframed to help people consider their predicament differently, helping them to cope better on a day-to-day basis, while at the same time being realistic about the nature of HIV infection and its effect on relationships.
8 Patients are helped to consider how they may have coped with past difficulties and how they might cope in the future by exploring resources available to them.
9 The wider health care team is engaged whenever possible through team discussions, and by including nurses and doctors in interviews with patients and families. This helps to relieve stress on staff and avoid 'burnout'.

Systemic Theory in HIV Psychotherapy

Systemic theory from mental health practice (Campbell and Draper, 1985), family systems medicine (McDaniel *et al.*, 1992) and organizational consultation (Selvini Palazzoli, 1986) informs our clinical practice. It is not possible to describe the theory fully in this paper. Readers are referred to previous publications (Miller and Bor, 1988; Walker, 1991; Bor *et al.*, 1992) for a more comprehensive account of the application of systemic theory to HIV-related psychotherapy. The key features are summarized below.

While HIV disease is, at one level, a medical and social problem with profound implications for personal relationships (both social and sexual), contrary to some popular wisdom not all people with HIV have psychological problems arising from adjustment to illness. Furthermore, for those who do experience psychological and social problems, their nature, severity and duration may vary and change over time through the different stages of illness (Bor *et al.*, 1992). Defining the so-called 'problem', and for *whom* the problem is *most* a problem, is an important task in family systems medicine (Bor *et al.*, 1989c). Psychological problems arise from ideas and conversations pertaining to 'normality' and 'dysfunction' (Maturana *et al.*, 1988). This is particularly relevant in HIV care, where the level of provision of psychological and social support is almost without precedent in health care. The extent of support services for people affected by HIV may inadvertently lead some people to feel that they *ought* to have problems (Bor *et al.*, 1989b).

The 'problem' that therapists choose to deal with is a matter of perception. Some counsellors and therapists have adopted the traditional approach of focusing on the individual and his or her symptomatic behaviour (Miller, 1987; Green and McCreaner, 1989). Their aim is to alleviate symptoms of distress that may manifest as depression, anxiety, sleeplessness, low esteem, low sexual desire and so on. A family systems approach addresses symptoms of distress in the context of relationships and beliefs, while taking into account the stage of illness the patient has reached, and life cycle developmental themes (Selvini Palazzoli *et al.*, 1980; Miller and Bor, 1988). Some of the relationships and beliefs that are discussed with patients are as follows:

Relationships
1 The patient's view of himself or herself with an illness.
2 Who is defined as the 'family'?
3 The patient's relationship with his or her biological family or family of choice.
4 The relationship between the family of origin and family of choice.
5 The relationship between the patient and the caring system, for example medical and social care systems.
6 The relationship between the families of choice and origin and the caring system.

Beliefs
1 What beliefs about illness and treatments does the person have?

2 What ideas about the person arise from this particular medical condition?

3 What ideas in the family are challenged by illness in general, and HIV in particular?

4 What might it mean for this family that a child might die before his or her parents?

5 What ideas do they have for attending to the needs of the sick family member, while at the same time acknowledging the need to proceed with 'normal' daily life events?

6 What will help to keep everyone going? What resources does this family bring?

Using this approach, the therapist extends the patient's view of the implications of his or her illness to include other relationships and what this may mean for the patient's beliefs (Jones, 1993). The therapist may seek to reframe the problem by addressing the complement of any aspect of a theme or idea (Bor *et al.*, 1992). For example, secrecy-related problems can be discussed in terms of openness, protection, loyalty, boundaries and obligations in relationships. Talking to the patient about hope addresses both sides or the complement of a particular theme, such as hope and hopelessness, which is the basis of a systemic reframe (Campbell and Draper, 1985). For example, 'Who holds hope? What do they hope for? What effect does it have on a relationship that Steven holds more hope than Julie?' In most therapy approaches related to HIV disease the emphasis is on one side of the problem, such as death and loss (Green and McCreaner, 1989; Hildebrand, 1992). By addressing the complements of life and gains, the therapist may be able to amplify, add complexity to and ultimately reframe the patient's view of his or her problems (Bor *et al.*, 1992). The complement can be introduced by asking hypothetical and future-oriented questions of the patient and others, such as: 'How might it affect your relationship with your boyfriend if your parents were to become more involved in your care?'

There are a number of recurring themes that arise in therapy whether the infected person is a child or an adult, or whether the person is heterosexual, homosexual or bisexual, or whether the infection was due to sexual activities, drug use or contaminated blood. These themes pertain to loss, isolation, secrecy, hopelessness, despair, fear of disfigurement, disablement, death and dying, stigma, sexuality, hope and hopelessness and roles in the families and other contexts (Bor *et al.*, 1989d, 1992).

It is not possible in this paper to discuss the full range of psychological and social problems arising from HIV disease. Instead we have chosen to illustrate some of the most common recurring themes and the dilemmas that these pose for the therapist through two case examples.

CASE EXAMPLES

Two case examples are given to illustrate themes of secrecy, protection and control, and some approaches used to reduce the dilemmas for therapists working with families with HIV. The overall aims, in both cases, were to find a balance that would enable the family members, and families as a whole, to prepare for the future but to go on living with HIV as well as possible in the present. This was done by identifying if there was a problem, for whom it was most a problem, and how each person in the family wanted to resolve or reduce the effects of the problem.

Genograms were used to provide a map and a sense of relationships. They affirmed non-traditional relationships, as between gay men. Using genograms helped to open up discussion about who had and had not been told about HIV in the family system and the wider network, and to address the effect of secrets. Genograms enabled patients and their families to look at their available support network.[2]

Case 1: Secrets in a Family

Families come for therapy at different stages of HIV illness and for different reasons. The Green family have been seen regularly at the Haemophilia Centre for 15 years because the child has haemophilia. Discussions about the risk of HIV infection began before a diagnosis was possible. We have chosen to focus on the effects of secrets on this family. Although the secret has now been revealed to the boy with HIV, the stresses of the secret remain because his sister is still excluded. It is possible that John's death will be followed by the end of the family as a unit. His mother has said that 'He is my whole life to the exclusion of everyone else.' His parents have been growing more distant from each other, so they may part. The daughter would be left to fend for herself unless some way could be found for her mother to see that the daughter has a future that could be contained in the continuation of the family. Figure 16.1 gives the genogram for this family.

Barry and Rose knew before their marriage that Rose was possibly a carrier of haemophilia because she had two haemophilic brothers. Their first child, John, was tested for haemophilia soon after his birth. The results revealed that he suffered from severe haemophilia, thus also confirming that Rose was a carrier. They decided to request prenatal diagnosis in her second pregnancy, planning to have selective termination of a haemophilic child. As the baby was female (females are potential carriers, males potentially infected) they decided to continue with the pregnancy and John's sister Mary was born when he was two years old. She was investigated when she was six and found not to carry haemophilia.

Haemophilia centres offer comprehensive care to patients, which includes treatment for bleeding episodes and any other medical conditions. Most centres recognize that haemophilia also affects the whole family, and psychological and social support is offered, either at the time of regular six-monthly reviews or when requested by the patient or his family.

The Green family required considerable support in the early years after John's diagnosis – initially in coping with his bleeding problems and then in decisions about having a second child. Barry and Rose had very different perceptions of the problems arising from haemophilia. Rose had experienced the death of two

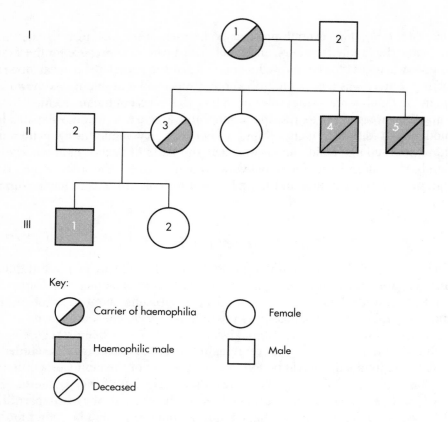

Key:

⊘ Carrier of haemophilia   ◯ Female

▨ Haemophilic male   ☐ Male

⊘ Deceased

Figure 16.1 Genogram of case 1, the Green family

younger brothers who were haemophilic – one very young when she was five years old and the other in his teens, when she was 19. Her greatest fear was that John, too, would die young. Barry tended to dismiss her fears, saying that the treatment given to John had not been available when her brothers were young. While this was true, he seemed unable to accept that there were still many restrictions on the activities considered safe for a haemophilic boy and he was unsympathetic to her fears. They were seen as a family at six-monthly intervals with Barry, Rose and Mary all coming with John. Rose gradually learned to cope with her fears and when John was five she learned to treat his bleeds at home. The distance between Barry and Rose was increased while she became more enmeshed with John at the expense of Mary, whom Rose acknowledged had been relegated to second place. Barry and Mary stopped coming with Rose and John to review appointments.

In 1985, when John was eight, the test for the antibody to HIV virus became available. He was found to have been infected with the virus as a result of blood product treatment. Testing of stored plasma samples showed him to have been infected two years before testing was possible. His parents were informed and several lengthy counselling sessions followed. Barry's first reaction was disbelief in the accuracy of the test, followed by a determination to believe that the disease would not progress. Rose was convinced that John would die within five years. Both agreed that they did not wish John to know his diagnosis.

After a year the family resumed the old pattern of Rose bringing John to the haemophilia centre without Barry or Mary. Rose requested time on her own at each visit, where she could be given the most up-to-date information on prognosis, treatment and advances in research into HIV. She remained adamant that John's HIV diagnosis be kept secret from him. She feared breaches of confidentiality and resulting stigma. She said that knowing that he had HIV would 'destroy' John and that her life would end if anything happened to him. He had asked once whether he had AIDS, to which she had answered 'no'. In her view this was a 'white lie'. Both parents later said that they would tell John about HIV 'if he asked' but he did not ask again, apparently secure in the knowledge that he did not have AIDS.

Haemophiliacs have their health closely monitored at regular six-monthly reviews. It is the policy in UK haemophilia centres for HIV-positive patients to be put on prophylactic therapy against pneumocystis pneumonia and candida infection (thrush) as well as antiviral therapy with AZT if their CD4 counts fall below 200 on two consecutive occasions (indicating a decline in the effective working of the immune system). Rose and Barry were aware of this and she always telephoned after blood tests to ask for his results.

The main concern of the parents was to keep the secret of John's HIV diagnosis from being revealed. While struggling to come to terms with the loss of a future for John they attempted to make him 'normal', allowing him to indulge in activities such as ice skating, which carried risks of serious injury for someone with haemophilia. The parents' relationship continued to deteriorate with only John's HIV and the desire to maintain the secret keeping them together.

The aim of the therapists was to help the parents to consider and deal with the implications of maintaining and disclosing the secret, and to support the family in mobilizing the resources that would allow them to prepare for the future while living as well as possible in the present.

The therapists explored with Rose ways in which she might tell John about his HIV. She was asked when she thought it would be the best time – while he was well or if he became ill. Who should tell him? Would they tell Mary? Should he know before he began to start relationships with girls? Who else needed to know?

Hypothetical and circular questions were used to help the parents make decisions about when, if, how and who to tell about John's HIV. They were also used to help the parents consider their fears of the effects of disclosure on John, and his sister, and of upsetting the balance that they had achieved in living from day to day. Examples of questions used over time to address the effects of secrets in the family included:

> What would be the worst thing that would happen if you told him?
>
> If Mary knew about John and had worries who would she talk to about them?
>
> If Mary knew about John what difference do you think it would make to their relationship?

How does keeping the secret affect your relationship with John?

Do you think that Mary has guessed that you are worried about John?

What effect might it have on John when you do tell him?

Although the therapists respected the parents' wishes about keeping the diagnosis of HIV from John, they were becoming increasingly concerned that John, now almost 15, might unknowingly put others at risk. HIV and sexual transmission were discussed with John in general terms. Rose said that they had emphasized the need for him to protect himself when he reached the stage of starting a sexual relationship. After this Barry came to a session with Rose where they were again seen on their own while John was receiving treatment for his haemophilia and having blood tests.

Once again, ways of telling John were rehearsed with them. They hoped that they could tell him together, while he was well and 'when the time was right'. Pressed to say when the time would be right they answered 'When he asks or when he seems to be interested in girls'.

Shortly before his sixteenth birthday and the beginning of his GCSE exams he was found to have a CD4 count just above 200. A repeat test was requested and it was arranged that the blood would be taken after a dental appointment at the hospital the next week. Rose did not tell John about the blood test until he reached the hospital. In the car on the way home John was very angry and demanded to know what was going on. Thinking that he suspected the diagnosis Rose told him that he was HIV-positive and that his count was falling, which might mean that he needed treatment. John was stunned by the news, having suspected nothing since he believed that he had not been infected. The second blood count was below 200 and they agreed to come to the centre together to discuss John's treatment.

Barry, Rose and John came without Mary, whom they had decided should not be told. This was to protect her and also to prevent the diagnosis being revealed outside the family. John's health was discussed openly and arrangements were made for him to start his prophylactic and antiviral treatments. John sat between his parents, who seldom looked at each other. Rose and John were tearful but Barry appeared detached. The immediate effects of revealing the secret were:

1 Involving John in decisions about his health care.
2 Re-engaging Barry in the therapy sessions.
3 Relieving stress on staff who felt bound to respect the parents' wishes while being concerned about their responsibility to others who might be put at risk by John's ignorance of his condition.

Questions were designed to relate the family to past events and to help them draw on previous experience to find ways of coping with illness and death. For example:

How did your mother tell you that your younger brother might die?

How did your brothers' haemophilia affect your relationship with your parents and your sister?

How did the deaths affect your parents' relationship?

In spite of careful planning of how they would tell John together, the pressure of keeping the secret had become too much for Rose. Barry's first reaction was anger that she had told him on her own and that this was shortly before his examinations. He maintains what may be unrealistic hopes for John to finish school and complete a university education 'to equip him for the future'. Rose is convinced that John will become steadily worse and die. Neither has any plans for including Mary or offering her support.

The original hypothesis was that the parents' greatest need was to keep the secret of John's HIV infection from the children to protect them all from breaches of confidentiality because of their fear of the repercussions of stigma and discrimination. They feared that if John knew the diagnosis he would be 'destroyed'. They feared that John would not be able to cope with the loss of a future they were struggling to accept themselves. Revealing the secret of HIV forced the parents to confront the loss of a future for John, who has been the focus of their energies because of his haemophilia. Their attempts to see him as normal had been shattered. His sister, Mary, may have to become a protector of her parents, ending her adolescence abruptly. John's threatened death may raise issues between the parents relating to blame of transmission of haemophilia and may end a fragile marriage.

Future therapy will be aimed at helping all of them to prepare for deterioration in John's health while maintaining some hope. Mary has become a source of greater concern for the team since she is being excluded from a central event in the family and is possibly being prevented from raising her own concerns for John, herself and her parents.

This family and the next case to be discussed are linked to therapy through the health care system: case 1 through haemophilia and HIV, and case 2 through HIV alone. When the index patients die, the families are unlikely to remain in contact with the hospital therapists. Both families will be offered bereavement counselling if they wish to come to the hospital. Neither family is likely to be able to disclose the cause of death openly and both will probably use liver disease as the explanation. They will not have support from their natural networks of friends and even some family members will be excluded because of the diagnosis. However, this is not the same for all families where there is an HIV death. Some openly disclose the diagnosis and become actively linked to other systems through HIV.

Case 2: Defining Who Is Protecting Whom

The family described in the next case might never have come for therapy if HIV had not become a problem for them. The dynamics of relationships in the family were challenged by events and processes at different stages of the patient's disease.

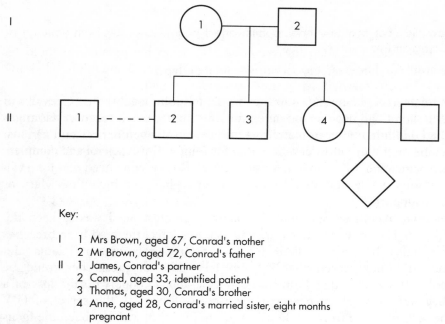

Key:

I 1 Mrs Brown, aged 67, Conrad's mother
   2 Mr Brown, aged 72, Conrad's father
II 1 James, Conrad's partner
   2 Conrad, aged 33, identified patient
   3 Thomas, aged 30, Conrad's brother
   4 Anne, aged 28, Conrad's married sister, eight months
      pregnant

Figure 16.2 Genogram of case 2, the Brown family

Themes of protection and control of one family member by another emerged in therapy sessions. The genogram is shown in Figure 16.2.

Conrad, a 33-year-old gay man, sought an HIV test through the hospital because he suspected that he was infected with HIV. Over the past year he had noticed symptoms that he connected with HIV infection. Conrad recognized his risk for HIV as being high because he had been a sex worker who had had unprotected anal intercourse with other men in the past. The problem that first brought him in contact with a therapist was a needle phobia, which had to be overcome in order for him to have a blood sample taken for an HIV test. A psychologist in the team (R.B.) helped reduce his anxiety in order for testing to proceed. The test result confirmed that he had been infected with HIV, a result which he had anticipated. The next few months were characterized by a period of adjustment. Conrad was determined to look on the bright side and to be optimistic about his prognosis. Conrad's needle phobia waned and he was able to have his blood tests, while psychological support was gradually reduced.

Six months after his diagnosis he was admitted to hospital on Christmas Eve with an acute lung infection. He asked to see the therapist because of his anxiety about what to tell his elderly parents, who lived in a small village outside London. He did not want them to know about his admission to hospital or about his diagnosis of AIDS, which he believed might be the news that would kill them. They knew he was gay, and that he was running a successful male escort agency, but had never discussed HIV with him. Conrad did not want to be viewed by his parents as the son who was different and who led a 'low' life. To compensate for this, he had provided them with financial assistance to give them a lifestyle that they would not have had without his support. The family were expecting to spend Christmas Day together. He decided to keep the secret of HIV from his parents, but told his younger brother, Thomas, the diagnosis so that he could attend to Conrad's business affairs. His married sister Anne was also informed.

Conrad enlisted his brother's support in corroborating a story that Conrad was going on holiday. Thomas's concern about the immediate crisis over Conrad's health forced him to respect his wishes. The use of hypothetical and circular questions enabled Conrad to consider that keeping secrets might be difficult for Thomas. For example:

> What effect do you think it will have on Thomas that he knows something about you that he cannot tell your parents?
>
> What might help Thomas to keep the secret?
>
> How long would you want Thomas to keep the secret?
>
> What would be the reaction from your parents that you would fear the most?

The last two questions helped Conrad to think about when and how he might disclose his HIV infection to his parents, and to identify his main concerns for himself and his parents if they were to know about his diagnosis.

Conrad decided to disclose his diagnosis to his parents a while after he went home, to protect them from seeing him as ill or vulnerable. Soon after disclosure he sought help from the therapist, saying 'HIV is not a problem for me, but supporting and counselling my parents is a burden which I can do without.' He maintained that he was coping well but wanted the therapist to see his parents without him. He sought to protect his mother, in particular, from the reality of his situation – that of declining health and early death. He wanted the therapist to inform his parents about his diagnosis, but to keep them optimistic and hopeful. He feared that increasing his mother's worry about his health would escalate the number of telephone calls she made enquiring about him. He viewed these phone calls as intrusive and disturbing, as they would increase his feelings of impotence about placating her worries. The diagnosis of AIDS compelled Conrad to ask for help, threatening his view of himself as coping with HIV and controlling communication between himself and his parents. Conrad resumed control by arranging the appointment, bringing them to the hospital to introduce them to the therapist, and then leaving.

The initial dilemmas for the therapist were twofold: first, how to respond realistically to questions about Conrad's prognosis, without giving him 'bad news'; second, whether to encourage Conrad to attend sessions with his parents, or to comply with his wish for them to be seen separately. Seeing the family together would enable them to express and hear each other's views, which might not be possible in conversations outside therapy. Allowing Conrad to feel he could control the closeness and distance of relationships was at that time deemed to be more important than seeing him with his family. Nevertheless, by using a systemic approach, some interventions could be made which helped to prepare the family for Conrad's death without breaching confidentiality. The therapist clarified with Conrad, his parents and his siblings that no medical or other details about Conrad would be given without him being present. Separate meetings would remain confidential, although HIV infection in general could be discussed. This engaged the family members and preserved some neutrality. It was possible to elicit from the parents what they considered to be Conrad's main concern, and how their concerns might affect their relationship with him and with their other children.

Conrad's parents were seen on their own four times, twice with Conrad's sister and brother, and twice with Conrad. Like Conrad, his parents were ambivalent. They needed to know his prognosis, while at the same time not wanting to know the 'truth' in order to protect themselves and each other from the full implications of Conrad's death. The therapist's task was to help Conrad and his family to keep the fine balance between maintaining hope and living as well as possible within the realities of his life-threatening condition. For example:

Therapist: Mrs Brown, you ask whether Conrad will die from his HIV infection. Mr Brown, how might you answer your wife's question?

Mr Brown: We are hopeful that it will not be soon. I know that there is no cure.

Therapist: How do you think that your wife will manage from day to day knowing this?

Mr Brown: She is stronger than she appears.

Therapist: Mrs Brown, do you agree with your husband's view of you?

Mrs Brown: Yes. I am more worried about how Conrad manages.

Therapist: How do you think Conrad would tell you he is managing?

Mrs Brown: He would say that I am not to worry, and that he has managed his life so far.

Despite describing themselves as a 'close family' they had communication difficulties, as each tried to protect themselves and others from the reality of AIDS by not talking about it. An aim of the therapy was to help the different members of the family to talk to each other about issues that they might need to settle, such as where Conrad wanted to be buried or how much to ask him about his health. Questions helped to address these issues. For example:

Therapist: Conrad, your father says that he has some worries for the future. Do you know what they might be?

Conrad: Perhaps what to tell the neighbours if I die.

Therapist: Do you agree with this, Mr Brown? Is it your main concern?

Mr Brown: We would like to know what to say, but I am more worried about what Conrad want us to do for him, and what he wants his 'friend' to do.

After a few sessions alone with the parents the fine balance of family interactions had been upset. As the parents appeared to become close to the therapist, or perhaps as Conrad felt excluded from the therapy, he conveyed that there was nothing more that she could do for his parents, thereby controlling the interactions between the parents and the therapist. The previous pattern of control was resumed. He achieved this by restricting his parents' phone calls and visits to him, and they acquiesced to these requests. His mother kept control over Conrad by letting him see or hear her anxiety, which brought him rapidly to protect her. Her anxiety protected him from having to face her disapproval of his lifestyle and her disappointment that he would not fulfil her wish for grandchildren. Conrad's father kept control of his emotions in order to protect himself and Conrad from getting too close and risking discussions about his sexuality that might have implications for both of them. Conrad wanted his father to accept the reality of his being gay by acknowledging that his partner, James, was his lover and not just a 'friend'.

As Conrad's health deteriorated, he asked for psychological help for himself for the first time. His main anxiety was that he would become physically and mentally dependent on others, and that he was 'going mad'. He accepted a referral from the doctor for a psychiatric opinion, which reassured him that he was not going mad. Soon after this he was readmitted to hospital with a serious eye condition that could lead to blindness. Again he asked the therapist to deal with his parents' panic. His own anxiety about becoming blind was addressed in therapy through the use of hypothetical, future-oriented questions and through metaphor. For example: If he thought that he was at risk of becoming blind, how might he best prepare himself for this? How would he see things for himself if he became more dependent on his boyfriend? What views of his parents would he want to preserve? What images would he want to remember from his relationship with his parents and his brother and sister?

Conrad arranged to meet his parents in the therapist's office to protect them from seeing other patients on the ward dying with advanced HIV disease. Soon after the start of the session the therapist invited Conrad to join his parents. The immediate aim was to help them engage with each other to discuss whatever issues they wished, by asking each of them circular questions about main concerns. Conrad did not want to see or hear his mother's worries for him. His mother did not want him to suffer from pain. His father wanted Conrad to know that they were 'there for him'. Their anxieties were reframed as protecting each other. The family members started talking directly to each other. At this point the therapist decided to leave the family alone to give them the opportunity to continue the conversation that they had started and to use the limited time that Conrad had made available to his parents without having the therapist to protect them. Conrad kept control by specifying that he had to return to the ward in 30 minutes. The remaining weeks of Conrad's admission were without adverse emotional events. He reported that his parents were much calmer despite having seen him at home on a day when he was quite incapacitated. They were also preoccupied with his sister, who was expecting a baby.

The main aims of therapy in this case were to respond to crises, while at the same time weaving into the sessions some preparation for the future, which meant addressing loss. Some examples of questions used to achieve this are:

> If Conrad did become ill and you were not immediately informed, how would that affect you?
>
> If Conrad did not get any better how might you cope?
>
> What might you tell your friends if Conrad did become very ill and died? (The parents many months after this discussion came up with the suggestion of liver disease.)

Conrad was given the support that he felt he needed in adjusting to and living with HIV disease. A focus was kept on main concerns, whether these were for Conrad or for the family as a whole, which gave the sessions a structure and helped to 'control' reactions of the family members to Conrad's deteriorating health. Therapeutic interventions reframed the problem of AIDS as a problem of communication, which has been brought to light for this family by AIDS. Mrs Brown's anxiety about Conrad's health, his ability to cope and the secret kept the family together. Mr Brown tried to protect his wife from the reality of Conrad's imminent death by asking questions about the prognosis, and at the same time construing any medical information as optimistic. Mr Brown and Conrad protected each other and other family members in this way. Some secrets seemed appropriate, such as protecting the parents from stigma and isolation in the future by not disclosing the diagnosis in the village where they lived. Conrad rarely visited his parents at home. The therapist maintained some neutrality, while enabling the family to discuss, in a controlled environment, issues that they were unable to raise alone, such as Mr Brown's prejudices about same-sex couples.

A challenge for the therapist was to balance the realities of the hopelessness of this family's situation with some hope. Themes of protection and control emerged early. Conrad's injunctions to keep his parents informed about his health and at the same time to maintain an optimistic view were a protection as much for himself as for his parents. Conrad knew that his condition was deteriorating. Time pressures of a shortened life expectancy, compounded by the complexity and number of issues, made it important to consider carefully appropriate approaches to therapy with this family. Brief therapy at points of crisis and appreciation of life stage transitions helped to reduce crises, and prepared the family members for the next stage of HIV disease. Having small goals, identified early in sessions, enabled Conrad to keep a sense of achievement.

The perturbations caused in this family system by HIV were: coping with a child dying before parents; accepting the consequences and conflicts of an alternative lifestyle in a conventional family; managing the disruptions caused to entrenched patterns of communication; and dealing with secrets.

CONCLUSION

The mode of HIV transmission was different in the two case examples. Despite this, once a family member was infected with HIV similar themes of secrets, hope, hopelessness and protection emerged for the families in both cases. The therapy sessions provided a safe and neutral place to discuss secrets and issues that might be difficult to raise without the presence of the therapist. The sessions were a place to challenge views and help patients and families to take another view of the problem, thereby maintaining hope in the face of life-threatening illness.

Conventionally, therapy for people with acute or chronic life-threatening illness addresses issues of loss, bereavement and 'coming to terms with illness'. HIV can complicate the conventional approach because of some of the special features, such as the stigma and secrets. Some patients would not go to therapy if not for HIV, which then makes them focus on problems arising for relationships. For others, problems from the past are either overshadowed or masked by HIV. Patients with HIV infection come to therapy in different ways. They seldom come saying that the family is in crisis; rather, a symptom, such as needle phobia, is the entrée to help for the family. Stress due to anxiety or the complexity and severity of the diagnosis may force individuals and families to seek help. Sometimes it is the overwhelming number and complexity of issues that health care staff perceive patients to experience that precipitate a referral for therapy. In a systems approach no assumptions are made about whether or not HIV is a problem for an individual, the nature of any problem and how, if at all, the individual wants to solve his or her problem.

One of the specific challenges to therapists is to remain neutral and to be able to let go. There may be a strong emotional pull to protect and rescue those who experience isolation due to the stigma associated with HIV. A systems approach helps to militate against being drawn too much into the patients' dilemmas and to help them join with their natural networks. A team also helps to share responsibility for some of the difficult dilemmas facing therapists, such as dealing with dual responsibility to the index patients and others.

In using a family systems approach to a medical problem the authors are concerned not only with the patient and his or her relationship with the many overlapping systems described, but also with how to use the approach in a conventional medical setting. Sometimes health care professionals can experience what is referred to as 'burnout' owing to the pressure of too many cases as well as the stressful nature of dealing with terminal illness in a young population. A systems approach has been found to reduce staff stress by enhancing the skills of a range of health care workers. The principles and techniques of the systemic approach are demonstrated by team meetings and by including nurses and doctors in sessions with patients.

NOTES

1 The authors use the word psychotherapy in preference to counselling to distinguish information-giving and primary support from psychological interventions aimed at relieving stress. The authors believe that irrespective of whether one is giving information or discussing psychological problems, the intervention itself should aim to be therapeutic.

2 To preserve confidentiality the names and details used in the case examples have been changed.

REFERENCES

Bor, R. and Miller, R. (1988) Addressing 'dreaded issues': a description of a unique counselling intervention with patients with AIDS/HIV. *Counselling Psychology Quarterly*, 1, pp. 397–406.

Bor, R. and Miller, R. (1990) *The Internal Consultant in Health Care Settings* (London, Karnac).

Bor, R., Miller, R. and Perry, L. (1988) Systemic counselling for patients with HIV/AIDS infections. *Family Systems Medicine*, 6, pp. 49–67.

Bor, R., Miller, R., Goldman, E. and Kernoff, P. (1989a) The impact of AIDS/HIV on the family, *Practice*, 3, pp. 42–48.

Bor, R., Miller, R. and Perry, L. (1989b) When the solution becomes a part of the problem in the psychosocial management of an AIDS patient. *British Journal of Guidance and Counselling*, 17, pp. 133–137.

Bor, R., Perry, L. and Miller, R. (1989c) A systems approach to AIDS counselling: defining the problem, *Journal of Family Therapy*, 11, pp. 77–86.

Bor, R., Perry, L., Miller, R. and Salt, H. (1989d) Psychosocial and behavioral aspects of AIDS, *Sexual and Marital Therapy*, 4, pp. 35–45.

Bor, R., Miller, R. and Goldman, E. (1992) *Theory and Practice of HIV Counselling: A Systemic Approach* (London, Cassell).

Bor, R., Miller, R. and Goldman, E. (1993) HIV/AIDS and the family: a review of research in the first decade, *Journal of Family Therapy*, 15, pp. 187–204.

Campbell, D. and Draper, R. (1985) *Applications of Systemic Family Therapy: The Milan Approach* (London, Grune & Stratton).

Carter, B. and McGoldrick, M. (1980) *The Family Life Cycle: A Framework for Family Therapy* (New York, Gardiner Press).

Engel, G. (1992) How much longer must medicine's science be bound by a seventeenth century world view? *Family Systems Medicine*, 10, pp. 333–346.

Green, J. and McCreaner, A. (eds) (1989) *Counselling in HIV Infection and AIDS* (Oxford, Blackwell).

Hildebrand, P. (1992) A patient dying with AIDS, *International Review of Psychoanalysis*, 19, pp. 457–469.

Jones, E. (1993) *Family Systems Therapy* (London, Wiley).

Karpel, M. (1980) Family secrets. 1. Conceptual and ethical issues in the relational context. 2. Ethical and practical considerations in therapeutic management, *Family Process*, 19, pp. 295–306.

Kernoff, P. and Miller, R. (1986) AIDS-related problems in the management of haemophilia, in: D. Miller, J. Weber and J. Green (eds) *The Management of AIDS Patients* (London, Macmillan).

McDaniel, S., Hepworth, J. and Doherty, W. (eds) (1992) *Medical Family Therapy* (New York, Basic Books).

Maturana, H., Coddou, F. and Mendez, C. (1988) The bringing forth of pathology, *Irish Journal of Psychology*, 9, pp. 144–172.

Miller, D. (1987) *Living with AIDS and HIV* (London, Macmillan).

Miller, R. and Bor, R. (1988) *AIDS: A Guide to Clinical Counselling* (London, Science Press).

Rolland, J. (1984) Toward a psychosocial typology of chronic and life threatening illness, *Family Systems Medicine*, 2, pp. 245–262.

Selvini Palazzoli, M. (ed.) (1986) *The Hidden Games of Organizations* (New York, Pantheon Books).

Selvini Palazzoli, M., Boscolo, L., Cecchin, G. and Prata, G. (1980) Hypothesizing, circularity, neutrality: three guidelines for the conductor of the session, *Family Process*, 19, pp. 3–12.

Walker, G. (1991) *In the Midst of Winter* (New York, W. W. Norton).

SEVENTEEN

A Multilevel Intervention Approach for Care of HIV-Positive Haemophiliac and Thalassaemic Patients and Their Families

John Tsiantis, Dimitris Anastasopoulos, Margarita Meyer,
Dionysia Panitz, Vassilis Ladis, Helen Platokouki, Sophie Aroni
and Christos Kattamis

INTRODUCTION

In this paper we describe the psychosocial intervention and services to patients suffering from chronic haematological conditions, such as haemophilia and thalassaemia, and to their families. The intervention was carried out by the mental health team of the Department of Psychological Paediatrics of a general children's hospital. Our objective was to assist the patients and their families to cope with the acute stress and the implications caused by HIV infection, a potentially lethal disease.

On another level, the intervention also took place in the thalassaemia and haemophilia care team in order to help the members gain better awareness and understanding of their intense feelings provoked by the seriousness of the condition of the affected children and the repercussions on their families. The psychiatric liaison team, through their regular meetings, identified and worked through the emotional strains created by the work with the affected children and their families as well as issues resulting from their collaboration with the staff of the units.

It has been estimated that up to approximately 17% of all the HIV-positive children have been infected by blood transfusions or the injection of blood products. Furthermore, it has been reported that in severe cases of haemophilia which require transfusions the rate of HIV infection is 75–90% in adults and 58% among children (Nelson and Album, 1987).

In early 1987, a telephone survey in Europe, Canada and Australia indicated that of more than 2,500 patients managed by haemophilia centres in those parts of the world approximately 51% of the Factor VIII deficient patients had seroconverted (Evant and Ramsey, 1988). In Italy, the percentage of thalassaemic patients infected with HIV through blood transfusions is reported to be between 11% (De Martino et al., 1985) and only 3–7% (Zanella et al., 1986). Politis et al. (1986) reported that in Greece the proportion of thalassaemic patients infected is between 2 and 4%. Leferer and Girot (1987) report the results of a study of the spread of the HIV virus among thalassaemic patients caried out in 36 centres in 13 countries before screening of blood donors became routine. The spread of infection varied between 0.003% in Algeria and 0.0095% in Israel. However, these findings seem rather low, probably because of under-reporting (Panitz et al., 1989).

It is expected that with blood screening and the heat treatment of Factor VIII there is unlikely to be an increase in the percentage of haemophiliac HIV-positive patients (Kernoff and Miller, 1986). It is also expected that with blood screening there is unlikely to be an increase in the percentage of thalassaemic HIV-positive patients.

Both haemophilia and thalassaemia are hereditary diseases, the first being transmitted as a sex-related recessive characteristic from the mother, as a carrier, to the son, as a sufferer; whereas thalassaemia is inherited through both parents – who are symptomless carriers – in a Mendelian recessive manner and can affect children of both sexes.

They are both chronic and life-threatening conditions, the first being treated with Factors VIII or IX replacement and the second, which is of the severest prognosis, with frequent blood transfusions and chelation therapy. Children, adolescents and young adults who suffer from the above-mentioned chronic haematological disease constitute a high-risk group for the manifestation of psychosocial problems and mental disturbance. Thalassaemic children, adolescents and young adults have been described as being anxious and depressed and over-dependent on their parents. Death anxiety has also been observed in them, whereas thalassaemic adolescents may become socially isolated and non-compliant to their treatment regime (Kattamis, 1989; Tsiantis et al., 1989; Woo et al., 1984). Haemophiliac children often display anxiety, phobic states, transient depression and dangerously accident-prone behaviour (Mattison and Agle, 1979; Meyer, 1980; Handford et al., 1985).

It is against this background of emotional, social and behavioural problems for the children and adolescents as well as of the repercussions caused by the chronic illness that infection with the HIV virus, another chronic condition, occurs.

The literature refers to the multiple requirements (medical, psychological, social and educational) of children and adolescents with AIDS and of their families. It also discusses the psychosocial and ethical issues which arise, together with proposals for how they may be dealt with and how these families may be helped (Miller, 1987; Miller et al., 1989; Report of Surgeons' General Workshop, 1987; Boyd, 1989). The stigmatization of the disease complicates the health and psychosocial care of the infected children, as in the majority of cases (approximately 80%) the infection is perinatal and their parents belong to the minority groups towards which there is already a negative attitude. In the particular case of children, adolescents and young people with chronic haematological diseases, there are some references to patients with haemophilia and fewer to patients with thalassaemia.

Some authors refer to the family's response to the initial diagnosis in terms of shock, disbelief and a state of crisis. They also note the resilience which some families display in the context of an added adversity set against a backdrop of chronic illness (Waters *et al.*, 1988). Miller and Bor (1988) describe some of the issues to be addressed in haemophilia, their families and health carers. Some of these issues are as follows:

- children at different developmental stages can be expected to be sensitive to different aspects of their situation;
- health care workers experience a role change from being saviours to feeling helpless and possibly guilty as well.

These authors stress the need for counselling and educational programmes to help cope with the stress and crises which affect the sufferers and their families. Miller *et al.* (1989) list some important principles that one has to take into consideration in counselling patients with HIV and their families.

Jones (1987, 1989) mentions the specific problems relating to HIV-positive haemophiliacs. More specifically, this author reports that the attitude of the public and of health care professionals towards these patients resembles the attitude generally adopted towards minority groups with AIDS and specific lifestyles. As a result, these attitudes affect the lives of the patients and their families, and consequently the counselling required. Jones (1989) also stresses the importance of comprehensive care and an interdisciplinary approach to AIDS in order to deal with the widely varying problems which arise when individuals who are connected with a previous chronic disturbance also contract AIDS. The literature refers to efforts to construct a set of innovative educational and skill-building programmes targeted at groups of haemophiliacs who have been infected with HIV, those at risk of infection with HIV, their families and friends, and health care professionals (Greenblat *et al.*, 1989).

It is therefore clear that there is a need to develop intervention models for specific populations who are suffering from infection or are at risk of it, their parents and the staff, health care professionals and institutions that serve them.

In this paper we shall be describing such an intervention model. It is currently being employed to care for and cope with children, adolescents and young people who have haemophilia or thalassaemia and who, in addition, have been infected with the HIV virus. The intervention also involves the families of such patients. We believe that the multilevel intervention used by the mental health team provides scope for an interdisciplinary approach to the multiple needs created by the effects of AIDS on children, their families and health care professionals.

THE SAMPLE

Our intervention involved 20 haemophiliac and HIV-positive children, adolescents and young people aged 7–21 years and their families, together with ten thalassaemic and HIV-positive children, adolescents and young people aged 8–23 years and their families. These patients were all in the care of the Department of Haemophilia and the Thalassaemia Unit of the First University Department of Paediatrics, Aghia Sophia Children's Hospital, Athens. These two units care for a total of approximately 70 haemophiliac patients and 400 thalassaemic patients. There was no selection of the sample, as all the infected patients were included in the intervention programme with the consent of the patients over the age of 16 and their families when the patients were under 16.

INTERVENTION – RATIONALE – STAGES

The intervention was carried out over a period of approximately one year, by an interdisciplinary psychiatric team consisting of one child psychiatrist, two social workers and two psychologists belonging to the Department of Psychological Paediatrics of the Aghia Sophia Children's Hospital, Athens. In the past three years, the Department has used liaison consultation psychiatry to build up a relationship of cooperation with the units where the children and their families are cared for, with the purpose of supporting the families and sensitising the medical and nursing staff.

When planning our intervention, we took into consideration the following factors: (a) the impact which, as noted above, the chronic disease has on the children and their families at a number of different levels – emotional, social, educational, economic – and the fact that the degree and extent of reaction depend on disease-related factors as well as on intrapersonal and environmental factors; (b) the fact that two years elapsed between the time at which the medical and nursing staff after testing became aware of the HIV positivity and their planning of the announcement to be made to the families, and three years until the announcements of the seropositivity in the families actually began to be made.

In this interim period, the doctors in the unit had made some attempts to give health education to the parents of all the children and adolescents who were receiving frequent transfusions on matters which included AIDS. It is interesting to note that none of the families approached the attendant doctors in order to discuss matters openly with them and ask whether their child was HIV positive. The same was true of the adolescents and young people. There were, of course, some indications of anxiety in the communications with the families of HIV-positive children, which showed that the parents and perhaps the children too had some latent awareness of the situation. In the same way, there were cases of families with HIV-negative children who feared that their children might be HIV-positive. Relevant to this is that in Greece when HIV testing was carried out for the first time approximately four or five years ago, there was not a generally accepted policy among clinicians concerning disclosure of serum-positive diagnosis to thalassaemic and haemophilic patients and to their families. This can be attributed to the lack of specific guidelines at that time set by the public health authorities and/or to the attitudes of and ethical dilemmas confronting clinicians, concerning disclosure of the diagnosis.

In the hospital units where chronic diseases are dealt with, special relationships are built up between the patients and the medical and nursing staff, who may come to believe that they, too, participate in the upbringing of the children. This is particularly true of the paediatricians, since they are in very regular contact with the children from very early ages. At the same time, the parents – and children – become involved in dependent relationships with the staff, on whom, and particularly the doctors, they often make quite considerable demands.

We also considered the impact that infection with HIV has on the family and on the staff of the units. More specifically, infection with HIV disturbs, or threatens to disturb the equilibrium of the family; it can revive conflicts from the past, can lead to stigmatization and rejection of the family and can also provoke a number of other reactions, which will be described below. On the other hand, the fact that the infection is iatrogenous may set up feelings of guilt in the medical and nursing staff. The medical and nursing staff also have to work under intense stress, since they not only have to disclose the seropositivity – for which they may feel responsible – but are also influenced by the death anxiety which permeates the atmosphere of the units. As a result, this atmosphere becomes highly charged and considerable involvement with the parent and the patient on the part of the doctor may be observed. It is also possible that the relationship of trust between the children and their parents, on the one hand, and the medical and nursing staff, on the other, may be disturbed.

The special problems which arise in the mental health team working with the HIV-positive children and adolescents and their parents were also considered. Among these problems may be mental exhaustion, the emergence of anger, frustration and self-criticism, with a trend towards defeatism as to what the mental health team can offer on the grounds that 'in any case his days are numbered', as well as tendencies to internalize the anxiety and avoid discussing it (Anastasopoulos, 1989).

The stages in the intervention were as follows:

1 Preparation and planning.
2 Disclosure of seropositivity.
3 Direct crisis intervention with the parents and children during the period of seropositivity and the new crisis which usually occurs when the patients develop symptoms. Intervention of this kind took place in the form of individual and family meetings and with parents' groups.
4 Indirect intervention with the provision of counselling and support for the staff of the units or in the course of work with groups of nursing staff. Further indirect intervention involved counselling work with the social services and the primary health care services.

Preparation and Planning

The preparation of the intervention consisted of the following.

Preparation of the mental health team responsible for the intervention was carried out, with an intensive schedule of meetings, case discussions and supervision and exploration of the feelings of the members of the mental health team and of the targets of intervention. The main targets of intervention in the case of the parents and the adolescents aged over 16 years (to whom the disclosure of seropositivity would be made directly) were as follows:

• acceptance of the reality of the situation;
• facilitation of the grief process;
• adaptation to the environment in the light of the infection with the HIV virus.

This stage was of great importance in planning the intervention, particularly with regard to the sharing of feelings and unconscious fears and prejudices among the members of the interdisciplinary team and also for setting realistic goals for the intervention.

Within the framework of the liaison–consultation psychiatry work with the haemophilia and thalassaemia units, weekly group meetings were held during the stage of preparation between the mental health team and the medical and nursing staff. In addition, individual consultation took place with the members of the medical and nursing staff in order to sensitize them towards issues of mental health and to develop a joint strategy. At these meetings, specific cases were discussed in order to develop a better understanding of family dynamics and to give the medical and nursing staff an opportunity to express themselves and share their feelings with the mental health team. The outcome of this work was the action research protocol described below, with its goals.

A psychosocial assessment of the families was made, using semi-structured interviews with parents and children, questionnaires, rating scales and projective tests. The purpose here was to draw up a broad psychosocial profile for each family, covering the identification of the protective and risk factors for each family, with the isolation of effective coping strategies and of the factors which would facilitate the family in adjusting to the effects of HIV/AIDS. Among other targets of the psychosocial assessment of each case was a long-term evaluation of the reactions of each family and of the ways in which the families coped with the problem of seropositivity or the development of AIDS symptoms. The assessment procedure has been described in detail elsewhere (Anastasopoulos and Tsiantis, 1989).

The intervention in each family was planned, on the basis of the coping strategies and weaknesses which had been identified.

APPLICATION OF THE INTERVENTION TO CHILDREN AND ADOLESCENTS AND THEIR FAMILIES

The intervention began with the disclosure of the diagnosis, to the parents in the case of children under the age of 16 years and in the case of older adolescents and young adults to the patients and their parents, separately, after individual assessment. The disclosure was made by the attending doctor, in the presence of a member of the mental health team with whom the family had already developed an acquaintance through the child and family assessment procedure that had preceded disclosure.

Care was taken to ensure that:

- there should be no pressure of time during the interview at which seropositivity was disclosed;
- the disclosure was not made just before public holidays or vacations;
- the mental health team were in a position to provide round-the-clock assistance during the days following disclosure;
- the member of the team who was present when the disclosure was made should follow up the case.

DISCLOSURE OF SEROPOSITIVITY: REACTIONS RECORDED

The description that follows is the qualitative assessment according to predetermined clinical criteria. This was carried out by the member of the mental health team who was present during the disclosure.

Most parents reacted to the disclosure with shock and intense feelings of despair, anxiety and mental pain. This was accompanied by refusal to accept the fact of infection with the virus and anger directed towards the attending doctor for failing to take the steps necessary to prevent infection. Later, the parents became dependent for support on the attending doctor and the mental health team and gradually came to accept reality. The reactions were similar to the mourning reactions observed after the disclosure of serious illness or imminent death.

When disclosure of seropositivity for a 12-year-old boy with haemophilia was made, the parents were devastated. The father became angry and said: 'We thought that we had started to breathe, now we have to start our struggle all over again.'

Transfusion-associated patients and their families often act out their anger and sadness within their relationship with health care professionals by being mistrustful and suspicious of them. For instance, the parents of a 12-year-old boy, after the disclosure of HIV positivity, decided to have their son tested again for HIV at another medical centre. The explanation they gave for their behaviour was that they had a relative in that particular centre who advised them to repeat the test.

The mother of a 15-year-old girl reacted with great sadness and fear as to what could happen to her daughter in the future. She expressed feelings of frustration that for 15 years she went through so many painful experiences associated with thalassaemia, and now she had to deal with the HIV – she was tearful as she said that 'you can never have future dreams for your child'.

Some parents reacted very intensely and developed transient psychopathological symptoms, such as depression, sleep disturbance, death anxiety, psychosomatic symptoms and ideas of reference (for instance, some parents felt that other people could tell that their child was infected with HIV).

The adolescents and young people developed anxiety, depressive symptoms and worry and guilt over what the disease would mean for their parents or their partners. Although thoughts and fantasies of acting out behaviour occurred, none of the patients went so far as to display such acute reactions. It is interesting that in no cases to date have the parents agreed to talk to their children aged 16 years and under about the seropositivity or the disease.

Many parents become over-protective and some of them manifested indirect rejection of their children. On the other hand, almost all of the younger children appeared to sense their condition, and this could be seen in their behaviour and in the content of interviews with them. One nine-year-old thalassaemic boy, for example, expressed his concern by saying that there is no cure for AIDS as there is none for cancer and that it would be better for AIDS patients not to know that they had the illness because their depression might bring death about more rapidly. At a later point he told his sister that he had AIDS and that she must be careful not to be infected by him. Many of the children were anxious and were concerned with the idea of death. All the families were dominated by a conspiracy of silence, which affected family relationships and prevented family members from supporting each other. As was expected, disclosure of the seropositivity reactivated old wounds and conflicts of the past, thus disrupting the equilibrium of the family.

Many of the mothers of haemophiliac children displayed guilt and intense self-criticism for having passed the disease on to their children, while in the thalassaemic families the conflict tended to revolve around the marriage which brought the couple together to have sick children.

It is interesting that in both groups of families the mothers displayed the more intense guilt feelings; we had expected that in the thalassaemic families the fathers would also have manifested intense guilt feelings, but this was not observed. This appears to bear a cultural connection to the state of relations between the sexes in Greece, but first and foremost, emotionally, to the fact that the mother carried and gave birth to the sick child, regardless of the genetic logic of the equal and joint contribution to the inheritance of thalassaemia. Our impression is that the families of the thalassaemia patients displayed acute reactions more frequently. This was to be expected, since in general the prognosis is more serious in cases of thalassaemia and the average life expectancy is shorter.

After disclosure, our intervention consisted of the following stages:

1 Intervention in the crisis caused by the disclosure.
2 Intervention during the stage of seropositivity.
3 Intervention when symptoms appeared and new crisis was at hand.

CRISIS INTERVENTION

All the members of the mental health team described earlier were included in the counselling during the crisis intervention period. Each member of the team was responsible for a number of families.

Our crisis intervention consisted of giving support on a round-the-clock basis. The counselling provided was intended to facilitate the parents in experiencing their grief, in expressing their feelings, which were chiefly of guilt and anger, and in regaining their balance. Counselling focused on helping the families to formulate questions relating to the disease, to identify issues and concerns regarding their situation and to explore ways of managing the crisis. Attempts were made to help the parents regain their control of the situation and to assure them that their reactions were natural and universal.

Intervention during Seropositivity

Crisis intervention was usually followed by a period during which the pace of family life returned to normal. However, most parents were frightened and anxious, with a tendency to social isolation, while the fear of social stigmatization was never far away. At the same time, they behaved in an over-protective manner towards the children, being unable to set limits and giving the sick child preferential treatment over his or her siblings. At this stage the parents were offered weekly or fortnightly meetings. In brief, the consultative and support intervention at this stage consisted of counselling of the parents and families with the following targets:

- to prioritize their needs;
- to reach a better understanding of what was happening;
- to relieve themselves from guilt and see that the illness was not an unjust punishment;
- to continue life as normal;
- to make use of the mental health services, the hospital and the social services;
- to maintain their adaptive defences;
- to facilitate the process of mourning, where it had begun, because of the revival of problems caused by the chronic disease.

Furthermore, the consultation was intended to help the parents concerning their attitude to the seropositive child and the healthy children, in their own relationship and in their relations with society in general.

One of the problems that has had to be dealt with in this stage (which is still continuing) is the difficulty of the parents in discussing seropositivity with the children. Some parents found it very hard to burden the child with the news of the HIV diagnosis and decided not to discuss the issue, whereas others felt unable to do so, probably owing to their guilt or need to maintain some control. As a result, there is a conspiracy of silence in the families, which exerts pressure on the family as a whole and particularly on the child, who senses the predominant tension and is called upon to shoulder the whole burden of the secret. During this period, the situation is assessed and if there are special indications the children or the parents are referred for more specialized psychiatric assistance (such as individual psychotherapy).

Intervention Once Symptoms Have Appeared

At this time the reactions during the initial crisis usually revive. The goal of our intervention has been to continue grief counselling and support the whole family in developing connections with the support systems in the community.

Parents' Groups

Apart from individual counselling, group work was also done with those parents of seropositive children and adolescents who agreed to take part in such groups. Both parents from four families are currently participating in the group. The group meets every two weeks and is coordinated by two psychologists from the mental health team. The targets of the group work are as follows:

The parents' group becomes a place where emotions and experiences can be exchanged, support provided and more profound problems in the family worked through. It is a place where problems can be projected without any risk of a 'boomerang effect', which would paralyse the participant concerned. It is a place where aggression towards the doctor or the hospital is permissible and will not destroy the participant's relationships with them.

Participation in the group is intended to help the individuals to modify the concept they have of the disease and perhaps, through the processes which take place in the group, the more general concept they have of themselves. Thus they are allowed to talk about their loss (death), which is impossible to incorporate into routine therapy and cannot happen against the background of silence concerning the fatal disease in both the family and the social environment.

The group also helps the unit staff, relieving them of the burden of the problems which involve the doctor–patient relationship. This frees the doctor of both unconscious guilt and his possible or probable feeling of omnipotence.

One direct consequence of the work with the parents' group is that their relationship with the patients develops further on a healthy basis, since there is now another repository for the negative emotions previously directed only towards themselves. This became obvious from direct clinical observation of their relationship with their children and from the coping style they have adapted before and after the group work. Prospects for the future include extending the parents' groups and setting up separate groups for adolescents.

INDIRECT INTERVENTION

The forms of indirect intervention used included:

- liaison and consultative work on the part of the mental health team with the paediatric haematologists;
- group discussions with the nursing staff;
- liaison work with schools, the social welfare services and primary health care services;
- health education in the school and the community.

Liaison and Consultative Work with the Paediatric Haematologists

Close collaboration between the paediatric haematologists and the mental health professionals in the thalassaemia and haemophilia units has inaugurated a new relationship reflecting awareness of the significant psychological component involved, for both patients and staff, in dealing with AIDS, the most challenging epidemic of our times.

Contacts between the mental health professionals and the haematologists took place almost every day. There were one or two official meetings each week, but informal meetings and discussions with the medical and nursing staff were much more frequent.

Realization that the medical management of young children and adolescents with HIV infection cannot be accomplished without considerable psychological upheaval, and that continuous attention to the psychosocial issues involved improved the quality of the experience for all the professionals concerned, fostered the integration of the mental health professionals into the thalassaemia and haemophilia teams.

Group Discussions with the Nursing Staff

The nursing staff group meeting took place once a week and lasted for 90 minutes. The two head nurses and the auxiliary nurses took part. The group was coordinated by a psychiatric social worker. The objectives of this form of intervention were as follows:

- To create an environment capable of enhancing the participants' ability to discuss concerns and issues relating to the HIV patients and to the thalassaemia and haemophilia patients in general.
- To facilitate communication and interaction, and to strengthen coping abilities in dealing with the realities of the situation.
- To increase understanding of the participants' own feelings about HIV. Theoretically, this could help them to accept the real situation and deal with their negative attitude to AIDS victims and their fears of contagion.

In this group the case of each AIDS patient was discussed separately so as to help the nurses gain greater understanding and knowledge of the psychosocial and ethical aspects of the disease. It was also possible for the nurses to identify the coping strengths and weaknesses of the family and observe how they adapted to the demands caused by the impact of AIDS.

The group meetings facilitated the grief process in the nursing staff, whose emotional involvement with the children and their parents dated back many years. This was intended to keep their attitudes to the children and their parents within the boundaries of their role, and at the same time relieve the nurses of some of their counter-transference feelings.

The two forms of indirect intervention we have described were of greater importance because we know that doctors, nurses and other health care staff involved in the treatment of AIDS patients are susceptible to occupational stress, fear, anxiety, prejudice and feelings of guilt. It is our impression that these reactions are more acute when the patients concerned are children and adolescents, particularly when infection has occurred through transfusion or infections with blood products. This intensity of the reaction could be attributed to the iatrogenous cause of the injection with its possible consequences on the caring staff, as has been already outlined earlier in this paper.

During the intervention, the work of the mental health team was rewarding. On the other hand, it was also a painful, tiring and draining experience. For that reason we believe that it is essential that there should be regular weekly meetings of the mental health team. These meetings provide an opportunity for the sharing of emotions, for mutual support and for clarification of the complex counter-transference reactions which emerge. Also of great importance is the supervision of the team by an outside supervisor. This process allows clarification of the counter-transference reactions, such as identification with the sick child or an attitude of omnipotence towards all the other professionals involved in the case.

Other Forms of Intervention

These forms of intervention concerned cooperation between the mental health team and the social welfare and primary health care services. One of the basic objects of these forms of intervention was that of health education.

In some cases, our intervention dealt with the school in particular, but only if the complex moral and ethical questions concerning confidentiality had been dealt with and on condition that the parents gave their consent. One such intervention on the part of the mental health team occurred when the seropositivity of two haemophiliac brothers was discovered by the other members of the small rural community in which the family resided. The parents of the other children in the community reacted by occupying the school to prevent classes. The family was in danger of complete ostracism and there was a considerable uproar in the local newspaper and radio. An on-the-spot intervention by two members of the mental health team, with community meetings and meetings with the staff of the school and with the local authorities, helped to overcome the crisis. The school reopened and the seropositive children were able to attend, while the family was helped with supportive counselling.

The overall programme for our psychosocial intervention can be seen in Figures 17.1 and 17.2 (Tsiantis *et al.*, 1990).

FOLLOW-UP AND CONCLUSIONS

A year after the programme has started, it appears that most of the families are coping satisfactorily with their situation, although a latent depression can be observed in them. Acute psychopathological reactions have manifested themselves

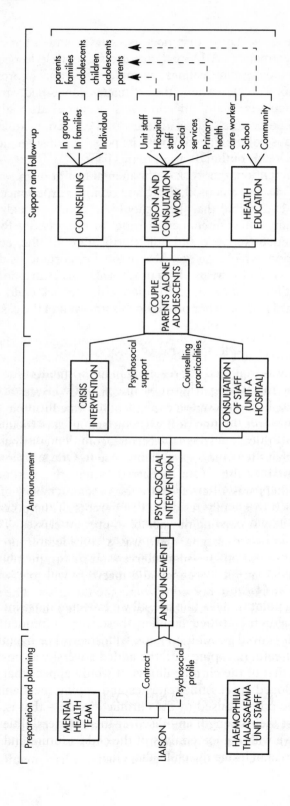

Figure 17.1 Programme of psychosocial intervention

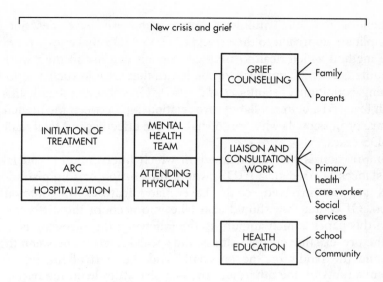

Figure 17.2 Programme of psychosocial intervention: new crisis and grief

in only two families. In one case, there was a reappearance of the father's manic-depressive psychosis, and in the other a latent psychosis in an eight-year-old haemophiliac boy was triggered off, resulting in his hospitalization.

Throughout the follow-up period subsequent to disclosure of the diagnosis, we have attempted to keep in contact with the families through regular meetings arranged on the basis of the needs in each case. In other cases, the follow-up has been combined with the family's planned visit to the thalassaemia or haemophilia unit, where care is taken to ensure that the mental health professionals and the staff of the units are available.

The factors that appear to have played a part in successful coping on the part of the families are cohesion between the family members, a good relationship between the parental couple and good relations between the parents and the child. On the other hand, the absence of a social support network appears to constitute a risk factor, as does previous mental disturbances in the child or in one of the parents. The detailed results of the analysis of the psychosocial assessments have been described elsewhere (Tsiantis *et al.*, 1990).

The interesting point is that while overall we expected more intense reactions on the part of the children and their families, these were infrequent. When they did occur, however, it proved possible to cope with them. We hypothesize that these families are resourceful in coping with the added adversity against a backdrop of a pre-existing one, that of the chronic illness. It would appear that these families in general had developed successful strategies and coping mechanisms to deal with the effects and the crises caused by the chronic disease – that is, they had had an opportunity to test their strength and discover their vulnerabilities. They may also have learned to live with the uncertainty of the child's future and they had already confronted the threat of losing the child altogether.

We believe that the multilevel intervention we have described and the interdisciplinary approach to the effects of HIV/AIDS make up a very helpful and effective method which health care professionals can use in their work of dealing with the intensity and complexity of the issues that arise in such a serious and life-threatening condition (Tsiantis *et al.*, 1989). On the other hand, this multilevel approach fostered a better collaborative relationship between the mental health and health care professionals who are so vital for the effective and total management of HIV/AIDS cases.

Our impression is that the manner in which intervention could take place in other instances of paediatric AIDS, where transfusion or administration of blood products are not involved, could have many features in common with that described. Of course, we should also take into account the differences outlined earlier in this paper, which amount to the following: the iatrogenous nature of the illness; the pre-existing chronic illness; the special relations between the child, the parents and the family on the one hand and the staff of the haemophilia and thalassaemia units on the other; and the negative attitude on the part of the public and the medical staff to the other cases of HIV-infected children, whose parents belong to minority groups (homosexuals, drug addicts). This may also affect the attitude of the caring staff in the thalassaemia and haemophilia units.

There is a need for follow-up studies to be carried out and for the effectiveness of intervention to be assessed, so as to allow identification of successful coping skills, strategies and other resources in the patients and their families. Such results would contribute to the planning and implementation of satisfactory modes of psychosocial intervention, with an overall emphasis on prevention.

REFERENCES

Anastasopoulos, D. (1989) Specific problems faced by professionals who provide mental health care to HIV-positive children and their families. Paper prepared for the WHO Regional Office for Europe, Mental Health Division (Copenhagen, WHO).

Anastasopoulos, D. and Tsiantis, J. (1989) A description of mental and psychosocial disorders displayed by HIV-positive haemophiliac or thalassaemic children and their relatives. Paper prepared for the WHO Regional Office for Europe, Division of Mental Health (Copenhagen, WHO).

Boyd, K. (1989) Ethical questions, in: J. Green and A. McCreaner (eds) *Counselling in HIV Infection and AIDS* (Oxford, Blackwell Scientific).

De Martino, M., Quarta, G., Melpigrano, A., Guadalupi, C., Vullo, C., Ferrucci, M., Saimot, A. and Vierucci, A. (1985) Antibodies to HTL VIII and the lymphadenophathy syndrome in multi-transfused beta-thalassaemia patients, *Vox Sanguinis*, 41, pp. 230–233.

Evant, B. L. and Ramsey, R. B. (1988) AIDS in the haemophiliac child: the need for a multi-disciplinary approach to prevention in AIDS in children, adolescents and heterosexual adults, in: R. F. Schirari and A. J. Nahmian (eds) *An Interdisciplinary Approach to Prevention*, pp. 245–251 (New York, Elsevier).

Greenblat, C. S., Katz, S., Gagnon, J. and Shannon, D. (1989) An innovative program of counselling family members and friends of seropositive haemophiliacs, *AIDS Care*, 1, pp. 67–75.

Handford, H. A., Dickerson, M. S., Bagnato, S. J. and Bixter, E. D. (1985) Relationships between variations in patients' attitudes and personality traits in haemophiliac boys, *American Journal of Orthopsychiatry*, 56, pp. 424–434.

Jones, P. (1987) AIDS-planning for our future, *Social Work Today*.

Jones, P. (1989) The counselling of HIV antibody positive haemophiliacs, in: J. Green and A. McCreaner (eds) *Counselling in HIV Infection and AIDS* (Oxford, Blackwell Scientific).

Kattamis, C. (1989) The child with thalassaemia, *Bulletin International Paediatric Association*, 4, pp. 19–29.

Kernoff, P. and Miller, R. (1986) AIDS related problems in the management of haemophiliacs, in: D. Miller, J. Weber and J. Green (eds), *The Management of AIDS Patients* (Basingstoke, Macmillan).

Lefrere, J. and Girot, R. (1987) HIV infection in polytransfused thalassaemic patients, *Lancet*, ii, p. 686.

Mattison, A. and Agle, D. (1979) Psychophysiological aspects of adolescence: haematological disorders, in: C. Sherman, Peter Feinstein, and L. and P. Giovarchini (eds) *Adolescent Psychiatry VII* (Chicago, University of Chicago Press).

Meyer, A. (1980–81) Psychiatric problems of haemophiliac boys and their families, *International Journal of Psychiatric Medicine*, 10, pp. 163–179.

Miller, D. (1987) *Living with AIDS and HIV* (New York, Macmillan).

Miller, R. and Bor, R. (1988) *AIDS: A Guide to Clinical Counselling* (London, Science Press).

Miller, R., Goldman, E., Bor, R. and Kernoff, P. (1989) Counselling children and adults about AIDS/HIV: the ripple effect on haemophilia setting, *Counselling Psychology Quarterly*, 2, pp. 65–72.

Nelson, L. and Album, M. (1987) AIDS: children with the infection and their families. A conference report, *Journal of Dentistry for Children*, Sept–Oct, pp. 353–358.

Politis, C., Roumeliotou, A., Germenis, A. and Papaevangelou, G. (1986) Risk of acquired immune deficiency syndrome in multi-transfused patients with thalassaemia major, *Plasma Therapy and Transfusion Technology*, 7, pp. 41–43.

Report of Surgeon General's Workshop (1987) *On Children with HIV Infection and Their Families* (1987) Office of Maternal and Child Health, US Department of Health and Human Services, National Maternal and Child Clearing-House, Washington, DC.

Tsiantis, J., Xipolita-Tsandili, D. and Papadakou-Lagoyannis, S. (1989) Family reactions and their management in parents' group with β-thalassaemia, *Archives of Diseases in Childhood*, 57, pp. 860–863.

Tsiantis, J., Kattamis, C., Aronis, S., Theodoridou, M. A., Meyer, M., Panitz, D. and Anastasopoulos, D. (1989) Paper presented at the International Conference on Children and Death, Athens, 30 October–4 November.

Tsiantis, J., Panitz, D., Meyer, M., Assimopoulos, H., Piperia, M. and Anastasopoulos, D. (1990) A model of multilevel intervention for HIV-positive haemophiliac and thalassaemic children, their families and health care professionals. Paper prepared for the WHO Regional Office for Europe, Division of Mental Health (Copenhagen, WHO).

Waters, B., Ziegler, J., Hampson, R. and McPherson, A. (1988) The psychosocial consequences of childhood infection with human immunodeficiency virus, *Medical Journal of Australia*, 149, pp. 198–202.

Woo, R., Giardino, P. and Hilpartner, M. (1984) A psychosocial needs assessment of patients with homozygous β-thalassaemia, *Annals of New York Academy of Sciences*, pp. 316–322.

Zanella, A., Mozzi, F., Ferroni, P. and Sinchia, G. (1986) Anti-HTLV III screening in multi-transfused thalassaemia patients, *Vox Sanguinis*, 50, p. 192.

EIGHTEEN

Sexual and Relationship Problems among People Affected by AIDS: Three Case Studies

Heather George

INTRODUCTION

Since 1982, when the first person was diagnosed with AIDS in the UK, there has been a great increase in the number and range of services developed for affected individuals. Emotional support has long been recognized as an essential part of AIDS service provision (Miller *et al.*, 1986); policies about pre- and post-HIV test counselling, and about providing longer-term support, have been adopted from well-established 'centres of excellence' by agencies throughout the country (Green, 1989).

General supportive counselling, with sensitive information-giving and advice about the nature of HIV and related illness, are central aspects of psychological care. More specialized approaches and interventions have been identified for different client groups, e.g. for 'worried well' people who perceive themselves as having HIV infection in the absence of evidence to support this (Hedge *et al.*, 1988), for drug users (Mulleady *et al.*, 1989) and for pregnant women (Sherr *et al.*, 1989).

An area of work relevant to all adult groups is psychosexual counselling and therapy (George, 1989). Sexual and relationship issues are central themes with clients affected by HIV.

'Worried well' people may present with an AIDS phobia, or request an HIV antibody test, but have underlying problems related to sexual orientation, or sexual guilt over some activity which they construe as transgressing their own sexual mores. The latter commonly take the form of having sexual contact outside their regular relationship, with a casual partner or as part of a long-term affair, or with a prostitute. Their sexual guilt may lead to a breakdown of communication with the regular partner; a sexual dysfunctional problem (typically loss or lack of pleasure, or inadequate arousal); a phobic disorder where they 'punish' themselves by obsessive thoughts about developing AIDS and dying; or all three of these. Alternatively, pre-existing relationship or sexual problems result in people having their needs met elsewhere, and guilt, anxiety and/or a phobia about AIDS develop as a consequence.

People with HIV infection frequently experience a loss of identity upon hearing their test results or diagnosis. They may feel sexually unacceptable and lose interest and confidence in having sexual contact, whether this is within an established relationship where the partner is aware of their HIV infection or, if they are 'single', with new partners. The strain of adjustment to their health status, anxiety and depression caused by living with the uncertainty of their future, and symptoms of or treatment for HIV-related disease, may obviously lead to disharmony in relationships and trouble with sex. Typically, sexual problems are very important and distressing to people when they are initially found to have HIV, and become less so as illness progresses. Difficulties also arise when one partner has AIDS and has lost interest in sex, and the other, physically well, partner feels rejected, frustrated and uncomfortable about having sexual drives. Furthermore, any existing sexual or relationship problems are usually aggravated and exacerbated by HIV.

Partners and significant others of people with HIV frequently seek help with coping with the stress of caring. They may cease to experience any pleasure from sexual contact with their partner who has HIV, either because of worries about infection (their own fears, or their partner's) or, more usually, because of their partner's loss of interest in and enthusiasm for sex. Where the relationship is ambivalent, the partner of someone with AIDS may feel the need to stay in the relationship out of compassion, and feel enormous guilt about planning time after the person's death and considering future sexual contact. When someone wholeheartedly wishes to devote all his or her time and effort to caring for a partner with AIDS, allowing little help from statutory workers, there can be great problems of adjustment after the death, including the establishment of new relationships.

The following case studies show the diversity and complexity of sexual and relationship problems presented by three people affected by AIDS. Each is based on an actual referral to the author, a clinical psychologist providing specialist services for AIDS/HIV and terminal care. Some aspects of each person have obviously been changed to ensure anonymity, but essential facts remain. Detailed case material is given to illustrate both the formulation of problems and the process and outcome of therapeutic interventions.

CASE STUDY 1: A 'WORRIED WELL' WOMAN, LINDA, AGED 36

Linda was referred to the psychology service at the Genito-urinary Medicine Department by her GP, who had been concerned about her because she had requested three HIV tests during the previous 18 months. The results to all these tests had been negative, but she remained extremely distressed and anxious about the thought of having AIDS.

During the initial psychology session Linda seemed to be relieved to find that her worries were being taken seriously. She became tearful when describing the development of her problem. She had first requested an HIV test when she became pregnant with her third child, Matthew, and had told her GP that she was concerned about AIDS because of having had a blood transfusion during surgery, over two years prior to her pregnancy. She had been told of the negligible risk of infection, but convinced her doctor that a negative test result would allay her fears. Indeed, Linda was reassured for seven months, but then her obsessive thoughts about AIDS returned. By this time Matthew had been born, and after some weeks he was admitted to hospital. Meningitis was suspected, and he was barrier nursed until the cause of his symptoms – a very common urinary infection – was diagnosed. The barrier nursing triggered Linda's fear about AIDS and she returned to her GP for a second test, informing him that her fears were really due to having had an extramarital affair with Don, a man she believed to be bisexual.

Over the following year Linda continued to ask questions about AIDS every time she visited her GP. She worried about having infected Tom, her husband, and the children, as well as being preoccupied with her own health. Finally her GP agreed to her having a third HIV test, on the condition that she attended psychology sessions or saw a psychiatrist.

Formulation and Intervention

Linda attended psychology sessions for 20 months. The following were discussed as factors related to the development of her phobia.

Long-standing relationship and sexual problems with her husband

Linda had never enjoyed sex with Tom, and always felt that he did not appreciate her, but she loved her children and liked being a mother, and was materially well provided for by Tom's employment as a manager in a motor manufacturing company. She had low expectations of marriage – her parents' marriage, her mother had told her, was maintained through habit and fear of living without a spouse.

Guilt over having engaged in and enjoyed sex and attention from men other than her husband

Tom was Linda's first boyfriend – they had met when she was 15 and he was 17. She had become pregnant at 18, but Tom had not wanted to marry. She had a termination, and the relationship with Tom ended. Linda had two other sexual relationships before meeting Tom again. They married when she was 22. Within three years she had two miscarriages, but later had two children. Linda was pleased to be a mother, but she felt that Tom paid too little attention to herself and their children. He frequently worked late and at weekends, and then stayed out drinking with colleagues and friends. Linda had met Don, who was also married, and found him attentive and kind. They shared interests and enjoyed conversation, and Linda found sex with Don 'wonderful'. Their affair ended after two years, when both decided that it was unfair to their respective partners.

Tom always assumed that he had been her only lover, and Linda had never told him of her former boyfriends, nor about Don. Although she found sex with Tom boring, she was pleased to become pregnant with Matthew. However, at this time she heard that a friend's brother had died with AIDS, and there was a great deal of media coverage on HIV. She began to suspect that Don was bisexual, although she had no grounds on which to base this.

Low self-confidence and esteem

Linda had never felt happy about her appearance or abilities. She had worked as a receptionist before marriage, and then as a part-time care assistant in an old people's home, but she felt insecure when mixing with people and believed herself dull.

Compulsive behaviours, repeated because of the temporary reduction in anxiety, and obsessive thoughts, maintained to 'punish' herself for her guilty secrets

Linda had confided in her sister and one friend, and daily would telephone them or AIDS helplines for reassurance. She also read magazine and newspaper articles about AIDS, and checked her body for symptoms of illness. These behaviours reduced her anxiety until fears about being 'found out' by Tom recurred.

A phobia that gained her attention and masked the difficulties she had with her husband

Tom knew only that Linda was frightened of AIDS because of the blood transfusion. Although he generally dismissed her worries, he would occasionally discuss them and help her when she became panicky.

Linda was told that her history was classic for someone with an AIDS phobia; that her sexual guilt and events such as Matthew's barrier nursing and high media coverage were reasons for her maintaining her fear; and that there were well-established approaches to providing solutions to her problems.

During the initial session she was taught a breathing technique to help with her panicky feelings and thoughts. The technique involved counting, which distracted her from thoughts about AIDS. After several sessions a distraction cassette tape was made, where the psychologist said phrases which had been useful during the sessions, e.g. 'There is no evidence to show that you have HIV', 'You are a fit and physically healthy woman'. Linda used this with a personal cassette recorder whenever she had the urge to telephone her sister, friend or AIDS helplines for reassurance. Linda was encouraged to save her questions about AIDS until the psychology sessions. These were initially answered by the psychologist, but in later sessions there was role reversal, where Linda answered her own questions aloud by taking the role of the psychologist. In this way she was able to find her own answers to questions such as 'Should I have another HIV test?' or 'How likely is it that Don was bisexual?'

Linda was asked to find tasks that would distract her from thoughts about AIDS, while providing structure and enjoyment to her, such as compiling a list and programme of activities for herself and her children during the Christmas holidays. She was asked to write a self-description, including positive as well as negative aspects, and to write about the person she would like to be. Some tangible aims which she could work towards were identified, such as taking physical exercise to improve her appearance, confidence and self-respect. In addition, she was able to express her feelings about being a good mother.

Linda's guilt about sexual contact with men other than Tom was examined and discussed with reference to the reality of the situation, i.e. that extramarital affairs were extremely common, particularly when one partner failed to meet the other's needs, as in Tom's case. Her fears about Tom's leaving her and the children were aired, and it was suggested that she needed to feel confident that she could cope without him before she could be sure of positively choosing to maintain the marriage, rather than staying with Tom to avoid being alone. Work on her self-confidence and examining the reality of coping as a single parent allowed Linda to reach a point where she could suggest to Tom that he also attended sessions; Linda knew that joint sessions would involve exploring separation as the solution to the couple's problems.

Tom agreed to attend, and nine joint sessions examined communication and sex. Linda was able to tell Tom of her former boyfriends – but not about her affair with Don – and that although she felt that she had a lower sex drive than Tom, she felt that sexual pleasure together could be greater.

A sensate focus programme (Masters and Johnson, 1970) enabled Linda and Tom to increase their sexual satisfaction. Time was planned for sexual contact, instead of its occurring last thing at night when both were tired and the baby often took time to settle. Linda was able to say that she felt that time together generally was more important than the money Tom earned from his overtime. Tom agreed to limit his working hours, leaving more time for activities as a family and for Tom to look after the children while Linda saw her friends.

Linda attended two further sessions alone after the joint work. She felt that her relationship with Tom was much improved, both emotionally and sexually. Her AIDS worries had diminished, and she found that she was able to read articles or watch television programmes in a 'neutral' manner, without the need for reassurance or morbid interest.

CASE STUDY 2: A MAN WITH HIV INFECTION, JOHN, AGED 49

John was a gay man who had been HIV antibody-positive and physically well for two years before he reported having panic attacks to the physician at the Genito-urinary Medicine Department. These occurred in a variety of situations. As an architect, John frequently travelled by public transport to offices and sites in central London, and he felt panicky even approaching his local station and so uncomfortable in crowded tube and overground trains that he had missed several appointments because he could not face the journey. He also felt apprehensive in gay clubs and bars, and had experienced such a loss of confidence that he was no longer able to attend an amateur drama group, which had been his main interest outside work. Tranquillizers had been prescribed as a short-term solution.

Formulation and Intervention

John attended 12 psychology sessions over seven months. The initial sessions concentrated on a systematic desensitization programme (Wolpe, 1973) for controlling John's panic attacks, but as time went by he began to talk more about his past, and about fears he had about his future. The following factors were identified as pertinent to the development of his problems.

Worries about ageing and establishing relationships

There had been one long-term affair in John's life. He had lived with Bob, ten years his junior, for seven years, until the couple had decided both to be tested for HIV. They were both found positive. John had reacted calmly, since he had suspected that he had HIV infection – he and Bob had an 'open' relationship and each had had a high number of sexual contacts. Bob, however, felt that he needed to change his lifestyle, and to realize goals and ambitions he had not achieved. Bob said that he felt the relationship with John had become routine, and left him for a younger partner.

John had felt shattered by the changes in Bob. He had believed the relationship was basically stable, and when they had discussed being tested for HIV they agreed to stay together and look after each other if found positive. Since Bob had left, John had been to gay clubs and bars, but was increasingly aware of his age and of the emphasis placed on physical attractiveness on the gay scene. He believed that he would never establish another long-term relationship, having a 'track record' of only one affair which lasted longer than a few months, about which he now felt very ambivalent. He felt that, despite having lived with Bob for years, he had not really 'known him' because of all the hidden plans and resentments Bob had only revealed before the breakdown of the relationship.

Erectile problems and premature ejaculation

Since breaking up with Bob there had been several short-term and casual contacts with men. These had all been in public places or on single nights with a partner at home. In the past John had always felt he had adequate control during sex, and had no erectile problems, but over the past two years since being alone he had difficulty establishing and maintaining an erection and, at times, experienced premature ejaculation, i.e. he reached orgasm much more quickly than in the past, so that his partners were not satisfied – some had commented on this. He feared being ridiculed, and had started to avoid sex. He found that he started to become anxious if he felt someone was showing any sexual interest in him.

Guilt about the possibility of infecting others with HIV

For several years, John had kept to safer sex (anal intercourse with condom and lubricant, or manual stimulation) with all partners except Bob, but he always felt worried about infecting his partners. He tended to prefer younger men (in their 20s to 30s) and was always flattered when younger men were interested in him, but he worried about infecting them with HIV. He had known about 20 friends die with AIDS-related illness, many of them younger than himself.

Fears about developing AIDS and coping alone

For several years, John had considered the possibility that he might develop AIDS. It was something he had frequently discussed with Bob. He felt that it would be easier for him to adjust to illness and death than for his younger friends, but he feared having to cope with illness and dependency alone. With Bob having left, and both parents dead, he felt that there was no one to turn to, and had fantasies about dying alone and in distress.

The systematic desensitization programme had been highly effective in decreasing John's fears of crowded places and transport, so that his worries had significantly decreased and he had stopped using the tranquillizers. There had also been some improvement in his confidence generally. Much session time was then used to allow John to express his worries, and to validate and make sense of them, e.g. to reassure him that concerns about changes in appearance through ageing or development of HIV-related illness were common on the gay scene. It was acknowledged that developing long-term relationships was not easy, but that sexual problems such as erectile difficulties were possible to deal with while he was without a regular partner.

Systematic desensitization was used to create a programme concerned with 'performing'. Initially John was given cassette tapes where, once he was relaxed, he imagined himself on stage, where his appearance and behaviour were appreciated by an audience. In subsequent tapes guided imagery related to being approached by an attractive younger man; having successful conversation with him; discussing safer sex, including that this need not lead to penetration; disclosing having HIV; and having mutual manual stimulation or intercourse with an adequate erection and orgasm. In addition, John was advised to masturbate with his non-dominant hand (to obtain greater feelings of feedback and changes in his erection than with the dominant hand) with a positive fantasy of an encounter with a new partner.

In parallel with this structured programme, session time was used to examine John's past achievements and goals in life. He was given information about AIDS support services, including about how illness was managed at home and in hospital, and about self-help groups and 'buddying' (befriending) schemes available, as well as discussing the importance of close and lasting friendships in his life and identifying people to whom he could turn in the event of illness.

By the final session there was great improvement in John's panic attacks in all formerly feared situations – he felt at ease in crowds, at his drama group and in gay clubs. There was moderate improvement in his sexual problems. He felt he could achieve adequate erections even when sex occurred in difficult situations, but he still felt he ejaculated too quickly at times. He was finding solo masturbation more enjoyable and felt less guilty about having sex with others, having decided to tell any potential partner about his HIV status before any sexual contact. He reasoned that rejection was better than the risk of infecting a partner unaware of his having HIV. He had not established a new partnership, but had kept in touch with two sexual contacts whom he felt would become close friends. John felt that he valued friendship more highly than in the past, felt less inferior and inadequate about failing to be in a long-term relationship, and was able to feel he could cope with the support of close friends if or when he became ill.

CASE STUDY 3: A PARTNER OF SOMEONE WITH AIDS, TONY, AGED 28

Tony was referred for psychology sessions by staff on the ward where his partner, Kevin, had been admitted on several occasions with AIDS-related illness. They were concerned about Tony's degree of commitment and devotion to caring for Kevin, who had been diagnosed as having AIDS 14 months previously. Kevin had been ill with a series of distressing infections and symptoms, including toxoplasmosis, a disease which had affected Kevin's central nervous system, leading to periods of confusion and fits before it was identified and treated. Kevin was on maintenance therapy for this and several other conditions, and had very low energy and wasting of his muscles, so that he required a good deal of help with basic skills, such as bathing and any activity that involved standing or walking for long periods.

Formulation and Intervention

During the 22 months over which Tony attended, the following problem areas were identified and discussed.

Dealing with Kevin's demands for time and attention, and his angry outbursts

When he first became ill, Kevin had said that he wanted Tony to care for him at home rather than having statutory or voluntary workers visit. Tony had agreed, as he had wished to be the primary carer, and his employers were sympathetic and his work as a graphic designer was flexible in terms of working hours. However, over time Kevin had become more demanding, refusing to see friends and demanding that Tony provide company and conversation as well as practical help, and that he do all the household chores. For periods of up to a week, Tony would be unable to do any design work or see any of his friends because Kevin would not allow him to leave the house. Kevin had always had a bad temper, but this had become worse and had been particularly bad during the periods of confusion prior to his toxoplasmosis being treated, when he had screamed and shouted at Tony to leave him, that there had never been anything good between them and that he would be better off alone.

Loss of pleasure and interest in sex

During periods of remission from acute illness, Kevin had had some sexual contact with Tony. Tony had never enjoyed anal intercourse, and had engaged in it only a few times, so that when Kevin had been found HIV-positive and Tony negative it had not been a problem to limit their sexual contact to manual stimulation and oral sex with ejaculation outside the mouth. However, Tony found that he did not really enjoy this contact. He did not consciously feel frightened about being infected with HIV, and he still found Kevin attractive, but he had no interest in sex and began to dread Kevin's suggestions or physical advances for sex. Although he remained physically affectionate and demonstrative to Kevin, Tony found it a relief that Kevin was too ill with acute symptoms to suggest sexual contact, and when his interest in sex waned as illness progressed over time.

Sexual orientation difficulties

Kevin had been Tony's second male partner – formerly, until he was 25, he had sexual relationships with women. He had met Kevin only four months prior to the AIDS diagnosis being made. Tony had found Kevin very attractive and by that time the couple were living together. His previous contact with a man had been very brief, and Tony had begun to have doubts about his sexual orientation. He did not feel sexually excited by women, and neither did he by men – he felt his interest in sex was so low that he described himself as 'asexual' – but when he considered his future without Kevin, this was with a female rather than a male partner. Tony had 'come out' to his family and close friends, who had been accepting and supportive, but he was beginning to feel that perhaps his contact with men had been a period of experimentation. His sexual contact with women had been quite limited, but he had good and close friendships with both men and women. He had gay and heterosexual friends and colleagues, and he reported that it had seemed 'natural' but exciting to become sexually involved with men.

Guilt about considering the future without Kevin

Tony frequently thought about how life would be after Kevin's death. He believed that it would be like 'returning things to normal', but he suffered extreme guilt when he realized that he was looking forward to Kevin's death as a relief.

Coping with a new life after Kevin's death

Tony had lost contact with some of the friends he had known before living with Kevin, and his output at work had dropped dramatically. He had left his own flat and moved away from his old neighbourhood when Kevin suggested he moved in with him. He had never felt comfortable on the gay scene, but his social circle included a higher number of gay friends than in the past. He worried about how he would cope with life as a single person after the intense emotional involvement with Kevin, and how people would react if he said he no longer believed himself to be gay.

The first three psychology sessions allowed Tony to express his ambivalence towards Kevin. He worried that Kevin's true feelings had been expressed when he was confused, that there was no love left between them and that they only stayed together because of Kevin having AIDS. Discussion aimed at giving Tony permission to have what he considered to be negative feelings, and looked at the ambivalence inherent in relationships, at finding a way of coping with Kevin's confusion and angry comments (by labelling them as evidence of Kevin being 'not himself') and at the natural need to consider life without Kevin, which were private thoughts and not necessarily something to share with him.

Tony came to realize the needs for others to help in Kevin's care as he became increasingly ill and dependent. In one joint session, Tony and Kevin were encouraged to examine how much care Tony could provide, and how much others could help. Kevin identified his mother and two sisters as emotionally close and others who lived sufficiently near to visit regularly, and he agreed to accept some help from home care nurses so that Tony could return to work on a part-time basis and spend more time with his friends. In addition Kevin agreed to see someone for his own psychological support (a therapist he had seen in the past for emotional difficulties).

Tony had not felt that he could discuss his sexual worries or his thoughts about life after Kevin's death in the joint session, which had essentially been 'bargaining' about how the couple spent their time. Kevin did talk a little about Tony's expectations of his future following a session he had discussing his death with his therapist. Tony began to feel more relaxed and to enjoy time at work and with his friends. Very shortly after this, however, Kevin's illness progressed, and Tony decided that he wanted to provide most of Kevin's care at the end of his life. Kevin continued to accept help from his family and from home care nurses, but for the last two months of his life Tony was present almost every hour of the day.

After Kevin's death regular weekly psychology sessions resumed. Tony felt pleased to have cared for Kevin and viewed their relationship positively, but he was very depressed after the death. He felt unable to believe that life would hold any pleasure or enjoyment. Bereavement therapy (Worden, 1983), aimed at helping Tony to face the death and begin to invest energy in other relationships, was the main focus for sessions over the following four months, after which Tony began to take on freelance work, moved out of Kevin's flat and began to consider his previous sexual problems.

Using a cognitive approach, Tony was encouraged to challenge the view of himself as sexless by considering the following suggestions:

1 The 'normal' state is not to be ever ready for sex, and a loss of libido is usual during bereavement, returning gradually and concurrently with general interest in life.
2 Potential sexual partners – whether male or female – are probably always anxious about a first contact.
3 Sexual relationships with men or women need not inevitably lead to penetration.

4 Many men who consider themselves gay have had sexual contact with women, and many who consider themselves straight have had contact with men.
5 Aspects of our sex lives may be considered private and need not be shared with partners, particularly in short-term affairs – typically, as a relationship develops, more information about our past is disclosed.
6 Safer sex is relevant to both gay and heterosexual sex, and responsible partners do not reject someone for suggesting the need to consider HIV infection.

Tony felt ready to explore his sexuality, and followed a modified sensate focus progamme (Masters and Johnson, 1970) where he gradually caressed more parts of his own body, to induce relaxation and to focus on the pleasure of this experience. During this programme he reported having sexual fantasies about women. The final stage was to incorporate fantasies about successful sexual activity with female partners. By the last psychology session, over a year after Kevin's death, Tony felt he had adjusted to the death and had no conscious regrets over the relationship with Kevin. He remained in contact with most of his gay friends, who accepted that he considered himself heterosexual, and he felt confident about starting relationships with women.

CONCLUSION

In the clinical setting it is rare for people to present with simple problems for which there are straightforward interventions. Experience of work with people affected by AIDS has clearly demonstrated that sex and relationship ('marital') therapy commonly forms part of the intervention, whether the client or patient is worried about having HIV, is actually infected or is the carer and/or partner of someone with AIDS. The case studies here illustrate that emotional support services for this client group must allow for flexible treatment approaches to complex problems and circumstances. For example, Linda's obsessive-compulsive and phobic disorder occurred within long-standing sexual and relationship difficulties with her husband. John wanted sex therapy as well as help with fears of crowds and travelling on public transport, but had no regular gay sexual partner. Tony and Kevin had been sexual partners, but after Kevin's death Tony was obviously without a sexual partner, and also experienced a complicated bereavement reaction following an ambivalent relationship and sexual orientation worries, which had in fact been present before Kevin's death.

Implications from such clinical work are, first, that although people may present with problems for which general supportive counselling and therapy will be appropriate, sexual and relationship problems may well be on the agenda as underlying or coexisting difficulties. Counsellors and therapists need specifically to assess for such difficulties in a non-threatening and supportive way. Second, it appears that a large number of people who may have previously had no or little access to therapeutic support are receiving help with sexual and relationship problems via the AIDS care services. This seems to be particularly the situation for gay couples who would have been unlikely to present to GPs or sex therapists with their difficulties. Third, interventions may include structured marital/relationship or sexual assignments in parallel with supportive techniques and therapists. Eclectic therapists like many clinical psychologists, may be able to offer complete therapeutic interventions, but for many AIDS counsellors and therapists networking with and referral to specialists in sexual and relationship work are essential to provide for the range of problems presented by people affected by AIDS.

REFERENCES

George, H. (1989) Sexual problems among people referred for AIDS counselling. Paper presented at the Association of Sexual and Marital Therapists, Birmingham, 15–16 September.

Green, J. (1989) Counselling for HIV infection and AIDS: the past and future, *AIDS Care*, 1, pp. 5–10.

Hedge, B., Acton, T. and Miller, D. (1988) The worried well: a cognitive-behavioural approach, presented at the IVth International Conference on AIDS, Stockholm, 13–16 June.

Masters, W. H. and Johnson, W. E. (1970) *Human Sexual Inadequacy* (London, Churchill).

Miller, D., Green, J. and McCreaner, A. (1986) Organizing a counselling service for AIDS-related problems, *Genitourinary Medicine*, 62, pp. 116–122.

Mulleady, G., Hart, G. and Appleton, P. (1989) Injecting drug use and HIV: intervention strategies for harm minimization, in: P. Appleton, G. Hart and D. Davies (eds) *AIDS, Social Representations and Social Practices* (London, Falmer Press).

Sherr, L. and Green, J. (1989) Counselling and pregnancy, in: J. Green and A. McCreaner (eds) *Counselling in HIV Infection and AIDS* (Oxford, Blackwell Scientific).

Wolpe, J. (1973) *The Practice of Behaviour Therapy*, 2nd edn (Oxford, Pergamon).

Worden, J. W. (1983) *Grief Counselling and Grief Therapy* (London, Tavistock/Routledge).

Index

self-esteem
  and coping strategies 98–107
  and drug users 132, 136
  low 192, 267
self-protection 53
services used
  by drug users 136
  by informal carers of gay men in UK 118,
    123–4
  unmet needs 124–6
  see also medical treatment
sexual and relationship problems and counselling
    case studies 264–75
  gay men 265, 268–74
  'worried well' 264, 265–8, 274
sexual behaviour
  gay men's partner choices 188–92
  see also gay men: open relationships
    maintained; sexual and relationship
    problems; sexual risk behaviour
sexual risk behaviour among women in
    Kampala 208–26
  cultural background 211–12, 215–16
  epidemiology of AIDS in Africa 209
  policy implications 220–1
  response to AIDS 216–17
significant others
  and drug users in Australia 129–40
  of gay men, disclosure to 45–57
    demographics 49
    discrimination fears 45–6, 52–3, 55
    patterns of 49–50
    psychological distress 46, 49, 51–3
    reasons for non-disclosure 45, 48, 52–4,
      56
silence, conspiracy of 170, 180
  see also non-disclosure
single-parent families 3, 26, 37–8, 175
sociability of gay men in UK 112, 115
social institutions and non-traditional
    families 10–18
social integration among gay men in UK
    110–17
  disclosure of sexual orientation 111–12, 115
  other gay men 113–15, 116
  practical support 113, 115–16
  sociability 112, 115
  social support 112–13, 116
social support 79–97
  changing concepts of family 7–8, 10–18
  current studies 84–7

drug users, *see* drug users: and significant
    relationships
extended family in rural Uganda 141–7
future studies 90–1
gay men 192
  see also coping; informal carers; social
    integration
  and health 80, 82–4, 130–1
  major findings 88–90
  seeking as coping 99–107
  significant others of gay men 45, 55
  theory 79–82
  see also carers
spiritual values, *see* beliefs and values; religion
status of relationship and gay men's partner
    choices 189–92
stigma, *see* isolation and social stigma
stress, *see* psychological distress
suicide, assisted, *see* euthanasia
symptoms
  children 170
  gay men 188–9, 271–2
  Kampala family 67–8

talking
  about casual sex among gay men 196, 200,
    201, 202, 205
  about HIV/AIDS, *see* disclosure
testing for HIV/AIDS and gay men's partner
    choices 187–92
thalassaemics, *see* multilevel intervention
therapy, *see* counselling
threesomes in gay sex 200, 203
traditional medical care in Africa 23, 30–7
transmission, *see* vertical (perinatal)

Uganda 26
  rural, extended family in 141–7
  see also Africa: children; Kampala
under-five mortality in Africa 151, 152, 154–6,
    160–2, 163–4
United Kingdom, *see* Europe; informal carers
    and gay men; social integration among gay
    men
United Nations and Africa 36
  children 152–5, 156, 157–8, 159, 165
United States
  children 153, 154, 155, 169, 180
  gay men's choice of partners 187–94
  social support 80–1, 86, 89–90
  see also ABRP; changing concepts of family